RADIATION THERAPY IN CANCER MANAGEMENT

In Memory of Simeon T. Cantril, M.D.   1908–1959

RADIATION THERAPY IN CANCER MANAGEMENT

Franz Buschke, M.D.

Professor of Radiology
University of California at San Francisco

Robert G. Parker, M.D.

Professor of Radiology
University of Washington

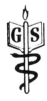

Grune & Stratton
New York and London

Grune & Stratton, Inc.
111 Fifth Avenue
New York, New York 10013

Library of Congress Catalog Card Number 73-164520
International Standard Book Number 0-8089-0725-5
Printed in the United States of America

Thanking Ruth and Nadine for their tolerance

CONTENTS

PREFACE

As clinical medicine becomes more complex, the need for understanding and communication between physicians increases. Although therapeutic radiologists are involved in the care of a majority of patients with cancer, medical students and consequently most physicians have had little, if any, useful introduction to a medical method (therapeutic radiology) which should be helpful to many of their patients. Recent improvements in medical school curricula have provided a somewhat cursory introduction of subject and student. While there are several good textbooks about therapeutic radiology, these have been written for the radiologist. This text is written for the medical student, the trainee in other medical specialties, or the practitioner who desires a general understanding of therapeutic radiology, but who has no interest in the sophisticated details of application.

If the reader gains enough information to answer the review questions at the end of each chapter, he will be more knowledgeable about therapeutic radiology than most contemporary physicians and should find clinical application of value to his patients.

If the reader develops an interest exceeding the bounds of this text, further information is available in the references listed in the bibliographies or in the many good textbooks available.

Franz Buschke

Robert G. Parker

Read not to contradict and confute;
nor to believe and take for granted;
nor to find talk and discourse;
but to weigh and consider.

Francis Bacon

1
RADIATION THERAPY
AS A CLINICAL SPECIALTY

Radiation therapy is a clinical medical specialty in which ionizing radiation is used in the treatment of patients with neoplastic diseases.

Ionizing radiation is characterized by its mechanism of energy dissipation, namely, by ionization (and excitation) of atoms and molecules of the absorbing material. This radiation is electromagnetic (x-rays, gamma rays) or corpuscular (electrons, protons, neutrons, alpha particles, mesons) and is of natural (gamma rays from radium) or artificial (x-rays, gamma rays from cobalt-60 or cesium-137) origin. It is assumed that these radiations act on living tissue by the ionization and excitation produced during absorption. Thus, the basic physical mechanism of action of all forms of ionizing radiation is the same. Differences in effects produced are explained by differences in spatial distribution and time of delivery of the absorbed radiation.

In clinical radiation therapy, use is almost exclusively limited to x-rays and gamma rays. Treatment by radioactive beta emitters or by external high-energy electron beams has been useful in a limited number of clinical situations.[1] Use of other ionizing radiations (protons, neutrons) is still being investigated.

Clinical radiation therapy occupies a unique position among medical specialties. Although some are defined anatomically (gynecology, otolaryngology, dermatology, urology) and others by the therapeutic method used in a number of clinical situations (surgery, internal medicine), radiation therapy is the only clinical specialty which uses one method in the treatment of one group of diseases. With a definition so restricted, it may be questioned whether radiation therapy deserves the status of a clinical specialty. Indeed, many physicians consider radiation therapy a technique to be used on prescription.

Radiation therapy as we understand and practice it should be considered "clinical radiotherapeutic oncology.[3, 7] This presumes a comprehensive understanding of medical radiation physics, biological effects of ionizing radiation, and the biology of neoplastic diseases in all their complexity.

Close cooperation between radiation therapists and *medical radiation physicists* is essential, resembling that between surgeons and anesthesiologists. However, the radiotherapist must have a sound knowledge of medical radiation physics, so that he may adjust the appropriate technical procedure to the specific individual problem (treatment planning).

An understanding of *pathology* is necessary for several reasons: (1) The therapist must understand the gross and microscopic changes in different tissues caused by ionizing radiation. He must be able to relate these to the quantity of radiation and its distribution in space and time. The pathologist may be familiar with generally recognized radiation effects, but he has little appreciation of the more important relationship of radiation-produced tissue effects and the technical details of irradiation. (2) In addition to knowledge of gross and microscopic tumor pathology, the therapeutic radiologist must be aware of the biologic behavior of various neoplastic diseases. For example, in treatment planning it is important to know that a primary carcinoma limited to the true vocal cord does not spread to regional lymph nodes, whereas a carcinoma of the false cord has a high incidence of lymphatic spread; or that a carcinoma of the tonsil, because of anticipated spread to regional lymph nodes, requires concomitant irradiation of the primary site and ipsilateral neck, although a carcinoma originating on the neighboring anterior tonsillar pillar can be included in a small treatment volume, thus permitting the necessary higher dose of radiation. (3) The therapeutic radiologist, like other clinicians, must be aware of the intricacies, difficulties, and limitations of histologic diagnosis in order to allow a proper appreciation of the pathologist's report.[8]

The diagnosis of epidermoid carcinoma usually is unequivocal. The diagnosis of mesenchymal neoplasms may be a matter of doubt even among experienced pathologists. Yet the therapy and prognosis may depend on such specific differentiation. Integration of the histologic findings with the gross pathologic findings and clinical details may permit a correct diagnosis, with its decisive implications for the patient. If the pathologist's diagnosis does not correlate with the clinical situation, the radiotherapist should challenge the diagnosis or obtain additional consultation.

The need for training in medical radiation physics usually is acknowledged, although the importance of an understanding of pathology frequently is not appreciated. A lack of understanding of the gross and microscopic appearance and biological behavior of tumors may result in a form of mechanical radiation therapy which is a physically well planned and executed, but biologically ineffective or even harmful, introduction of radiation energy into a human phantom instead of an intelligent adjustment of treatment to a human with disease.

Recently there has been an increasing emphasis on radiobiology. The term *radiobiology* currently is ambiguous. However, two major functional divisions can be recognized: (1) radiation effects at the cellular level; and (2) radiation effects at the tissue level. The latter is of practical importance to the clinical therapeutic radiologist, as mentioned in the discussion of radiation pathology. Radiobiology at the cellular level is of great interest and fundamental importance, but to date has contributed little to clinical radiation therapy as the specialty has developed empirically. As Kaplan[5] emphasized in his 1970 Failla Memorial Lecture, ". . . it is an ironic fact that they" (referring here to the classical experiments by Regaud and his collaborators, see p. 27) "are the only radiobiological experiments to date that have had a lasting and universal impact on the practice of radiation therapy."

The radiation therapist is concerned with tumors involving any organ or body structure. Consequently, he must have a working knowledge of the *diagnostic procedures* used in other medical specialties in order to evaluate the gross appearance and extent of tumor. This evaluation often is more important than the tumor histology in estimation of radiovulnerability and radio curability. The response of tumor and adjacent normal tissue during the course of irradiation must be used as a guide for treatment. Therefore, the therapeutic radiologist must be competent in the simpler endoscopic procedures, such as indirect laryngoscopy and nasopharyngoscopy. He should join the special examiner at bronchoscopy, esophagoscopy, or cystoscopy in order to assess the gross appearance and extent of tumor, the response to treatment, or radiation-produced change. An estimate of the gross appearance and extent of the tumor and the condition of the adjacent normal tissues, necessary for the planning and administration of treatment, can be obtained only by inspection and palpation. No detailed report can substitute for this first-hand examination. In addition, the physician, knowledgeable in other medical specialties, does not appreciate the importance of seemingly minor details, which may be useful therapeutic and prognostic guides. The therapeutic radiologist need not be competent in these technical procedures, but he must appreciate the possibilities and limitations of the examinations to foster the necessary close cooperation with the participating specialist.

The radiotherapist must understand the possibilities and limitations of *modern cancer surgery* to enable necessary close cooperation with the surgeon in evaluating the relative merits of surgery and radiation therapy in each situation. Great progress in cancer therapy in the last decade has resulted from the appreciation of the need for cooperation, rather than competition, between surgeon and radiotherapist.

The therapeutic radiologist must have considerable interest in and understanding of *cancer chemotherapy* to promote effective cooperation with the chemotherapist. This rapidly growing medical specialty deserves the tolerance and understanding only recently afforded radiation therapy.

As medicine currently is practiced in the United States, physicians caring for cancer patients in special medical centers are seeing an increasing number with persistent or "recurrent" tumor following inadequate initial treatment. The problems of radiation therapy of these previously inadequately treated patients are numerous and complex.[6] Radiation therapy with intent of sterilization of cancer is a radical procedure. Such treatment cannot be repeated following initial failure. Inadequate irradiation also can preclude later optimal surgery. Therefore, initial patient selection, treatment planning, and treatment implementation must be done carefully. *The patient's fate often is decided by the initial therapeutic attempt.* Errors rarely can be corrected.

Nearly all radiation therapy as now practiced requires a substantial overall application time, for example, two months for the treatment of a patient with cancer of the cervix. Although such long treatment periods have inherent disadvantages, they provide an unparalleled opportunity for the physician to become involved in the interaction of a life-threatening disease and a concerned human host. During this period, the therapeutic radiologist is the physician primarily responsible for the total care of the patient. This responsibility, essential during treatment, frequently is continued on the insistence of the patient and is strengthened by the necessary close post-treatment follow-up.

Optimal therapy for patients with cancer is most likely in special institutions or departments because: (1) There is a need for a wide range of closely cooperating medical specialists. (2) Decentralization makes it impossible for the isolated physician to accumulate adequate experience or even maintain skills previously mastered.

There are about 3,000 new diagnoses of cancer per million general population per year. *By current standards, about 40 percent of such patients should receive radical radiation treatment as the initial therapeutic gesture, while about 70 percent of patients with cancer will receive radiation therapy at some time.* (3) Adequate diagnostic and treatment facilities are expensive and should be fully utilized without wasteful duplication. (4) Adequately trained radiation therapists are presently so scarce that they are found only in special institutions or departments. The current number of about 400 can be contrasted with the estimated need of about 2,000.[2] This rationale for the centralization of personnel and facilities for the treatment of the patient with cancer was documented by Regaud as early as 1927.[9] Such centers have developed throughout Europe, Canada, and parts of Asia, but remain infrequent in the United States.

From this survey, it is clear that radiation therapy, if understood as "clinical radiotherapeutic oncology," deserves status as an independent clinical medical specialty. Yet it has become recognized very slowly in the United States.[7] In many places it still is considered an adjunct to x-ray diagnosis. There are several reasons for this slow recognition. Radiation therapy developed from two separate sources: One source was roentgen therapy initially performed by the "roentgenologist" as an adjunct to x-ray diagnosis; the other source was the surgical techniques used for radium implantation as developed by surgeons and gynecologists. Only slowly has it been recognized that *all radiotherapeutic procedures must be integrated as part of a uniform method of treatment and consequently must be performed by a single specialist.* Another reason for slow recognition is that because of the essential alliance of the few radiotherapists with specialized institutions, often exclusive of medical schools, there has been minimal interchange between radiotherapist, practitioner, medical student, and trainee.

REVIEW QUESTIONS

1. What is the basic physical characteristic of the radiation energy used in the treatment of the patient with cancer?

2. What are the two major physical forms of ionizing radiation? Give examples of each.

3. What are the two general origins of ionizing radiation? Give examples of each.

4. What specific types of radiation are currently used in clinical radiation therapy?

5. Why is clinical radiation therapy similar to, but different from, surgery or internal medicine as a medical specialty?

6. Why must the radiation therapist have an understanding of medical radiation physics? of tumor pathology? of radiation biology?

7. Therapeutic radiology has been described as having a transverse rather than a vertical structure as compared to most other clinical specialties. Can you explain?

8. Surgeons, chemotherapists, and radiation therapists should be cooperating partners rather than competitors in the care of the patient with cancer. Explain.

9. What are the advantages of special medical centers (i.e., cancer hospitals) in care of the patient with cancer? What are the disadvantages?

10. Do you believe that the trend should be toward such specialized medical centers?

BIBLIOGRAPHY

1. BOTSTEIN, C., and SCHULZ, R. J. Experience with high energy electron beam therapy. In: *Progress in Radiation Therapy*, Vol. II. F. Buschke, Ed., Grune & Stratton, New York, 1962, chapter 2.
2. BUSCHKE, F. Introduction: *Progress in Radiation Therapy*, Vol. II. Grune & Stratton, New York, 1962, page 7.
3. ————. What is a radiotherapist? *Radiology*, 79:319-321 1962.
4. ————. Introduction: *Progress in Radiation Therapy*, Vol. III. Grune & Stratton, New York 1965, pp. 10-14.
5. KAPLAN, HENRY S. Radiobiology's contribution to radiotherapy: Promise or mirage? *Radiat Res*, 43, 460-476, 1970.
6. KRAMER, S. Re-irradiation: Indications—Technique—Results. In: *Progress in Radiation Therapy*, Vol. II. F. Buschke, Ed., Grune & Stratton, New York, 1962, chapter 12.
7. LAMPE, I. The radiation therapist in contemporary medicine. *Radiology*, 43:181-183, 1944.
8. RAMBO, O. The limitations of histologic diagnosis. In: *Progress in Radiation Therapy*, Vol. II. F. Buschke, Ed., Grune & Stratton, New York, 1962, chapter 13.
9. REGAUD, C. What is the value and what should be the organization and equipment of institutions for the treatment of cancer by radium and x-rays? *Surg, Gynec Obstet*, 44:116-136 (Supplement 2), 1927.

2

THERAPEUTIC RADIOLOGY: PAST, PRESENT, AND FUTURE[7]

Medical students and young physicians interested in therapeutic radiology as a career ask questions which have been recurrent for many years. What is the future of therapeutic radiology? What happens to them if "a cure" or "preventive measures" are discovered? What is the possibility that other medical specialists will usurp the functions of today's radiotherapist? What are the job opportunities? What are the health hazards? What changes are predictable in therapeutic radiology, and how should training programs anticipate these? Considering the cost of facilities and the need for sizable numbers of patients, what does the future hold for private practice? What will be the extent of the "influence" of government?

Answers to these questions and others can be framed in a reference to the short history and current status of therapeutic radiology.

HISTORICAL PERSPECTIVES

The use of ionizing radiation in medicine dates to Röentgen's[22] discovery of a "new kind of ray" (x-ray) on November 8, 1895 and to the Curies' discovery of radium in 1896.[20] The short life-history of medical use, the necessary early empiricism, the delayed appearance of unrelentingly progressive, undesirable sequelae, and perhaps even the mysticism of a powerful biologic agent, which cannot be detected by the usual human receptors, have influenced and continue to influence the attitudes of physicians and others toward use of ionizing radiation in medicine. Unfortunately, some attitudes, based on misconceptions and misinformation, adversely influence today's medical care.[6]

A predictable sequence of reactions followed the discovery of this powerful agent which could cause marked biologic change. The first reaction was that of overenthusiasm, when ionizing radiation was reported as a "cure" for most previously incurable diseases. When such impossible predictions failed to materialize, there was a counterreaction of pessimism and despair, and ionizing radiation was claimed incapable of any beneficial effect. The ultimate realistic appraisal is that *ionizing radiation is a unique agent, beneficial in selected circumstances*, and, thus, is similar to other medical agents.

Clinical therapeutic radiology had a long and frequently painful gestation

6

period[7] from 1895 to the early 1920s. During this period, most radiation therapy was done, and thus influenced, by surgeons, as they were the physicians most interested in the patient with cancer. Unfortunately, the resulting basic philosophy was that ionizing radiation was a caustic agent to be used to produce a "slough in lieu of excision."[7] This "brutal form"[7] of radiation therapy, used in single, massive doses, resulted in disastrous consequences. Clinical radiation therapy was nearly stillborn, and today's youngster still bears the scars of this period. Some physicians, even today, consider ionizing radiation as a cauterizing agent rather than as a *subtle instigator of chemical change* which produces selective responses in cells, tissues, organs, and whole mammals.

Much of lasting value developed during this gestation period. Even prior to the famous inadvertent, first radiobiologic experiment (non-grant supported) by Becquerel in 1901,[3] when he noted a burnlike sore on his abdominal skin adjacent to a vest pocket in which he carried a glass tube of radium salt, medical therapeutic attempts were reported.[8]

E. H. Grubbe, a Chicago layman manufacturer of vacuum tubes, claimed to have treated a patient with carcinoma of the breast in January, 1896.[17] Voigt, in Germany, treated a patient for pain relief about the same time.[24] Despeignes, in France, treated a patient with gastric cancer in July, 1896.[14] Most physical infirmities, including blindness,[15] were treated and reported to respond favorably. Techniques of application were inconstant and nonreproducible.

Although indications for use and techniques of application continue to change, it soon became apparent that ionizing radiation was primarily beneficial in the treatment of patients with cancer and that definite conditions of application were a prerequisite for use.

Technological advances were more rapid than accumulation of basic biological knowledge. By 1913, Coolidge[10] had developed an x-ray tube with a heated tungsten filament, a tungsten target, an effective vacuum, and a peak energy of 140 kv, thus providing the foundation for external roentgen teletherapy. By 1922, 200 kv x-ray tubes were available for "deep therapy."[10]

During this same period, radium has been used in containers in the uterus (Margaret Cleaves, 1903[9]) and interstitially (Robert Abbe, 1905[1]). Later it was developed as a teletherapy source (Finzi, 1911[8]; Kelly, 1920[8]; Regaud,[8]; Forssell[8]; Cutler[8]; Quick, 1955[19]).

Clinical radiation therapy was born in 1922, when Regaud, Coutard and Hautant presented evidence to the International Congress of Otology in Paris,[21] that advanced laryngeal cancer could be cured without disastrous, treatment-produced sequelae. Thus, for the first time the method was used by physicians (radiotherapists) interested in its development rather than by surgeons who considered ionizing radiation as a minor adjuvant to be used as a caustic agent.

During this period of French and Scandinavian influence, the treatment philosophy was to avoid tissue necrosis and sloughing through distribution of radiation in time and through use of sources with short wavelengths.[7] By 1934, Henri Coutard[11] had developed a *protracted-fractional method* which remains the basis of current radiation therapy. A few radiotherapists, primarily in France, Scandinavia, and England, had developed techniques for the treatment of patients with cancers of the larynx and cervix *prior* to the definition of a unit of radiation dose in 1928. These techniques, with minor variations, are valid today!

The next period of development was physical. Ionizing radiation was quanti- tated and qualitated. These units and measures (roentgen = radiation quantitated by measurement of ionization of air; rem = roentgen equivalent mammal; rep = roentgen equivalent physical; rad = radiation absorbed dose; half value layer = a measure of quality; interstitial dose schemes of Paterson-Parker and Quimby) were standardized throughout the world. Treatment planning and delivery became accurate and reproducible.

The leaders in this growth phase were the British. Use of British-developed treatment techniques and dependence on British-trained physicists and dosimetrists continues throughout the world today.

There was coincident enrapture with apparatus, as if cancer cures were as close as the development of ever more "powerful" radiation sources.

X-ray generators operating at 800–1,000 kv were installed for medical use as early as 1932.[5] These were followed by cyclotrons, synchro-cyclotrons, betatrons, bevatrons, linear accelerators, and nuclear reactors. Cobalt-60 and cesium-137 succeeded radium-226 as isotopic teletherapy sources. Yet cancer cures remained elusive.

Today, major interest has returned to the biologic responses induced by ioniz- ing radiation and to the biology of cancer in the human. Recent explosive growth of radiobiology at times has resulted in a failure of communication between basic- science–oriented and clinically oriented workers, with consequent inattention to problems of immediate clinical importance and even to production of data conflicting with long-established empirical observations. Development of an understanding of radiobiological responses and correlation with the necessary knowledge of human cancer biology should be the major thrust during the foreseeable future.

CURRENT STATUS

"Radiation therapy as a specialty has been accepted very reluctantly and is still far from being generally accepted throughout the country. Most of the radiation therapy was and much still is performed as an annex to x-ray diagnosis by the general radiologist, although in Great Britain, France, and the Scandinavian countries, radia- tion therapy has long been accepted and practiced as an independent specialty."[7] As early as 1938, Forssell stated[16] "Roentgen diagnostic and radiotherapy demand different scientific training, and the investigation of each belongs to different spheres of medicine. The conditions necessary for their practical utilization are also very different. . . . Radiotherapy's task of treating about two-thirds of cancer patients alone or in cooperation with surgery has, even from a mere practical point of view, made it impossible for one and the same man to satisfactorily direct both the roentgen diagnostic work and the radiotherapy of a large hospital, if he is not a genius."

Yet as late as 1955 the transcript of the Annual Conference of Teachers of the American College of Radiology[2] included the following statement: "In our system of free enterprise, it is readily apparent that the bulk of radiologic practice will continue to be carried on by radiologists who must assume the responsibility for both diagnosis and therapy. Any other method would require transportation of many patients to centers large enough to support *adequate specialized therapy equipment and personnel.*" This seems a curious position in an age when people travel hundreds of miles for recreation and thousands of miles for committee meetings, and perhaps partially explains why as late as 1948 a delegation from the British Empire Cancer Campaign found only three institutions in North America (including one in Canada) practicing radiotherapy equivalent to that practiced in England.[4] This gap between prevalent and optimally obtainable cancer treatment was noted by Steiner in 1952[23] and still exists today.

Regardless of the inherent scientific integrity of any medical specialty, its success depends upon its disciples. In 1960, Kaplan[18] estimated that, by 1970, 1,400 to 1,700 therapeutic radiologists would be required to adequately care for the U.S. population with cancer. The number of full-time, active radiotherapists in the U.S. increased from 111 in 1959 to 295 in 1968,[12] but remains less than 400 at present. Therefore, the potential for growth in the immediate future exceeds the recent rapid growth.

The number of trainees in "straight" radiotherapy was 25 in 1960, 84 in 1968, and is estimated to be 150 in 1970.[13] In 1969, 29 therapeutic radiologists were certified by the American Board of Radiology. Therefore, the number of newly qualified radiotherapists only slightly exceeds the attrition rate and makes little inroad on the existing demand. A major problem for therapeutic radiologists is choice of a job from among many offered. This situation is the basis of a form of "occupational musical chairs" which involves all radiotherapists.

Although the number of institutions offering this training has increased from 29 to 66 in the decade 1960–1970, only about one-half of the available positions are filled. This healthy growth of trainees in radiation therapy has been accompanied by a proportional increase in straight diagnostic radiology trainees, thus reducing the number of general radiologists tempted to do radiotherapy.

Although the American Board of Radiology has offered certification since its inception in 1934, the American Medical Association has certified training programs independent of diagnostic radiology only since April, 1969. The first Department of Therapeutic Radiology in a U.S. medical school was established only a few years ago. By July, 1970, 15 to 20 such independent departments should exist.

Such developments as independent training and certification and the establishment of vigorous departments in U.S. medical schools will be followed by more widespread recognition of therapeutic radiology as a legitimate medical specialty. This can only result in a period of quantitative and qualitative growth unknown to date.

ATTEMPTED ANSWERS

There are multiple indicators that the foreseeable future for therapeutic radiology is one of continuing rapid growth. Today's requirement for a four- to fivefold increase in the number of radiotherapists to manage patients with cancer may be intensified by the rapid reduction in the training of general radiologists, the limited number of radiotherapy trainees, and an inherent appeal of the method whenever adequately demonstrated.

In the unlikely but hoped for event that unforeseen curative agents become available during our lifetime, therapeutic radiologists, because of their unique background in clinical oncology, will be the best qualified to master new techniques and continue their involvement with the cancer patient. If "cancer preventatives" are developed, radiotherapists can become medical administrators.

Inasmuch as increased understanding of radiation use and increased complexity of application have led to the development of a special physician, the radiation therapist, it is unlikely that other physicians will usurp the function of the radiation therapist as the methods become even more complex. Indeed, today few surgeons use radioactive materials for implantation, and the number of gynecologists applying radium is decreasing, because today's gynecology trainee realizes his limitations.

Much of the data on short- and long-term radiation effects in humans was provided by early radiologists as inadvertent experimental objects. These physicians, martyrs to ignorance, suffered from an increased incidence of skin cancer, leukemia, cataract, and perhaps life shortening. Today's radiation therapist should receive little exposure to ionizing radiation, certainly less than the diagnostic radiologist doing fluoroscopy. With good practices based on current knowledge, risks should not exceed those to any physician.

Future changes are not easily predictable. However, it is unlikely that new radioactive agents or equipment will result in revolutionary changes. As in surgery, there is much work to be done in understanding, refining, and applying existing methods. However, ever-increasing knowledge of basic biology might revolutionize the specialty. For example, if cancer cells could be synchronized and irradiated when most sensitive, or if chemicals could selectively sensitize cancer cells to irradiation, today's methods might be quickly outmoded. Training programs can anticipate such unforeseen developments by encouraging the trainee to be a life-long student.

The private practice of all medical specialties is rapidly changing. The private practice of therapeutic radiology, never well developed, is no exception. Requirements of expensive facilities and a large number of patients always have encouraged location in medical centers and organization in groups inclusive of specially trained physicians, physicists, dosimetrists, technicians, and nurses. Trends toward physician group practices in other specialties may make these activities similar to what has been commonplace in radiation therapy.

It is important to emphasize that therapeutic radiology can legitimately compete economically in today's marketplace, despite the high cost of facilities. Many excellent private groups attest to this in all parts of the U.S.

Cancer programs in the U.S., as in other countries, have been influenced by government at all levels. The National Cancer Institute, the first institute in the National Institutes of Health, has been constructively involved in meaningful programs in cancer prevention, detection, treatment, training, and investigation. This participation has contributed to the health of our citizens through encouragement of all cancer workers.

BIBLIOGRAPHY

1. ABBE, R. Radium and radioactivity. *Yale Med J,* p. 433, June, 1904.
2. American College of Radiology: Annual Conference of Teachers of Clinical Radiology, 1955.

3. BECQUEREL, H. On various properties of the uranium rays. *C R Acad Sci* [D] (Paris) 123:855, 1896.

4. British Empire Cancer Campaign: Report by a delegation from the campaign on a visit to Canada and the United States, 1948.

5. BUSCHKE, F., CANTRIL, S. T., and PARKER, H. M. *Supervoltage Roentgentherapy*. Charles C Thomas, Springfield, Ill., 1950.

6. BUSCHKE, F. Common misconceptions in radiation therapy. *Amer J Surg*, 101:164–171, 1961.

7. BUSCHKE, F. Radiation therapy: The past, the present, the future (Janeway Lecture), *Amer J. Roentgen*, 108:236–246, 1970.

8. CASE, J. T. History of radiation therapy. In: *Progress in Radiation Therapy*, Vol. I, F. Buschke, ed., Grune & Stratton, New York, 1958.

9. CLEAVES, M. A. Radium therapy. *Med Rec*, 64:601, 1903.

10. COOLIDGE, W. D., and CHARLESTON, E. E. Roentgen ray tubes. In: *Medical Physics*. Otto Glasser, ed., Year Book, Chicago, 1950.

11. COUTARD, H. Principles of x-ray therapy of malignant disease. *Lancet*, 2:1–8, 1934.

12. DEL REGATO, J. A. Introduction, Roster, Amer. Soc. Ther. Radiol., 1968.

13. DEL REGATO, J. A. Survey of training in radiotherapy, 1970.

14. DESPEIGNES, V. Observations on a case of carcinoma of the stomach treated with roentgen rays. Lyon Med, July, 428; Aug., 503, 1896 (in French).

15. EDISON (THOMAS A.), MORTON, SWINTON, and STANTON. Discussion: The effect of x-rays upon the eyes. *Nature*, 53:421, 1896.

16. FORSSELL, G. Role of radiology in medicine. *Radiology*, 30:12–18, 1938.

17. GRUBBE, E. H. Priority in the therapeutic use of x-rays. *Radiology*, 21:156–162, 1933.

18. KAPLAN, H. S. Report to the National Advisory Cancer Council, 1960.

19. QUICK, D., and RICHMOND, J. A. Preliminary experiences with a 50 gram converging beam radium unit. *Amer J Roentgen*, 74:635–650, 1955.

20. QUIMBY, E. H. The first fifty years of the American Radium Society, 1916–1966.

21. REGAUD, C., COUTARD, H., and HAUTANT, A. Contribution au traitement des cancers endolarynges par les rayons-X. X Internat. Congr. d' Otol. 19–22, 1922.

22. RONTGEN, W. C. Uber eine neue Art von Strahlen. Erste Mitteilung. Sitz gsber. physikal.—med. Gessellschf. zu Würzburg, pp. 132–141, Dec. 28, 1895; zweite Mitteilung, March 9, 1896.

23. STEINER, P. Evaluation of the cancer problem. *Cancer Res*, 12:455–464, 1952.

24. VOIGT, A. Behandlung eines inoperablen Pharynxkarzinoms mit Röntgenstrahlen. Arztlichen verein. i. Hamburg, Nov. 3, 1896.

3

FUNDAMENTALS
OF CLINICAL RADIATION
THERAPY

TECHNICAL MODALITIES

The technical modalities used for clinical radiation therapy may be divided into three major groups (Tables 3–1 and 3–2):

1. *External (transcutaneous) irradiation:* Irradiation from sources at a distance from the body (x-ray; teletherapy with radium-226, cobalt-60, or cesium-137).
2. *Local irradiation:* Irradiation from sources in direct contact with the tumor.
   a. *Surface irradiation with applicators* loaded with radioactive material (molds for the treatment of certain oral and skin tumors).
   b. *Intracavitary irradiation* with radioactive material (most commonly radium-226, cobalt-60, cesium-137) in removable applicators which are inserted into body cavities, such as uterus, vagina, or maxillary sinus.
   c. *Interstitial irradiation* by removable needles containing radium-226, cesium-137, or cobalt-60; by nonremovable "seeds" of radioactive gold-198 or radon; by small radioactive iridium-192 sources in nylon suture; or by radioactive tantalum-182 wire.
   d. *Direct roentgen therapy* to epithelial lesions by means of cones (ie., transvaginal, intraoral).
3. *Internal or systemic irradiation:* Irradiation by radioactive sources (i.e., ^{32}P, ^{131}I) administered intravenously or parenterally.

During the past three decades, improvement in facilities for external irradiation has made the use of local techniques less important. In our own practice, local techniques are limited to intracavitary treatment of certain gynecological cancers (cervix, vagina, uterus) and some carcinomas of the bladder, to interstitial and mold treatment of some carcinomas of the tongue and floor of the mouth, and to occasional transoral and transvaginal roentgen therapy.

External Irradiation

For irradiation of neoplasms from external sources, roentgen rays generated at voltages between 85 kv and 35 mv and gamma rays from radium-226, cobalt-60, cesium-137 currently are used clinically. The energy (and penetrating power) of

Table 3-1. Modalities for Clinical Radiation Therapy

External Irradiation	Local Irradiation			Internal or Systemic Irradiation
	Surface	Intracavitary	Interstitial	
See Table 3-2	Radium-226 and strontium-90 in plaques (skin) and in needles and tubes for use in molds (skin, lip, floor of mouth)	Radium-226, cobalt-60, and cesium-137 in needles and tubes for use in special applicators for the cervix, vagina, uterine cavity, bladder, paranasal sinuses	Radium-226, cobalt-60, and cesium-137 needles, tantalum-182 wire, and iridium-191 seeds in a ribbon for temporary (removable) implantation	^{32}P ^{131}I
		X-ray through a cone in the vagina or oral cavity	Radon and gold seeds for nonremovable (permanent) implantation	
		Isotopes, i.e., colloidal ^{198}Au, or ^{32}P for instillation in serous cavities		

ionizing radiation increases as the photon wavelength decreases. Differences in the physical characteristics of the radiation are of great importance in therapeutic radiology. Although these physical characteristics gradually change over the energy spectrum, arbitrary gross grouping within broad energy ranges have been made for clinical use. The clinically important changes occur with radiation generated in a range between 400 and 800 kv. Above this energy, the advantages are: reduced absorption of radiation in bone, less damage to the skin at the portal of entry, better tolerance of the vasculoconnective tissue, greater radiation at a depth relative to the surface dose, and reduced lateral scatter of radiation in the tissues.

Table 3-2. Modalities For External Irradiation

Term	Voltage	HVL	Source
Low voltage (superficial)	85–140 kv	1–3 mm Al	X-ray
Medium voltage (orthovoltage)	180–400 kv	0.5–3 mm Cu	X-ray
Supervoltage	500 kv–8 mv	4–15 mm Cu	X-ray Radium-226 Cobalt-60 Cesium-137
Megavoltage	Above supervoltage energy		Specific generators, e.g., betatron, synchrotron, linear accelerator

Generally, ionizing radiation of sufficient energy to have these characteristics is termed *supervoltage radiation,* even though it need not be electrically generated (^{60}Co, ^{137}Cs, ^{226}Ra), whereas ionizing radiation generated at lower energies and not having these characteristics is termed *orthovoltage radiation.* The lower energy radiation usually is further subdivided into "superficial" (85–140 kv) and "deep" or "medium" (180–400 kv). The term *megavoltage* has been introduced for radiation generated at very high energies by current standards. However, the demarcation from supervoltage remains obscure despite liberal use of the term (see Table 3–2 for these general groupings).

"Skin Sparing" and Relative Depth Dose

The reduced skin effect of supervoltage radiation as compared with ortho-voltage radiation is based on the physical fact that, with higher energy radiation, forward scattering (in the direction of the primary beam) of radiation in the absorber is greater and lateral scattering less. With supervoltage radiation the maximum ionization occurs below the level of the epidermis. For example, with

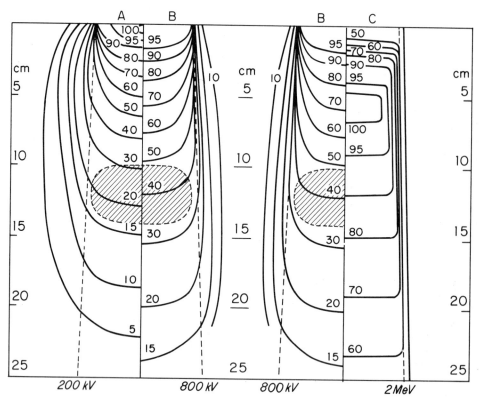

Fig. 3-1. Comparison of isodose curves in a large volume of tissue with 200 kv (A), 800 kv (B), and 31 Mev (C). Field size 7.5 cm diameter. Focus-skin distance, 100 cm. Note the reduction of lateral scattering with 800 kv and 31 Mev compared to 200 kv radiation. Dotted line indicates the geometrical beams. (Constructed by P. Wootton based on data by H. M. Parker, from Buschke, Cantril, Parker: Supervoltage Roentgenotherapy, Springfield, Ill.: Charles C Thomas, 1950, and from G. Joyet and W. Mauderli: Brown Boveri Rev, 28:281, 1951).

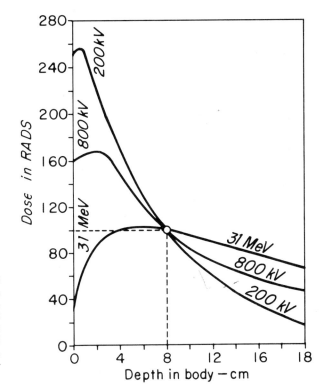

Fig. 3-2. Depth dose curves in water or tissue for 200 kv, 800 kv, and 31 Mev x-rays, indicating the necessary skin dose for the delivery of the same dose of 100 rads at 8 cm depth. (From F. Buschke: 31 Mev Rontgentherapie, Oncologia, 6:225, 1953.)

cobalt-60 teletherapy, maximum ionization occurs about 5 mm below the surface, while the surface dose may be only 40 percent of this maximum.

As the energy of radiation increases, it becomes "more penetrating." As photons and resultant electrons become more energetic, they travel a greater distance into the absorbing material. Therefore, the percentage of radiation at any specific depth, compared to the surface dose, increases as the energy increases (see Figure 3–1).

The greater penetration into tissue and the better skin tolerance of higher energy radiation permit the introduction of a significantly higher dose through each field of application. For example, the delivery of a dose of 100 rads at 8 cm depth requires a skin dose of 250 R with 200 kv radiation (HVL* 0.9 mm Cu), 160 rads with 800 kv (HVL 9.1 mm Cu) and 40 rads with 31 mv (Figure 3–2). Since it may require a single dose of 1,000 rads with 1,000 kv, compared with 680 R with 200 kv (dose includes back scatter), to produce a threshold skin erythema, it is possible to introduce through an individual field at least twice the physical dose at 10 cm depth with supervoltage than with medium-voltage radiation.[1]

This advantage of supervoltage is of critical importance in the treatment of tumors when the introduction of a sufficiently high dose with medium-voltage radiation is difficult or impossible (carcinoma of the bladder, esophagus, bronchus).

*HVL (half value layer) is a gross measure of radiation quality represented by the thickness of a specific material required to reduce radiation intensity 50 percent.

For example, in order to introduce 6,000 rads into a carcinoma of the thoracic esophagus at 12 cm depth through a field measuring 8 $\times$ 14 cm, a skin dose of about 20,000 rads would be required with 200 kv radiation, but a skin dose of only 12,000 rads would be needed with 2 mv.[1] Since the skin tolerates 6,000 to 6,500 rads in six weeks with supervoltage radiation, the entire tumor dose can be directed through two treatment fields, whereas, with a maximum skin tolerance of 5,000 rads for medium-voltage radiation, at least four skin fields are required. The greater number of fields necessary for the introduction of large doses of radiation to the tumor include some which are anatomically undesirable. To compensate for the difficulty of accurately directing radiation through multiple fields, the fields usually are enlarged. The greater lateral scatter of medium-voltage therapy adds still further to the total tissue volume irradiated. Thus, a greater volume of normal tissue is treated unecessarily, with the consequent increase of normal tissue damage and systemic effect.

The greater relative depth dose and better skin tolerance often permit the introduction of the entire tumor dose through a single field. This has proved advantageous in certain tumors of the oral mucosa (those in gingival ridge, gingival-buccal sulcus, buccal mucosa, and anterior faucial pillar).

Radiation Absorption in Bone

In the supervoltage range, absorption of radiation in bone approximates that in water or soft tissue per unit density, whereas with medium-voltage radiation absorption is considerably greater in bone than in soft tissue. The vasculoconnective tissue immediately adjacent to the bone around the Haversian channels receives a significantly higher dose because of scattered radiation than it would if surrounded by soft tissue. This higher radiation dose increases the risk of bone necrosis by destruction of the osteoblastic elements and damage to the vascular tissue. Furthermore, preferential bone absorption leads to a reduction in dose at the point of interest when thick bone must be transversed by the radiation. For example, Wootton[8] has demonstrated that when 200 kv radiation is introduced through lateral fields, the dose in the nasopharynx is 20–25 percent lower than calculated from soft tissue measurements, whereas with 2 mv radiation the measured dose in the nasopharynx corresponds to the dose expected from measurements in soft tissue. This makes it possible, with supervoltage radiation, to introduce an adequate dose into the nasopharynx through opposing lateral fields, while with medium-voltage radiation, because of the preferential absorption of radiation in bone and the risk of bone necrosis, the nasopharyngeal tumor dose from opposing lateral fields must be complemented either by additional, less desirable fields, or by complicated intracavitary radium application.

It is apparent that supervoltage radiation has a decisive advantage in the treatment of practically all neoplasms about the head when bone is included in the treatment volume.

Tolerance of Soft Tissue

It has been observed clinically that, as the radiation energy increases, similar tumor effects can be produced with less damage to important adjacent normal structures. The incidence and severity of mucosal and skin reactions are reduced and, most important, there is less damage to the vasculoconnective tissue.

This is explained, in part, by the more favorable physical distribution of radiation through the tissues, allowing the irradiation of smaller, anatomically more favorable volumes.

In part, the reduced soft tissue effects of supervoltage radiation may be related to the lesser "relative biological efficiency" (RBE)[4] of the same measured dose compared to medium-voltage x-ray (the RBE decreases with decreasing wave length). From clinical experience, radiation in the million volt range is estimated to be approximately 20 percent less "efficient" than 200 kv radiation. This difference in RBE may be explained by the different pattern of so-called "specific ionization." The primary electron liberated by the introduced quantum of radiation energy in turn liberates secondary and tertiary electrons along its path as it passes through tissue. The number of clusters of ion pairs along the path of an electron liberated by a quantum of low energy is greater and the distance between the clusters shorter than for electrons liberated by a quantum of high energy. Thus, the average number of ions per micron of tissue (so-called "mean linear ion density") for x-rays produced at 1,000 kv is about 15, with an average distance between clusters of 0.2 μ, as compared with a density of 80 and an average distance of 0.04 μ between clusters for 200 kv x-rays.[2]

These physical considerations, however, do not completely explain the clinical observation of better tolerance of the vasculoconnective tissue to supervoltage radiation with doses producing equal effects on tumor. As Lederman has expressed it: "The radiation is kinder to the tissues."

Some experimental observations indicate that the recuperative power of a biological object increases with decreasing density of ionization. As the tolerance of the vasculoconnective tissue is greater than that of some tumors when the dose is protracted, it is possible that this difference becomes even more pronounced for radiation with lesser ion density.

It has been our experience throughout the last 30 years that, for comparable tumor effect, the damage to the vasculoconnective tissue is appreciably less with supervoltage than with medium-voltage irradiation. For example, in the treatment of patients with extensive carcinomas of the lip and skin, we have been able to introduce tumoricidal doses without objectionable late changes in the vasculo-connective tissue (even when the dose was increased to allow for the reduced RBE) whereas with medium-voltage irradiation such doses would likely have led to tissue necrosis.[6,7]

The greater tolerance of the vasculoconnective tissue to a high dose of properly protracted supervoltage radiation therapy is one of the factors that now permits the planned combination of radical preoperative irradiation with radical surgery without increasing the surgical risks beyond those associated with surgery alone. These combined procedures are being used more frequently in the treatment of carcinomas of the oral mucosa, esophagus, bronchus, and bladder. Such combined treatment was not safely possible with medium-voltage irradiation.

Constitutional Tolerance

"Radiation sickness" can be related to the size of the daily radiation dose and the size of the tissue volume irradiated. The greater relative depth dose and lessened scattering outside the geometric beam with supervoltage radiation permit reduction of the total tissue volume irradiated, thus resulting in better constitutional tolerance than is possible with orthovoltage radiation. With properly conducted supervoltage radiation therapy, "radiation sickness" is negligible.

Supervoltage external therapy has now passed the test of more than 30 years of clinical experience.[3] In its early use, emphasis usually was placed on the better skin tolerance and the greater penetration of the radiation with consequent better depth dose. However, the most important advantages of supervoltage therapy are the reduced bone absorption and the better tolerance of the soft tissue. The disadvantages of lesser depth dose and skin tolerance with medium-voltage radiation can be overcome, in most situations, by technical maneuvers, such as crossfiring or rotational therapy. However, the greater tolerance of bone and vasculoconnective tissue for supervoltage radiation cannot be compensated by any technical maneuver.

Although the superiority of supervoltage radiation therapy is acknowledged by all who have used it, the use of medium-voltage equipment in radiation therapy unfortunately remains widespread. Medium-voltage x-ray therapy must now be considered part of history. Unless otherwise specifically indicated, the discussion of external radiation therapy in the following chapters implies use of supervoltage radiation therapy. We should emphasize that, because of the extensive use of medium-voltage x-ray therapy over a long period of time, most of the older publications are based on this obsolete technique. Consequently, such publications in earlier text-books and journals must be interpreted with the appropriate criticism of both accomplishment and radiation hazards.

Radiation in the megavoltage range has certain advantages, but these are less important when compared with the use of supervoltage radiation than those of supervoltage radiation when compared with medium-voltage radiation. X-ray radiation generated at voltages of 15 to 50 mv at times facilitates more elegant treatment, but its use is a tidbit for the radiologic gourmet.

The use of high energy electrons generated by megavoltage equipment has certain advantages, but experience is too limited for a textbook discussion.

Local Irradiation

The localized application of radiation permits very high doses to restricted tissue volumes. The physical principle that the intensity of radiation rapidly decreases with distance from the radiation source is used to advantage in specific clinical situations. Criteria for application include: a small tumor with well-defined limits; a desire to restrict the volume of tissue irradiated; need for a larger dose than that easily delivered from an external source, even if the dose is nonhomogeneous; accessibilty for mechanical introduction of the radiation sources.

Sources of Radiation

Radium has been the most frequent source for local application. It has been chosen either as a source of high energy gamma rays or beta rays by means of filtration through various materials (usually platinum, brass, silver). These filtering materials usually are in the form of needles or tubes, which must be carefully constructed and frequently inspected because of the serious danger of leakage of radon gas or the powdered radium salt ($RaCl_2$, $RaSO_4$).

Small, custom-made "seeds" containing radon gas (a disintegration product of radium) or consisting of ^{198}Au have been used for nonremovable implantation. These materials have the disadvantages of difficulty of preparation, rapid radio-active decay, inhomogeneity of dosimetry, and danger of radioactive contamination, with few compensatory advantages.

In recent years, many other materials (^{60}Co, ^{137}Cs, ^{192}Ir, ^{182}Ta) have been available for local application. Many of these have specific advantages over radium: They may be incorporated in solid materials such as ceramics, and they do not form gas and so may be heat sterilized. However, radium continues to be the standard for use because of a long and admirable performance record.

Mechanics of Application

Local irradiation techniques include temporary (removable) or permanent (nonremovable) applications. The radiation sources, placed in highly specific containers, may be applied to a body surface (molds for application to the skin, lip, or oral mucosa; intracavitary applicators for insertion into the uterine cavity, vagina, maxillary sinus, or urinary bladder) or may be inserted directly into tissue (needles or sutures containing radioactive sources for interstitial application).

X-rays, generated by standard methods, may be directed for very short distances through cones. In these circumstances (transvaginal treatment of tumors of the cervix, peroral treatment of tumors of the oral cavity) the principles of local application pertain.

Dosimetry

If radiation intensity decreases rapidly with increasing depth in tissue, that tissue adjacent to the radiation source may be treated adequately without harmful irradiation of the underlying structures. This optimum situation may result from (1) use of a quality of radiation which will be absorbed near the surface (beta rays, electrons, low-energy x-rays) or (2) placement of the radiation source close to the surface to be treated to utilize the physical principle of proprtionately larger "fall off" of dose close to the radiation source.

For these same physical reasons, the dosimetry of localized applications, particularly of multiple discrete sources, will be less homogeneous than that with irradiation from external sources distant from the body. However, extensive experience has resulted in the formulation of rules for local application, such as those of Paterson and Parker,[5] which limit variations in dose to ± 10 percent from the mean. Applied in this manner, there is no clinically significant necrosis from "hot spots" or accountable tumor persistence from "cold spots."

Clinical Application

The use of local irradiation will be discussed under treatment of specific tumors. Such use can be predicted from the advantages (localized high dose; minimal irradiation of tissue adjacent to the tumor; more rapid treatment than with external irradiation) and the disadvantages (difficulty of application, i.e., may be a major operative procedure; inhomgeneity of dose; potential danger to personnel).

Internal or Systemic Irradiation

Early enthusiasm for the medical potential of sytemically administered radioactive materials was based on the highly specific attraction of radioactive iodine (^{131}I) to the thyroid and radioactive phosphorus (^{32}P) to tissues and tumors with great cellular activity. In the intervening 25 years, the use of ^{131}I and ^{32}P in the treatment of malignant tumors has become very restricted, and new materials have been of little clinical importance.

Although radioactive iodine has become a standard agent for the diagnosis and treatment of noncancerous thyroid disorders, it has been therapeutically useful in less than 10 percent of patients with thyroid cancer. This limitation is based on the failure of most thyroid cancers to accumulate iodine.

Use of ^{32}P is limited by its poor specificity of action, with consequent undesired side-effects in normal tisues which have a rapid cell turnover (intestinal lining, bone marrow).

REVIEW QUESTIONS

1. What are the three major groups of technical modalities? Give examples of each. Which modality currently is used for the radiation treatment of most patients with cancer?

2. What is the physical definition of "supervoltage" radiation? Can nonelectrically generated radiation, i.e., ^{60}Co, be considered "supervoltage"?

3. List four advantages of "supervoltage" radiation over medium-voltage radiation. Which are the most important of these advantages?

4. What is the physical basis of skin sparing with "supervoltage" radiation? This skin sparing is present at the surface of entry of the radiation beam. Does skin sparing exist at the surface where a supervoltage beam leaves the body (exit field)? Why?

5. What is the clinical advantage of skin sparing?

6. Explain the concept of relative depth dose. Why is this value higher as the radiation energy increases?

7. What are the clinical disadvantages of the preferential absorption in bone of low- and medium-voltage radiation as compared with supervoltage radiation? At what approximate energy range does the preferential absorption of radiation energy in bone disappear?

8. Undesirable constitutional response to radiation ("radiation sickness") can be related to what factors? Can you suggest how "radiation sickness" can be avoided?

9. Physically measured doses from supervoltage sources more than 20 percent larger than those from medium-voltage sources may be better tolerated by soft tissues. What is a possible explanation?

10. Why are most of the radiation treatment data in textbooks and other older sources of limited value?

11. What is the physical principle exploited in localized applications of radiation? What are the clinical advantages? What diseases frequently are treated by local irradiation? Why aren't these techniques used more frequently?

12. What are the limitations that restrict use of systemic irradiation?

BIBLIOGRAPHY

1. BUSCHKE, F. Clinical application of supervoltage radiation. *The Cancer Bulletin*, Texas, 8:12–18, 1956.
2. BUSCHKE, F. Fundamental radiobiology. *The Cancer Bulletin*, Texas, 8:2–7, 1956.
3. BUSCHKE, F., CANTRIL, S., and PARKER, H. *Supervoltage Roentgentherapy*, Charles C Thomas, Springfield, Ill., 1950.
4. KOHN, H. The relative biological effectiveness of external beams of ionizing radiation. In: *Progress in Radiation Therapy*, Vol. I. F. Buschke, Ed., Grune & Stratton, New York, 1958.
5. PATERSON, R., and PARKER, H. M. Dosage system for gamma ray therapy. *Brit J Radiol* 7:592–632, 1934.
6. PARKER, R. G. and WILDERMUTH, O. Radiation therapy of lesions overlying cartilage. I. Carcinoma of the pinna. *Cancer*, 15:57–65, 1962.
7. PARKER, R. G. Tolerance of cartilage and bone in clinical radiation therapy. In: *Progress in Radiation Therapy*, Vol. II. F. Buschke, Ed., Grune & Stratton, New York, 1962.
8. WOOTTON, P., and CANTRIL, S. T. Comparison of the use of standard depth dose data at 250 KVP and 2 MV by direct measurement of tumor exposure dose in vivo. *Radiology*, 72:726–734, 1959.

EFFECTS OF IONIZING RADIATION ON CELLS AND TISSUES

The basic physical and chemical changes produced in matter by ionizing radiation of any type are fundamentally the same, although each type of radiation may initiate biological responses through a broad spectrum. The physical changes are sufficiently well understood to provide a basis for exacting qualitative and quantitative measurement and, thus, for well-controlled clinical application. The chemical changes and biological responses, although the subject of intense study, are less well understood, and thus provide an inadequate basis for replacement of clinical empiricism by scientific application.

Physicochemical Effects

When ionizing radiation interacts with matter, deposition of energy in the absorbing material initiates chemical and biological responses. Although the physicochemical changes are practically instantaneous (10^{-4} to 10^{-12} sec)[17], the observed biological effects may be delayed for long periods (15 years or longer for human carcinogenesis, generations for genetic changes). The energy transfer is mostly through *ionization,* but also through *excitation* of the molecules of the absorber. If the primary radiation is either photon energy or uncharged particles, secondary charged particles are formed by the transfer of kinetic energy through collision with molecules of the absorbing material. The ejected electrons and the ionized and excited molecules rapidly are transformed into new stable molecules or reactive molecular fragments. These reactive chemical products initially are clustered in high concentration along the paths of the charged particles, where they may interact among themselves or diffuse throughout the absorbing material before reacting. Vitally important structures in a cell may be damaged by these reactive chemical products (*indirect effect*) or by direct intracellular energy transfer with resultant ionization or excitation (*direct effect*).

The highly complex physical and chemical changes induced by radiation are beyond the scope and purpose of this book. The interested reader is referred to the many good textbooks of medical radiation physics and radiation chemistry and to a summary article and bibliography by Boag.[4]

Biological Effects

The biological effects of radiation are proportional to the amount of energy absorbed (dose). There is no evidence of biological specificity of action related to wavelength of radiation. Differences in observed gross effects in controlled test objects following absorption of photon radiation of different energies (wavelength) can be explained by differences in the distribution of physically absorbed energy. Thus, any apparent biological differences produced by "supervoltage" radiation (i.e., cobalt-60, cesium-137) compared with "medium-voltage" or "orthovoltage" (250 kv) radiation are not radiation-quality specific, but can be related to differences in the physical pattern of absorption and the distribution of energy in tissue.

The selective destruction of certain tumors by ionizing radiation without consequent intolerable damage to adjacent normal structures is based on one of nature's whims whereby certain cells, tissues, and resultant tumors have greater radiovulnerability than others. The utilization of a differential in radiovulnerability between tumor and adjacent normal tissues (*therapeutic ratio*) is the foundation of clinical radiation therapy. All radiotherapeutic techniques must exploit this differential, and improved results can be expected only from techniques which increase it. Theoretically, the differential can be enlarged either by increasing tumor radiovulnerability or by decreasing the radiovulnerability of the adjacent normal tissues.

The ultimate response of any tissue/organ/tumor to ionizing radiation depends on: (1) the cellular response, (2) the response of the intercellular tissues, (3) the influence of the immediately adjacent tissue (tumor bed), (4) factors related to the organization and function of the tissue/organ/tumor, and (5) factors related to the host.

1. *Cellular Response.* Cell death may result from interference with the repetitive process of division (*reproductive death*) or from structural degeneration independent of progression through the cell replication cycle (*interphase death*).[7]

Reproductive cell death may be rapid within the current cell replication cycle or may not be detectable until the lethally damaged cells have completed several grossly normal cycles. Inactive cells, such as those of the liver parenchyma, may not show evidence of reproductive death until the cells are stimulated to attempt division. By this definition (reproductive death), cells which cannot sustain division are considered dead even though complex metabolic functions may continue.

Inasmuch as the critical radiation damage to the molecular structure of a cell probably is in its DNA,[13] the radiovulnerability can be correlated with phases of the replication cycle in which DNA is synthesized and the cell divides (Figures 3-3). For many mammalian cells, the DNA synthetic (S), postsynthetic (G_2), and mitotic (M) phases vary little in combined overall time (10–15 hours), although the post-mitotic phase (G_1) may vary from less than one hour to an indefinite period.[24] The radiosensitivity of a specific cell may vary throughout the cycle,[26, 27] but such differences are not detectable for a heterogeneous collection of cells distributed throughout all phases of the cycle.

The term *radiosensitivity* is used differently by various authors. Basically it means the susceptibility of the cell to lethal injury by ionizing radiation.[2] A conventional measurement of this susceptibility to damage is that dose required to reduce a viable (reproducing) cell population to 37 percent of its initial value on the exponential portion of the cell survival curve. This D_{37} or D_0 value for many aerobic mammalian cells ranges between 110 and 240 rads (using ^{60}Co radiation).[24] As visualized in Figures 3-4, 3-5, and 3-6, radiosensitivity increases as the D_{37} decreases (the slope of the radiation dose-cell survival curve becomes steeper).

The chance that a specific cell, in a population of cells, will be affected by an ionizing event can be calculated by the statistical rules of probability. (How many cells of a tumor population that must be killed to accomplish clinical eradication is unknown.) Thus, a specific radiation dose kills a constant fraction of those cells irradiated. The absolute number of cells killed depends on the number irradiated. Therefore, the initial dose of a series of equal doses kills the largest absolute number of cells (Table 3-3).

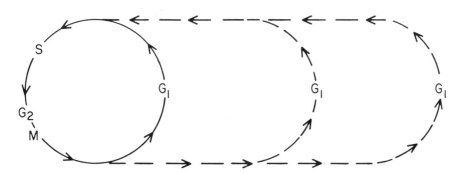

Fig. 3-3. Cell Replication Cycle.
S = period of DNA synthesis
G₂ = interval between DNA synthesis and mitosis
M = mitosis
G₁ = variable time after mitosis before DNA synthesis
Time for S + G₂ + M = 10–15 hours
Time for S₁ = varies from less than one hour to indefinite
The radiosensitivity measured by D₀ may vary by at least
50 percent at various positions in the cycle.

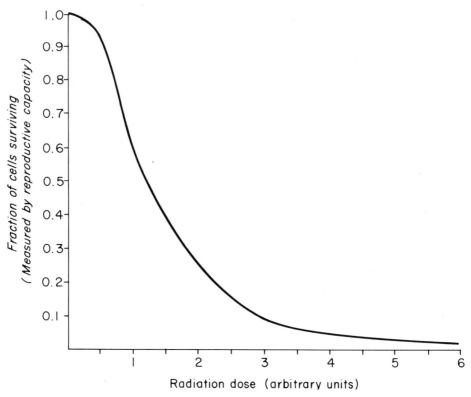

Fig. 3-4. Cell Survival Curve—Linear Plot. (Multitarget Response Viability Measured by Ability to Form Colonies.) This is a graph of a typical postirradiation cell survival curve. A specified radiation dose kills a constant fraction of the cells. The initial less steep portion is characteristic of cells having multiple critical targets.

Table 3-3. Number of Cells Killed per Dose Increment to Demonstrate Statistical Nature of Response

Accumulated Dose (rads)*	Dose in Increments	No. Variable Cells Irradiated	No. Cells Killed	No. Cells Surviving
400	400 × 1	10,000,000,000	9,000,000,000	1,000,000,000
800	400 × 2	1,000,000,000	900,000,000	100,000,000
1,200	400 × 3	100,000,000	90,000,000	10,000,000
1,600	400 × 4	10,000,000	9,000,000	1,000,000
2,000	400 × 5	1,000,000	900,000	100,000
2,400	400 × 6	100,000	90,000	10,000
2,800	400 × 7	10,000	9,000	1,000
3,200	400 × 8	1,000	900	100
3,600	400 × 9	100	90	10
4,000	400 × 10	10	9	1

90% of population irradiated killed by 400 rads
*Single increment doses—no recovery
After Suit[24]

24

Fig. 3-5. Cell Survival Curve —Log Plot. (Multitarget Response Viability Measured by Ability to Form Colonies.) This is a graph of a typical postirradiation cell survival curve. The exponential portion of the curve is a straight line (BC) on log paper. Extrapolation to the ordinate at A is a measure of the number of critical cell targets (N number). The D_0 dose, that which results in a surviving fraction of 0.37, is a measure of sensitivity.

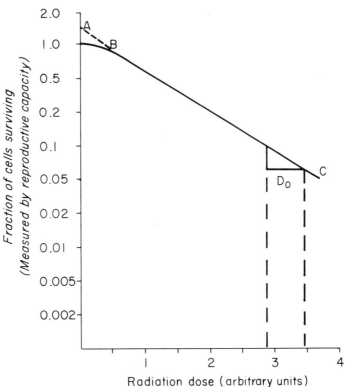

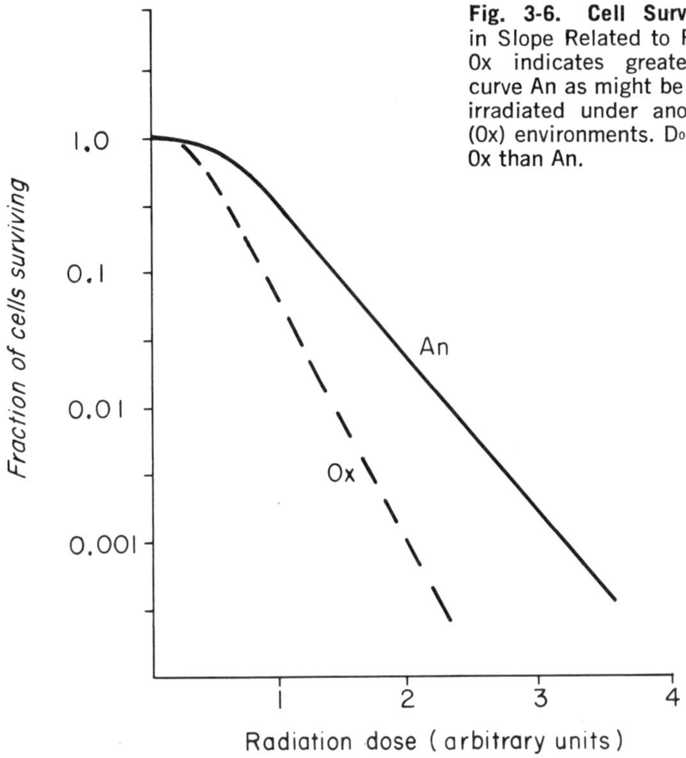

Fraction of cells surviving
(Measured by reproductive capacity)

Radiation dose (arbitrary units)

Fig. 3-6. Cell Survival Curve. (Variations in Slope Related to Radiosensitivity.) Curve Ox indicates greater radiosensitivity than curve An as might be found for same cell line irradiated under anoxic (An) or oxygenated (Ox) environments. D_0 would be less for curve Ox than An.

Fraction of cells surviving

Radiation dose (arbitrary units)

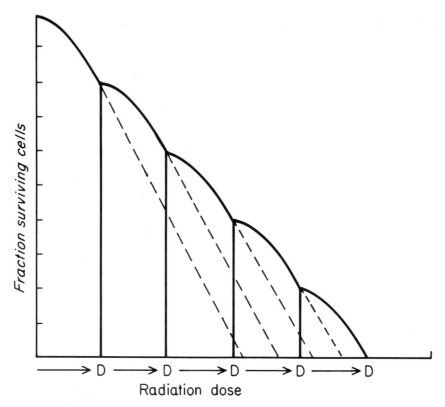

Fig. 3-7. Composite Cell Survival Curve for Fractionated Doses of Radiation.
This composite of several similar survival curves illustrates the overall effect of
multiple equal doses repeated at a fixed interval which allows complete cellular
recovery from the preceding dose but no increase in cell number from replication.

Radiation dose-cell survival curves are used to study various parameters in
cellular radiobiology. Most data conform to a survival curve consistent with the
following: All cells contain multiple critical targets of "uniform size"; a target is
inactivated by a single hit; and all targets must be hit to produce cell death.[24] Such
a "multitarget-single hit" survival curve is illustrated in Figures 3-4–3-6. The first
portion (shoulder) of the curve indicates an initial relative ineffectiveness of radiation, being indirectly related to intracellular "target" number and repair of sublethal
injury.[2] The data of particular interest to the clinical therapeutic radiologist, namely,
cell survival fractions in the range of 10^{-10} for fractionated applications of radiation
(Figure 3-7) are sparse. Also, some data are more consistent with "multihit-single
target" survival curves, yet another indication that the explanations for human
clinical responses are extremely complicated.

The ultimate response of a cell or cell population is conditioned by its ability
to repair sublethal injury. In mammalian cells, full repair of the reproductive capacity may be accomplished within four hours by processes which are considered bio-
physical rather than metabolic.[9-11] However, these "recovered" cells are likely to be
altered as measured by other parameters such as culture colony size, radiosensitivity,

cell volume, chromosome number, and intermitotic period.[21] Variations in recovery are especially important when the radiation is delivered in multiple fractions, as in clinical application, for differences in recovery between tumor cells and cells of adjacent structures may determine whether there is an exploitable therapeutic ratio. Although the division of a radiation dose into multiple fractions separated by intervals longer than a day lessens its absolute cell-killing efficiency (Fig. 3-7), variations in recovery between tumor cells and normal tissue may be favorably accentuated with consequent improvement in the therapeutic ratio.

Although modern cellular radiobiology dates to the development of mammalian cell culture by Puck and Marcus in 1956,[18] clinically important observations date almost to the discovery of radioactivity. The relationship between cellular reproductive activity and radiation responsiveness was described in 1904 by Bergonie and Tribondeau,[3] based on experimental investigation on the testis: "The sensitivity of cells to irradiation is in direct proportion to their reproductive activity and inversely proportional to their degree of differentiation." This statement frequently is referred to as the *"law" of Bergonie and Tribondeau*. This relationship of radiovulnerability to cellular reproductive activity and differentiation has been correlated with many clinical observations: (1) greater radiovulnerability of such rapidly reproducing tissues as testicle, bone marrow, and epithelium of the small intestine, as compared with skin or peripheral nerve; (2) greater radiovulnerability of the faster growing, more anaplastic tumors compared with the more differentiated variety of the same cellular origin; (3) greater radiovulnerability of the less differentiated and growing peripheral portions as compared with the more differentiated central portions of the same tumor.

In 1922, Regaud[19] demonstrated that variations in radiovulnerability between adjacent but different tissues and between cells of varying maturation within the same tissue could be accentuated by the fractionated application of ionizing radiation. Permanent sterilization of the Ram's testicle could not be produced by a single radiation dose without production of necrosis of the overlying skin and damage to the rectum. However, when Regaud fractionated the irradiation over one to two weeks, the total accumulated dose could be increased and permanent sterilization accomplished without significant damage to the normal structures through which the beam passed. This experiment was of great importance because it provided the rationale for the use of fractionated doses in clinical radiation therapy. This fractionated application of radiation over several weeks is known as the *Coutard method*.

The applicability of this technique varies with the type of tumor. For neoplasms such as lymphosarcoma, the time factor, within wide limits, is not critical. For other tumors with more rapid recovery rates (particularly epidermoid carcinoma), the time factor is important. The art of radiation therapy of tumors which have critical limits of radiovulnerability is based on a judgment of optimal fractionation and protraction of the total dose in order to exploit the maximal therapeutic ratio (relationship of tumor vulnerability and tolerance of normal structures included in the *critical·volume*).

In the treatment of tumors with a narrow margin between vulnerability of tumor and vulnerability of normal structures in the critical volume, the power of *repair* and *regeneration* of the normal tissues can determine whether radiation therapy can be used, and usually establishes the limit of radiation dose. Regeneration and repair must not be confused with cell recovery. In the process of regeneration, surviving cells replace those destroyed. This is readily observed in the healing of a moist skin reaction when regeneration occurs from normal cells at the periphery of the field and from islands of epithelial cells which have escaped destruction. Repair is the replacement of destroyed tissue by some other tissue, such as scar tissue. Satisfactory function and comfort following regeneration or repair will depend on the size of the treated volume and upon the anatomical site involved.

Permanent destruction of normal and neoplastic cells which repopulate from a cellular matrix by a process of differentiation (testicle, epidermis, epidermoid carcinoma) often depends upon the vulnerability of the cells from which regeneration takes place. These precursor cells may be more or less radiosensitive than their progeny. If the derived cells are less radioresponsive, they may live out their life cycle so that gross evidence of sterilization occurs after a period during which there has been no repopulation. As a result, the sterilization of a testicle becomes evident after about 30 days, and the epidermis is denuded after about 28 days. This may explain, in part, the slower visible regression of epidermoid carcinomas as compared with lymphosarcoma, in which the tumor cells are directly affected.

2. *Intercellular Substances.*   The effect of radiation on intercellular substances is particularly important in the "protection" of normal tissue. Irradiation of connective tissue is followed by an initial inflammation and later thickening of collagenous and elastic fibers. Clinically detectable fibrosis follows large doses. These changes progress long after irradiation has ceased and may not be clinically manifest until many years later. They are accompanied by permanent changes in the small caliber blood vessels: destruction of the endothelium; disintegration of the elastic elements; degeneration of the muscle, followed by thickening of the intima and obliteration of the lumen (radiation endarteritis). In contrast to the radiation-produced changes in cellular components of normal organs, which may be transient because of regeneration from unaffected elements, changes in the intercellular vasculoconnective tissue are irreversible and progress relentlessly after they have reached a certain intensity. These changes in intercellular vasculoconnective tissue are the basis of many serious late complications of radiation therapy (necrosis; fibrosis; obliteration of hollow organs, such as intestine).

The tolerance of the vasculoconnective tissue determines the limitation of the radiation dose in many anatomical sites. For example, moderate damage to the intestinal mucosa may be reversible, but fibrotic changes in the intestinal wall, once initiated, continue. These postirradiation fibrotic and poorly vascularized tissues are less resistant to mechanical injury and infection. Therefore, long after irradiation, minor trauma or infection may induce serious, and at times disastrous, complications in this compromised tissue.

3. *Tumor Bed.*   The condition of the tumor bed influences the radiovulnerability of the tumor. At times this influence is critical. An epidermoid carcinoma originating in the tonsillar mucosa, which overlies loose connective tissue, can easily be controlled locally, although a histologically similar carcinoma of the mucosa of the anterior pillar, growing in a tumor bed with dense stroma closely attached to muscle, often is not controllable. There is ample experimental and clinical evidence to demonstrate the importance of adequate vascularization. Decreased oxygen tension has been shown experimentally to decrease radiation response. Therefore,

a "radioresponsive" tumor in a poorly vascularized bed is less likely to be controlled than a similar tumor in a well-vascularized tumor bed. An epidermoid carcinoma in a tongue with syphilitic glossitis may not be controlled because of the poor vascularization secondary to the syphilitic endarteritis. The reduced vulnerability of a tumor following previous radiation therapy (Regaud's so-called radioimmunization) is probably not due to an inherent change in the radiosensitivity of the tumor cells, but to a reduced vulnerability caused by impairment of vascularity and fibrosis. This difficulty is further increased by the reduced radiation tolerance of the previously irradiated connective tissue and vessels of the tumor bed.

The difficulty in controlling metastatic tumor deposits in lymph nodes, even when a carcinoma can be controlled at its primary site (oral tongue, lip, pharynx, cervix), is well recognized and in part may be explained by the impairment of circulation within the node. If this explanation is correct, it should be possible to sterilize a lymph node containing minimal tumor which does not interfere with the circulation.

The presence of infection decreases the radiation response. Therefore, judicious use of antibiotics in association with radiation therapy can contribute to the curability of certain cancers.

4. *Tumor-related Factors.* Specific factors related to a tumor, as a collection of cells and intercellular substances, may influence the effectiveness of radiation.

The radiovulnerability of a specific tumor cell and consequently of a tumor often can be predicted by the responsiveness of the parent cell. Thus, the small-cell lymphosarcoma is highly sensitive as might be predicted from the response of the lymphocyte, whereas a well-differentiated squamous cell carcinoma is less radiovulnerable as predictable from the responsiveness of epithelium. However, the radiovulnerability of tumors is made less predictable by variations in tumor cell differentiation, a conglomerate content, i.e., Hodgkin's disease, varying amounts of intercellular substances, and differences in physiological status of the tumor cells and the surrounding tissues.

Within the same tumor type, there is correlation between the degree of histological differentiation and the radiovulnerability. This correlation varies considerably for different tumors. The importance of this observation, however, is overemphasized. The degree of histological differentiation of most epidermoid carcinomas is not a highly reliable basis for an estimate of radiological response, although the very undifferentiated epidermoid carcinoma may be most responsive. In contrast, the degree of differentiation is of clinical importance, and may determine the therapeutic approach, i.e., in carcinoma of the bladder or endometrium.

The structure of a tumor may influence its response to radiation in many ways. For example, tumors may consist of three zones[25]: a central zone of necrosis which is of no concern because the tumor is not viable; a peripheral zone of adequately oxygenated active tumor growth close to the supplying blood vessels; and an intermediate zone of reduced oxygen tension in which the cells are still viable but not actively dividing. Cells in the poorly oxygenated intermediate zone are less responsive (up to a factor of three times) to irradiation than are the cells in the well-oxygenated periphery. Adjuvant administration of oxygen under increased pressure (3 to 4 atm) has been used in an attempt to increase the radiosensitivity of cells in this intermediate zone by improving their oxygenation. The increased oxygen tension does not alter the optimal normal oxygenation of well-vascularized normal tissues, and therefore, does not significantly change the radiosensitivity of normal structures. In this way, it may be possible to selectively increase the radiosensitivity of the tumor as well as the differential between the radiovulnerability of the tumor and that of the surrounding normal structures (therapeutic ratio). Radiation therapy with concurrent administration of high-pressure oxygen is now in the process of clinical investigation.

Reduction of the radiosensitivity of both normal tissues and well-oxygenated parts of a tumor by rendering them hypoxic permits higher doses to both tumor and adjacent normal tissues. This maneuver, which might counteract the selective hypoxia within some tumors, is being investigated[22] by use of a tourniquet technique applied to tumor-bearing extremities.

Cellular radiosensitivity, and consequently tumor radiovulnerability, can be increased by incorporation of certain drugs at the time of irradiation. Analogues of the base constituents of DNA molecules have been used on the assumption that this is a primary site of the cell killing. However, such chemicals frequently are toxic to the human and so far have not improved the therapeutic ratio as compared to the use of radiation alone. Thus, after clinical trials of many chemicals (HN2, chlorambucil, amethopterin, actinomycin-D, 5-fluorouracil, 5 BUdR, TEM), "the therapeutic value of this form of combination therapy is yet to be proved."[14] (See Chapter 5, Chemical Modification of Radiation Effect.)

Although no tested method has been found to consistently and effectively increase the radiovulnerability of any specific tumor, at times the relative vulnerability can be increased by protection of adjacent normal tissue. It is necessary to differentiate between those tissues in the immediate neighborhood of the tumor which must be included in the treated volume (*critical volume*) and those tissues through which the beam passes on its way between the body surface and the critical volume (*extraneous volume*).

The protection of the extraneous volume is not a major problem. By changing the geometrical distribution of the beam (cross firing through multiple fields or rotational therapy) or by judicious utilization of different distributions of ionization associated with radiation of different wavelengths, it is usually possible to respect the radiation tolerance of the more important structures.

Protection of the normal structures in the critical volume is more difficult, and their tolerance often determines the limitation of radiation therapy. For instance, in the treatment of carcinoma of the cervix, the tolerance of the intestinal mucosa and the pelvic vaculoconnective tissue determines the maximum permissible dose. In carcinoma of the larynx, the tolerance of cartilage is a limiting factor.

There are two technical modifications that increase the differential radiovulnerability between normal and some neoplastic tissues: greater protraction of treatment and the use of radiation of shorter wavelength.

Inasmuch as the probability of inactivation of any specific cell by ionizing radiation is a statistical event, the dose required to reduce the surviving cell population to a small fraction should be larger for tumors with a greater number of cells. Although this is true within limits, the relative importance of this correlation in clinical tumor control is small when compared to other factors, i.e., cellular radiosensitivity and recovery, tumor bed effect, and host factors.

Tumor growth rate as a manifestation of cell replication may influence the response to radiation if the cell cycle time is less than the interval between the radiation dose fractions. Also the interval between treatment and clinical reappearance should be shorter for rapidly growing tumors if this growth rate is a reflection of cell cycle time.

The radiation response of tumor in its primary site often varies from that noted for its metastatic deposits. This probably reflects the influence of environment, i.e., oxygenation and nutrition, on the tumor cell.

A reliable correlation between the rate of tumor regression following irradiation and the probability of its local control would be a clinically useful indicator. Suit et al.[23] have found no such correlation in animal experiments or in studies of squamous cell carcinomas of the human oropharynx.

5. *Host Factors.* The least understood and possibly the most important factors are host related. Every experienced clinical oncologist has seen patients systemically thrive in the presence of large tumor masses, particularly when these are lymphomas or carcinomas arising in the kidney, breast, or ovary; or these patients may die within a short time of widespread metastases from a very small primary tumor, particularly one in the breast.

Females fare better than males with nearly all cancers. Pregnant females may do very well with Hodgkin's disease,[16] but they do less with cancer of the breast[12] or cervix.[5] Children do very well with thyroid cancer,[28] but badly with lymphosarcoma.[20]

Patients with Hodgkin's disease often develop immunological defects.[1] Occasionally documented cancers, especially neuroblastomas, "spontaneously" disappear.[6] Despite the ease of identifying cancer cells in the bloodstream, especially in patients with cancer of the bowel at the time of resection, the incidence of distant metastases is low.[8, 15]

These biological behavior patterns, as yet unexplained, should temper all observations of responses attributed to treatment.

REVIEW QUESTIONS

1. What are the two fundamental processes by which energy is transferred from radiation to matter?

2. Differentiate between direct and indirect action.

3. Can you explain the disparity between the "instantaneous" physicochemical reaction and a biological response not evident for many years?

4. What are two known methods of cell killing?

5. In radiobiology, cells are considered "nonviable" when they can no longer sustain proliferation, even though complex metabolism may continue. Can you give an example of a clinical situation in which this concept might be useful?

6. What is the cell replication cycle? What are its phases? Is a cell uniformly radiosensitive throughout the cycle? If not, at what positions is it most sensitive? Can this be exploited clinically?

7. Give three clinical observations that can be correlated with the relationship of cellular radiovulnerability to reproductive activity and differentiation.

8. What is the reason for the use of fractionated doses in clinical radiation therapy?

9. Are precursor cells or their derivatives more radiosensitive?

10. Why are changes in the intercellular substances important?

11. Describe the changes of radiation-produced endarteritis. What caliber vessels are affected? Are these changes reversible? What are the clinical consequences?

12. What is the basis of all radiation therapy techniques?

13. What determines tumor radiovulnerability?

14. Is there a correlation between radiosensitivity and cell of origin of a tumor? between radiosensitivity and histological differentiation of tumor? Which is the most reliable clinical guide?

15. What is the tumor bed? What is its clinical importance?

16. Can radiation therapy control tumor metastatic in a lymph node? If so, under what conditions? What is your clinical experience?

17. What is the basis of using oxygen under pressure (3–4 atm) in radiation treatment?

18. Do you know of any chemicals that increase cellular radiosensitivity? Are they of clinical value?

19. How can radiation damage to normal structures adjacent to tumor be minimized?

20. What role does postirradiation cellular recovery have in clinical radiation therapy?

BIBLIOGRAPHY

1. AISENBERG, A. C. Manifestations of immunologic unresponsiveness in Hodgkin's disease. *Cancer Res.*, 26:1152–1160, 1966.
2. ANDREWS, J. R. *The Radiobiology of Human Cancer Radiotherapy.* Saunders, Philadelphia, 1968.
3. BERGONIE, J., and TRIBONDEAU, L. Action des rayons X sur les spermatozoides de l'homme. *C R Soc Biol* (Paris) 57:595, 1904.
4. BOAG, J. W. Primary processes of deposition of radiant energy and initial radiochemical events. *Amer J Roentgen*, 90:896–908, 1963.
5. BOSCH, A., and MARCIAL, V. A. Carcinoma of uterine cervix associated with pregnancy. *Amer J Roentgen*, 96:92–99, 1966.
6. BOYD, W. *The Spontaneous Regression of Cancer.* Charles C Thomas, Springfield, Ill. 1966.
7. CHRISTENSEN, G. M., and JACKSON, K. L. Personal communication.
8. COLE, W. H. Dissemination of cancer of colon. *Gastroenterology*, 41:412–414, 1961.
9. ELKIND, M. M., and SUTTON, H. X-ray damage and recovery in mammalian cells in culture. *Nature*, 184:1293–1295, 1959.
10. ELKIND, M. M., WHITMORE, G. F., and ALESCIO, T. Actinomycin D: Suppression of recovery in x-irradiated mammalian cells. *Science*, 143:1454–1467, 1964.
11. ELKIND, M. M., ALESCIO, T., SWAM, R. W. MOSES, W. B., and SUTTON, H. Recovery of hypoxic mammalian cells from sublethal x-ray damage. *Nature*, 202:1190–1193, 1964.

12. HOLLEB, A. I., and FARROW, J. H. The relation of carcinoma of the breast and pregnancy in 283 patients. *Surg Gynec Obstet*, 115:65–71, 1962.
13. KAPLAN, H. S. Biochemical basis of reproductive death in irradiated cells. *Amer J Roentgen*, 90:907–916, 1963.
14. KLIGERMAN, M. M. Present status of combined radiation therapy and chemotherapy. In: *Progress in Radiation Therapy*, Vol. III. F. Buschke, Ed., Grune & Stratton, New York, 1965, pp. 183–199.
15. MOORE, G. E., and SAKO, K. The spread of carcinoma of the colon and rectum: A study of invasion of blood vessels, lymph nodes and the peritoneum by tumor cells. *Dis Colon Rectum* 2:92–97, 1959.
16. PETERS, M. V. A study of survivals in Hodgkin's disease treated radiologically. *Amer J Roentgen*, 63:299–311, 1950.
17. PLATZMAN, R. L. Basic mechanisms in radiobiology. U.S. Nat. Acad. Sciences Publ. No. 305, 1953.
18. PUCK, T T. and MARCUS, P. I. Action of x-rays on mammalian cells. *J. Exp. Med.*, 103:653–666, 1956.
19. REGAUD, C. Influence de la durée de radiation sur les effets determinés dans le testicule par le radium. *C R Soc Biol* (Paris) 86:787–790, 1922.
20. ROSENBERG, S. A., DIAMOND, H. D., DARGEON, H. W., and CRAVER, L. F. Lymphosarcoma in childhood. *New Eng J Med*, 259:505–512, 1958.
21. SINCLAIR, W. K. X-ray induced heritable damage (small colony formation) in cultured mammalian cells. *Radiat Res*, 21:584–611, 1964.
22. SUIT, H. D. Radiation therapy given under conditions of local tissue hypoxia for bone and soft tissue sarcoma. In: *Tumors of Bone and Soft Tissue*, Eighth Annual Clinical Conference on Cancer. Year Book, Chicago, 1963.
23. SUIT, H. D., LINDBERG, R., and FLETCHER, G. H. Prognostic significance of extent of tumor regression at completion of radiation therapy. *Radiology*, 84:1100–1107, 1965.
24. SUIT, H. D. Radiation biology: A basis for radiotherapy. In: *Textbook of Radiotherapy*. G. H. Fletcher, Ed., Lea & Febiger, Philadelphia, 1966.
25. THOMLINSON, R. H., and GRAY, L. H. The histological structure of some human lung cancers and possible implications for radiotherapy. *Brit J Cancer*, 9:539–549, 1955.
26. TOLMACH, L. J., TERASIMA, T., and PHILLIPS, R. A. In: *Cellular Radiation Biology*, Williams & Wilkins, Baltimore, 1965.
27. WHITMORE, G. F., GULYAS, S., and BOTOND, J. In: *Cellular Radiation Biology*. Williams & Wilkins, Baltimore, 1965.
28. WINSHIP, T., and ROSVOLL, R. V. Childhood thyroid carcinoma. *Cancer*, 14:734–743, 1961.

RECOMMENDED READING

1. SUIT, H. D. Radiation biology: A basis for radiotherapy. In: *Textbook of Radiotherapy*. G. H. Fletcher, Ed., Lea & Febiger, Philadelphia, 1966, pp. 65–97.
2. ANDREWS, J. R. *The Radiobiology of Human Cancer Radiotherapy*. Saunders, Philadelphia, 1968.
3. CASARETT, A. P. *Radiation Biology*. Prentice-Hall, Englewood Cliffs, N.J., 1968.

SIDE EFFECTS AND HAZARDS OF RADIATION THERAPY

Every effective therapeutic procedure has its undesirable, and at times dangerous, side effects. Progress in the medical use of ionizing radiation consists of finding techniques that minimize these side effects without reducing the desired effect on tumor.

Radiation therapy has matured from infancy to adulthood within one physician generation. Many physicians still remember the severe tissue damage caused by irradiation of normal tissues, when the risks were unknown or ways of avoiding them were not available. The frequent delay, for many years or decades, in the clinical manifestations of these severe radiation injuries has promoted the interpretation that such injuries are unavoidable, masking their true significance as a residual from the early times of treatment by trial and error. Thus, it is important to differentiate between the risks of modern radiation therapy and the sequelae of techniques that should no longer be used.

Many misconceptions of the hazards of radiation therapy result from lack of understanding of the relationship of tissue damage to radiation technique. It is important to recognize three different situations: (1) injuries produced under experimental conditions not comparable to any clinically used techniques (e.g., large single doses); (2) injuries following clinical therapy with techniques previously used, but now considered inappropriate; (3) injuries associated with therapy considered competent by present standards. This discusion usually will refer to the third type of radiation injury.

Radiation therapy is used in the management of patients with lethal disease. Therefore, certain radiotherapeutic side effects are acceptable, just as some severe surgically produced functional and anatomical defects are acceptable, in an attempt to preserve life (for example, a colostomy in the treatment of carcinoma of the rectum). Today, serious damage associated with technically correct radiation therapy is considerably less than that accepted for many major surgical procedures in the treatment of cancer.

The incidence of significant tissue damage varies with the individual therapist's treatment philosophy: Is he willing to risk serious damage in most patients in the hope of controlling tumor in a few more? We believe that the old clinical rule of "primum nil nocere" also applies to radiation therapy. Raising the dose above that which is known to be tolerated by most patients will at best lead to a minimal improvement of curative results, bought at the price of considerable damage to normal structures. Above known ranges of tolerance to irradiation, the risk of damage increases more rapidly than does the likelihood of cure. If control of a tumor can be obtained only with doses which cause extensive damage to normal structures, then radiation therapy is not the indicated method of treatment.

Radiation reactions and radiation hazards will be discussed separately. *Radiation reactions* are tolerable constitutional responses and local tissue changes associated with the absorption of ionizing radiation. *Radiation hazards* are risks of clinically unacceptable tissue damage.

Radiation Reactions

Early and late radiation reactions may be recognized. *Early reactions* occur during or immediately following treatment and include constitutional effects and transient local changes in irradiated tissues.

Radiation sickness may be initiated clinically by a few days of headache, followed by anorexia, nausea, and vomiting. The probable cause is absorption of breakdown products of the irradiated tissues. Consequently, the incidence and severity are related to the volume of tissue treated and the daily dose. Radiation sickness, like the toxic effect of other potent drugs, can be prevented or minimized, in most instances, by adjustment of the treatment technique (daily dose, tissue volume treated) to the tolerance of the individual patient. The initial symptoms of irradiation sickness indicate that the limits of the patient's constitutional tolerance to radiation therapy are near. Such warning signals should be heeded. To give these patients medication to suppress symptoms rather than adjust treatment is comparable to prescribing morphine for the pain associated with appendicitis. With modern techniques, good radiation therapy rarely causes radiation sickness except when an emotional patient has been prepared by the referring physician or by "friends" to expect such symptoms.

Early tissue reactions of consequence include those of the skin and mucous membranes. *Skin reactions* were common with use of low or medium voltage x-ray, and were used as a therapeutic guide, indicating local normal tissue tolerance to radiation. When medium-voltage radiation is administered daily for several weeks to a total dose of at least 4,000 R, the skin initially becomes erythematous, and a moist "radioepidermite" may develop by the twenty-sixth to twenty-eighth day. The exudative radioepidermite, localized to the radiation field, consists of a thin, glistening layer of fibrin covering a denuded dermis. More intense reactions may include sites of hemorrhage. In the absence of secondary infection, these lesions usually are painless. A lesser reaction is the dry or desquamative radioepidermite, characterized by an initial erythema followed by bronzing and scaling of the epidermis over the treated area. The severity of the radioepidermite from low- or medium-voltage irradiation depends upon radiation quality, pattern of application, intensity of delivery (daily dose), total dose, size of the field, and individual patient sensitivity. Following the maximum radioepidermite, about 4 weeks after the beginning of treatment, the reaction subsides and re-epidermitization of the denuded area progresses to completion in 10–14 days (regeneration). The radioepidermite may subside and the skin may heal during continuation of daily therapy. After the healing of a moderately severe reaction, the skin may appear grossly normal, but it is never biologically normal. Injuries or infections may cause reactions limited to the treated volume, indicating a biologic difference between irradiated and nonirradiated skin. Examples are the reappearance of an erythema in grossly normal skin following systemic treatment with actinomycin D, or the development, after many years, of a neuroepidermite limited to the treated but normal-appearing skin. When the radiation was intense, or the total dose was high, or the field was large, there might be late sequelae of atrophy, telangiectasia, and permanent epilation. The skin reaction varies in different anatomic locations. Skin over bone is particularly vulnerable because scattered radiation increases the total dose. Skin in body folds is prone to the early development of reaction because of increased absorbed dose and trauma with movement. Such reactions can be anticipated, and particularly sensitive regions often can be protected.

A radioepidermite should be differentiated from the unfortunate misnomer, *"x-ray burn."* The radioepidermite is a transient, superficial denudation of the dermis without significant alteration of the underlying vasculoconnective tissue. The term "x-ray burn" should be reserved for local necrosis, usually secondary to vascular damage, which resembles changes produced by cautery.

Since, with supervoltage radiation, maximum ionization occurs below the epidermis, skin reactions at the portal of entry usually are avoided unless the doses are very large. As used today, radiation therapy of almost all deep-seated tumors does not cause marked skin reactions because the tolerance of other structures limits the dose. Fibrotic changes occasionally may develop at the site of maximum dosage in the subcutaneous tissues beneath a grossly normal-appearing epithelium.

Ionizing radiation causes a characteristic *mucosal reaction,* first described by Coutard[13] in 1922. When a mucous membrane can be repeatedly examined (oral cavity, pharynx, larynx), the initial reaction noted is an enanthema, gradually progressing to a radioepithelite, characterized by a white, glistening membrane overlying the surface. Histologically, the radioepithelite is an accumulation of desquamated cells, leukocytes, and fibrin associated with the destruction and desquamation of the superficial layers of the epithelium.

The incidence and severity of the mucosal reaction are partly dependent upon the accumulated total dose but, more importantly, depend on the intensity of treatment, measured by the size of the daily dose and the pattern of treatment. For example, with a total dose of 6,000 rads protracted at 1,000 rads per week, a membranous reaction may be mild. If this same total dose is administered with the so-called split course technique (3,000 rads in 14 days, a two-week interval, and 3,000 rads in another two weeks), the early reaction will be more severe and will be visible by the time the first 3,000 rads have been delivered at the rate of 1,500 rads per week.

The time of appearance of a mucosal reaction is specific for different anatomic sites and can be predicted with remarkable accuracy. Thus, the radioepithelite over the squamous epithelium of the buccal mucosa may be visible after 16 to 18 days of daily therapy, but on the soft palate it may appear 10 to 13 days after the beginning of therapy. The radioepithelite on the vocal cords, covered by highly differentiated, keratinizing squamous epithelium, may appear after 27 to 28 days, similar to skin, whereas the reaction on the ventricular bands and subglottic mucosa, involving cells of a more cylindric type, may occur after about 40 days of irradiation.

The radioepithelite may subside about one week after its appearance, even though daily treatment is continued. If the reaction is very intense, the patient may be more comfortable if the daily dose is reduced or treatment is suspended for a few days.

Coutard originally believed that an epithelite was inevitable if a cancer, particularly an epidermoid carcinoma, was to be controlled. It is now recognized that the epithelite is a side effect related to certain techniques, but not necessary for the sterilization of the neoplasm.[1,10,28] Indeed, it may be preferable to use techniques which avoid such a reaction. For instance, Lederman[21] emphasized the rarity of late complications in the treatment of laryngeal carcinoma when a massive early mucosal reaction is avoided by prolongation of treatment to six weeks. "In no circumstances should a brisk or severe local reaction be callously regarded by a radiotherapist as the 'price' the patient has to pay for possible cure."[21]

The mucosal reaction is an important indication that the limit of radiation tolerance is being approached. It is fortunate that the radiosensitivity of mucosal epithelium is greater than the radiovulnerability of the underlying connective tissue and small vessels. Thus, by detecting the mucosal reaction, in visible membranes (oral cavity, larynx, pharynx, vagina) by frequent observation, and in those not visible (esophagus, intestinal mucosa) by recognition of symptoms and signs, it is possible to avoid damage to the vasculoconnective tissue, the basis of serious late complications. Our experience confirms Lederman's statement: "Generally the patient who does not suffer during treatment rarely encounters complications after treatment."[21]

When medium-voltage x-ray is used, these mucosal reactions are severe and may create morbidity that is serious because of interference with adequate nutrition. With the use of supervoltage radiation, mucosal reactions of such potential consequence usually can be avoided.

The appearance of the radioepithelite over the tumor may be an important guide to its radiosensitivity. If the surrounding normal mucosa reacts while the epithelium overlying the tumor does not, the radiosensitivity of the tumor may be less than that of the normal mucosa, and this tumor may not be controlled (Coutard's reaction "en couronne").

Late radiation reactions are separated from the time of treatment by intervals varying from months to years. The incidence and severity of these reactions are directly proportional to the incidence and severity of the early reactions. It is rare that a late reaction has not been antedated by an early reaction. There are no late sequelae of radiation sickness. Late changes of atrophy, telangiectasia, epilation, and fragility are permanent in skin and mucosa.

Radiation Hazards

"Radiation hazards" are risks of tissue damage beyond the tolerable side effects of properly conducted radiation therapy.

There are two types of radiation hazards, although the demarcation is not always sharp, i.e., that related to injury of the mesenchymal tissues (vasculoconnective tissue, cartilage, and bone) and that related to the injury of specific organs.

Because of the ubiquity of the vasculoconnective tissue, its lack of reparative power, and the irreversible and often disastrous late effects of severe fibrosis and vascular impairment, the radiation tolerance of the vasculoconnective tissue often determines the upper limit of radiation dosage. The dose of 6,000 rads (with a weekly dose which does not exceed 1,000 rads), which undeservedly has been honored by the term "cancerocidal", is the average limit of tolerance of the vasculoconnective tissue, and therefore the maximal "safe dose". In tissues which are particularly sensitive to impairment of the oxygen supply, such as the central nervous system, the average safe dose may be lower.

One of the most important steps in the progress of radiation therapy during the last 20 years is the better ability to minimize damage of the vasculoconnective tissue by the use of radiation of shorter wavelength, by longer protraction of the overall treatment time, and by the adjustment of treatment to the sensitivity of the individual patient through recognition of mucosal reactions as warning signals. The following discussion of the incidence of significant radiation injury to the vasculoconnective tissue is based on our policy[5] of using supervoltage therapy for the external irradiation of all major, deep-seated radiocurable cancers and of protracting the treatment over a period of not less than six weeks and frequently for eight to ten weeks(with a weekly dose of 800 to 1,000 rads). Hazards observed with techniques using protraction of less than five weeks (frequently found in the literature) are not considered here, except in the treatment of skin cancer. The comparable importance of longer protraction of local radium application in the treatment of cervical carcinoma in order to avoid intestinal injuries was demonstrated by Corscaden, Kasabach, and Lenz in 1938[12] and later by Kottmeier and Gray in 1957.[14,17]

The most important clinical manifestations of serious radiation damage to the vasculoconnective tissues are: the formation of fistulas (rectovaginal, vesico-vaginal, bronchoesophageal) caused by vascular damage resulting in necrosis; obstruction of hollow organs (rectosigmoid, esophagus, and ureter) due to fibrosis of the wall; pulmonary fibrosis; contracted bladder; fibrotic changes with vascular impairment which prevent or seriously complicate radical surgery in heavily irradiated tissues.

Because there is frequent misconception, the incidence of such damage following proper radiation therapy of frequently treated cancers (of cervix, larynx, esophagus, bladder) will be reviewed.

In 583 patients treated between 1939 and 1956 for carcinoma of the cervix and cervical stump,[4,7] there were 7 (1.2 percent) clinically significant bowel injuries. No patient was permanently incapacitated. There were three late bladder ulcerations (0.5 percent), all healing within one year. There was no vesicovaginal fistula or fracture of the femoral neck.

We attribute this low incidence of late complications to deliberate attempts to avoid or minimize mucosal reactions of the rectum and bowel during therapy. This is accomplished by protraction of dose and adjustment of the intracavitary and external radiation to individual tolerance, as manifested by symptoms and signs of rectal or intestinal irritation. Marked rectal reactions can be avoided. Significant late rectal, intestinal, or bladder complications rarely occur in the absence of early severe mucosal injury.

For treatment of carcinoma of the larynx, Lederman has used telecurie radiation therapy with a minimum protraction of six weeks. He emphasizes the comfort of the patient during treatment, as well as the rarity of late complications.[21] In his opinion, a severe local reaction should be avoided because a patient who has not experienced such a reaction usually does not suffer significant late tissue changes. In his experience, prolonged protraction has not compromised curative results in close to 1,000 cases.[21] In a study with Vaeth,[10,30] we have shown that by greater protraction of treatment, the mucosal reaction (and the late tissue changes) can be avoided without compromising the curability of laryngeal carcinoma.

The possibilty of fibrosis of the wall of the urinary bladder following radiation therapy still haunts some urologists. When the radiation tolerance of the bladder was not known, severe fibrosis was caused by excessive intracavitary or external irradiation.[6] Fibrosis may cause sufficient reduction of the capacity of the bladder so that patients need a permanent indwelling catheter or cystectomy, even in the absence of neoplastic disease.

The radiation tolerance of the bladder is now well established, both for intracavitary therapy[23] and external irradiation with supervoltage techniques. Since 1939 we have not observed clinically significant fibrosis of the bladder following technically correct external supervoltage irradiation.[8,16] In patients enjoying tumor control for as long as 22 years, normal bladder function has been maintained.

In carcinoma of the esophagus, there continues to be an excessive emphasis on the risk of bronchoesophageal or tracheoesophageal fistula following irradiation. With careful selection of patients and good treatment technique, such fistulas usually occur in the presence of uncontrolled tumor. In our experience, this has occurred in 10 percent of patients. Perforation rarely has occurred during or immediately following therapy. If imminent performation is not recognized prior to treatment, it can occur during treatment, and may even be hastened by therapy. The incidence of perforation increases if treatment is administered rapidly so that there is disintegration of tumor without fibroblastic replacement.

Radiation damage to cartilage and bone is of considerable clinical importance. An unjustified prejudice still exists that irradiation of overlying tissues subjects cartilage and bone to a high risk of necrosis. This prejudice has arisen from experience with poor treatment techniques, particularly use of soft radiation and insufficient protraction. With radiation in the lower- and medium-voltage ranges there is a relative increase in the absorbed dose in bone with resultant damage to the small vessels in the Haversian channels. Supervoltage radiation has overcome this difficulty because the absorption in bone is little increased per gram over the absorption in soft tissues. With adequate protraction, treatment of lesions overlying bone and cartilage is possible with medium-voltage radiation, although allowance must be made for the increased dose in bone. With the proper technique (quality of radiation and protraction), necrosis of bone and cartilage, not compromised by invading cancer or by infection, can be avoided. It is impossible, however, to control carcinoma that has invaded bone or cartilage without causing necrosis, regardless of the technique. Whether such necrosis is tolerable depends on the individual situation.

In 196 patients treated for lesions overlying the nose,[24] there were two instances (1 percent) of cartilaginous necrosis, both in patients with uncontrolled tumor. Following treatment of 39 carcinomas of the skin of the auricle,[25] there were three instances of cartilaginous necrosis, all associated with tumor invasion of the cartilage or with uncontrolled disease.

Our experience with radical preoperative irradiation of oral cancers followed by planned radical surgery[9] has been that the resected mandible appears grossly normal up to six months after having received doses as high as 8,000 rads. Free bleeding was encountered when the transection passed through heavily irradiated bone. Cordectomy through laryngofissure for radiation failures in cancer of the larynx has been possible without cartilaginous necrosis or other complications.[10]

Damage to the central nervous system is in part the indirect result of vascular and glial tissue changes, but in part results from direct effect on the cells of the central nervous system. The importance of potential damage to the spinal cord was first stressed by Boden,[2] who described the entity of "radiation myelitis" in 1948. He observed that radiation myelitis occurs in two clinical forms: transient and progressive. The transient form is reversible, and complete recovery is possible. It is manifest clinically as numbness or hyperesthesia in the limbs. The most typical symptom is an "electric shock" passing through the limbs (Lhermitte's sign), induced by anterior flexion of the head. These symptoms appear within one month to one year after irradiation, may last for a few months to a year before gradually disappearing, and are not accompanied by neurologic signs.[29]

Progressive myelitis is not reversible and is clinically manifest by a weakness or paralysis of muscles. It usually is preceded by the "transient" form, which may either gradually progress into the severe form or antedate it by several months, separated by a symptom-free interval. Once the neurologic signs and symptoms have become severe, they rarely disappear and may even progress to those of a partial cord transection.

The transient form probably results from demyelinization of the ascending pathways in the posterior and lateral columns, whereas the late progressive form is more likely due to damage to the vasculoglial tissue.

It seems from the reports in the literature[20] and from our experiences,[5] that a total dose of about 5,000 rads delivered no faster than 1,000 rads per week represents the average limit of radiation tolerance of the central nervous system. There are many individual differences, however, and radiation myelitis may occur after smaller doses.

In our own experience, the clinically significant forms of "progressive radiation myelitis" have been uncommon. Among 125 patients treated for cancer of the nasopharynx, tonsil, and pharygeal tongue between 1944 and 1956, six developed neurologic symptoms and signs attributed to cervical radiation myelitis.[5] All of these patients had rather complicated situations (such as re-treatment) and received, as calculated in retrospect, accumulated cord doses in the range of 7,000–8,000 rads in approximately 50 days. Three of the six patients recovered without residual symptoms, two had nonincapacitating symptoms until death five and eight years later, and one had symptoms persistent for 13 years. The relatively low incidence of progressive radiation myelitis in our experience is attributed to rather long protraction of treatment. This seems to be supported by Vaeth[29] in an analysis of cervical cord damage which documented an increase in risk with weekly doses exceeding 800 rads. An analysis of the radiation tolerance of the thoracic cord by Phillips and Buschke suggested "that the number of fractions is the most important factor in the determination of late radiation damage to the spinal cord . . . and that radiation myelitis can probably be prevented by avoiding an excessive total dose to the spinal cord and by planning treatment that does not deliver more than 200 rads per fraction."[27] With techniques using proper distribution of radiation anatomically and in time, it usually is possible to avoid serious damage to the central nervous system.

Some clinically important radiation hazards are associated with specific organ radiosensitivities rather than with damage to connective tissue and small vessels. The most important structures are the eye, ear, kidney, heart, and liver.

Damage to the lens or cornea may result from exposure of the eye to ionizing radiation. Radiation damage to the lens (*radiation cataract*) long has been of concern, although there is little risk under conditions of carefully conducted clinical radiation therapy. Many studies reported in the literature describe radiation cataract produced under conditions no longer prevailing in the clinical treatment of cancer. In a study of the incidence of radiation cataract under conditions of clinical therapy as we perform it,[26] "probably radiation-related lens changes" were found in 4 of 85 lenses, each following doses to the lens of 2,040 to 3,900 rads (in equal daily increments) over 46 to 85 days. Of 30 lenses that had received more than 500 rads in 32 to 93 days, 20 were without significant change, and 6 had equivocal changes 2½ to 15 years after treatment. Eight of 14 lenses that had received over 1,000 rads (1 in 32 days, 7 in more than 50 days) 5 to 13 years previously showed no significant changes, although 2 were equivocal. Most importantly, only 2 of 85 eyes had grossly diminished visual acuity probably related to radiation following doses of 3,570 to 3,900 rads for the treatment of carcinoma of the maxillary sinus. The alternative in these patients would have been orbital exenteration.

These findings have been reported in such detail to show that radiation cataract rarely occurs under optimal conditions of clinical radiotherapy for malignant disease. Damage to the lens has been emphasized because single doses as low as 400 rads have been reported as cataractogenic. With proper protraction, as used in the treatment of malignancies around the eye, the risk can be considerably reduced, and for practical purposes can be disregarded. In the treatment of lesions of the skin around the orbit, adequate protection of the lens and cornea is possible by the insertion of shields under the lids. When the eye cannot be protected without protecting tumor (i.e., carcinomas of the suprastructure of the maxillary sinus), the risk of cataract is relatively unimportant and should not influence the conduct of therapy.

The radiovulnerability of the cornea is a more important clinical problem. Damage to the cornea may result in ulceration and necrosis with severe pain. Extensive damage may necessitate enucleation. At times it is impossible to protect the cornea without protecting tumor in the orbit. In many situations, however, it is possible to conduct treatment so that the dose to the cornea is within tolerable limits. From our own observations of 23 patients who received direct irradiation to the eye (ranging from a D max* of 1,650 rads in 11 days to a D max of 6,000 rads in 29 days),[5] it appears that direct corneal exposure to supervoltage radiation doses as high as 2,000 to 2,500 rads D max has been tolerated.** After 3,000 rads D max, transient keratitis has occurred. Six patients who received corneal doses of 6,000 rads D max developed permanent corneal opacity, ocular phthisis, enophthalmos, and perforation in one instance.

It must be very carefully considered whether protection of the cornea may jeopardize control of the tumor. If so, preliminary enucleation of a good eye may be advisable. However, in general, it is our policy to protect the cornea after a surface dose of 2,500 rads D max or to risk corneal damage, avoiding enucleation unless it becomes necessary because of treatment-produced damage.

In the treatment of nasopharyngeal tumors, high doses are delivered to the external auditory canal, the middle ear, and the inner ear, but clinically significant permanent damage to the auricular structures is infrequent. When patients are systematically examined during and following radiation therapy, ear-related symptoms and signs can be detected in about one-half during or shortly after completion of treatment.[3] The findings of a sensation of fullness, moderate conductive hearing loss, earache, and tinnitus (symptoms of serous otitis media) are explained by occlusion of the eustachian tube by edema or mucus. Only in a small number of patients are these symptoms severe enough to cause spontaneous complaints by the patient. This "radiation otitis media" usually subsides in a few weeks. Permanent damage from necrosis of ossicles is occasionally observed in situations in which excessive doses have been delivered. This rare occurrence of permanent damage to the structures of the middle or inner ear need not influence treatment

---

*Site of maximum ionization in the absorber is 0.5 cm below the skin with cobalt-60 teletherapy.
**If the eyelids are open and the axis of the incident cobalt-60 beam is 90° to the corneal surface, the dose in the cornea will be only 40 percent of D max.

planning. There may be a marked reaction of the epithelium of the external auditory canal, particularly when "soft" radiation is used. Usually this can be avoided by the use of a better quality of radiation or by protection of the external canal by a small lead cylinder inserted in the beam.

Damage to the heart following irradiation of intrathoracic malignant disease occasionally has been observed. The most common cardiac complication is acute transient pericarditis which may occur during or after therapy.[11] In the Stanford experience,[11] it occurred in 3 of 117 patients treated for carcinoma of the breast (2.5 percent), and in 8 of 120 patients treated for mediastinal Hodgkin's disease (6.7 percent) with doses to the heart of 5,500 rads in five weeks and 4,000 rads in four weeks, respectively. The incidence was half that large (3.2 percent) in 93 patients irradiated with smaller individual fractions and a longer overall treatment time, at the University of California Hospitals.[28] In a prospective study in this institution,[31] no clinically significant radiation damage to the heart was detected in 20 patients carefully investigated during and following therapy, although in 2 patients electrocardiographic evidence of transient pericarditis was noticed during treatment. These changes did not interfere with the continuation of therapy and subsided by the end of treatment. More serious complications, apparently attributable to irradiation, have been observed so rarely that no detailed discussion is justified.[11]

The incidence of damage to the pericardium or the heart muscle may be somewhat higher than these figures indicate. In some instances the clinical symptomatology of radiation injury may have been misinterpreted as having been caused by neoplastic disease. However, radiation injury sometimes is assumed when the proximity of the disintegrating tumor is responsible for the cardiac damage and its symptoms. With modern radical radiation therapy, patients have been cured without clinically significant cardiac damage even when neoplasm was found to extend into the pericardium and heart muscle. It is also possible that with the frequent use of more radical radiation techniques (for instance, the treatment of large volumes in the chest of patients with Hodgkin's disease), the incidence of radiation injury to the heart may increase in the future.

Current knowledge of radiation damage to the heart should not be a deterrent to treatment of patients with intrathoracic malignant neoplasm, for the cardiac damage is prognostically less serious than progressing intrathoracic tumor.

In 1950, Zuelzer et al.[32] called attention to the possibility of radiation-produced glomerulonephritis. The problem was thoroughly investigated by Kunkler et al.[19] Since then, the radiovulnerability of the kidney has been considered in treatment planning.[18] If the entire renal parenchyma is included in the treatment volume, a dose beyond 2,000 rads is hazardous, although the individual tolerance varies considerably. In Luxton's carefully analyzed material[22] only one-third of the potential candidates developed radiation nephritis, and among these patients the syndrome varied in severity. Renal damage may present clinically as acute radiation nephritis (occurring 6 to 13 months postirradiation), primary chronic nephritis, benign hypertension, late malignant hypertension, or harmless proteinuria.[22] The incidence of renal radiation damage may be greater than is generally assumed because of failure of clinical recognition.

For practical purposes, two points should be emphasized: (1) The renal radiation tolerance must be properly appreciated in treatment planning. It is possible in most situations to adjust the technique so that at least one-half or one-third of one kidney is sufficiently protected so that it does not receive more than 1,500 to 2,000 rads. Clinically serious renal damage has been observed only when the entire parenchyma of both kidneys received doses beyond tolerance. (2) In some instances of hypertension caused by radiation damage of one kidney, removal of this kidney has been curative.[22]

The liver has been considered relatively "radioresistant." This tolerance need be related to radiation dosage and amount of liver irradiated. Because of its large functional reserve, radiation damage to portions of the liver does not create a clinical problem. However, changes in those segments of irradiated liver can be detected by isotope liver scan. Irradiation of the entire liver to doses above 3,500 rads in four weeks may cause changes which may be functionally important and histologically characteristic.[15] The need for such treatment is infrequent, being limited to certain circumstances in patients with cancer of the ovary, lymphoma, or hepatic metastases.

REVIEW QUESTIONS

1. Have you seen any serious sequelae of radiation treatment? Do you know the treatment conditions? Was the tumor controlled?

2. Have you seen any sequelae attributed to irradiation that you now know were not related? What are the clinical risks of such unfounded incorrect diagnoses?

3. If surgery is not possible following radiation therapy with "curative" objective, is more aggressive irradiation with higher risk of serious sequelae justified?

4. Differentiate between radiation reactions and radiation hazards.

5. Have you seen a patient with "radiation sickness"? Was the patient forewarned about the symptoms? Did the symptoms disappear during treatment? Did the radiation therapist alter the treatment?

6. Have you seen a radiation-produced skin reaction? Did it heal without sequelae?

7. What is the basis of local radiation-produced necrosis? Is "x-ray burn" an accurate term? Why?

8. Describe a radiation-produced reaction of the oral mucosa grossly and histologically. What does it indicate? How should this evidence be used clinically?

9. What is the long-term benefit of minimizing skin and mucosal reactions during treatment?

10. Of the two major types of radiation hazards, which is the most frequent clinical problem? Why?

11. What measures should be used to "protect" the vasculoconnective tissue?

12. What are some serious clinical problems secondary to damage of the vasculoconnective tissue?

13. What is the frequency of serious bowel and bladder injury following proper radiation therapy of patients with carcinoma of the cervix?

14. In a patient with carcinoma of mid-thoracic esophagus, is tracheoesophageal fistula more likely to be related to treatment or the progression of tumor?

15. Radiation therapy is preferable treatment for most carcinomas of the skin of the eyelid, nose, and ear, because of comparable effectiveness and better cosmetic and functional results than are possible by surgery. Have you heard that radiation therapy cannot be used in these sites because of the intolerance of the underlying cartilage? What is the evidence?

16. What is the magnitude of risk of damage to the CNS in clinical radiation therapy? What can be done to minimize this risk?

17. What is the magnitude of risk of damage to the lens in clinical radiation therapy? Should lens damage ever occur with proper radiation therapy of carcinoma of the eyelid? In the rare patient (average age 60–70 years) who develops a cataract many years following radiation therapy of cancer about the orbit, what is the consequence? What is the frequent surgical alternative in treatment of malignant tumors about the orbit?

18. In what tumors is radiation damage to the kidneys an important consideration? Can irradiation of the kidneys be avoided? What are the possible consequences?

BIBLIOGRAPHY

1. BACLESSE, F. Clinical experience with ultra-fractionated roentgen therapy. In: *Progress in Radiation Therapy*, Vol. I. F. Buschke, Ed., Grune & Stratton, New York, 1958, chapter 6.
2. BODEN, G. Radiation myelitis of cervical spinal cord. *Brit J Radiol*, 21:464–469, 1948.
3. BORSANYI, S. The effects of radiation therapy on the ear: With particular reference to radiation otitis media. *Southern Med J* 55:740–743, 1962.
4. BUSCHKE, F. Common misconceptions in radiation therapy. *Amer J Surg*, 101:164–171, 1961.
5. BUSCHKE, F. Predetermination of avoidable or unavoidable radiation hazards and complications—calculated risks. *Amer J Roentgen*, 89:649–653, 1963.
6. BUSCHKE, F., and CANTRIL, S. Roentgentherapy of carcinoma of the urinary bladder. *Staff J. Swedish Hospital*, Seattle, 1941 (Suppl. 2, pp. 77–94).
7. BUSCHKE, F., CANTRIL, S., and PARKER, H. *Supervoltage Roentgentherapy*, Charles C Thomas, Springfield, Ill., 1950.
8. BUSCHKE, F., and JACK, G. Twenty-five years' experience with supervoltage therapy in the treatment of transitional cell carcinoma of the bladder. *Amer J Roentgen*, 99:387–392, 1964.
9. BUSCHKE, F., and GALANTE, M. Radical preoperative roentgen therapy in primarily inoperable advanced cancers of head and neck. *Radiology*, 73:845–848, 1959.
10. BUSCHKE, F., and VAETH, J. Radiation therapy of carcinoma of the vocal cord without mucosal reaction. *Amer J Roentg*, 89:29–34, 1963.
11. COHN, K. E., STEWART, J. R., FAJARDO, L. F., and HANCOCK, E. W. Heart disease following radiation. *Medicine*, 46:281–298, 1967 (extensive bibliography).
12. CORSCADEN, J. A., KASABACH, H. H., and LENZ, M. Intestinal injuries after radium and roentgen treatment of carcinoma of the cervix. *Amer J Roentgen*, 39:871–894, 1938.
13. COUTARD, H. Sur les delais d'apparition et d'évolution des réactions de la peau et des muqueuses de la bouche et du pharynx provoquées par les rayons X. *C R Soc Biol* (Paris) 86:1140–1141, 1922.

14. GRAY, M. and KOTTMEIER, H. Rectal and bladder injuries following radium therapy for carcinoma of the cervix at the Radiumhemmet. *Amer J Obstet Gynec*, 74:1294–1303, 1957.
15. INGOLD, J. A., REED, G. B., KAPLAN, H. S., and BAGSHAW, M. A. Radiation hepatitis. *Amer J Roentgen*, 93:200–208, 1965.
16. JACK, G., and BUSCHKE, F. The role of external irradiation in the treatment of transitional cell carcinoma of the bladder. *Calif Med*, 106:12–16, 1967.
17. KOTTMEIER, H., and GRAY, M. Rectal and bladder injuries in relation to radiation dosage in carcinoma of the cervix. *Amer J Obstet Gynec*, 82:74–82, 1961.
18. KUNKLER, P. The significance of radiosensitivity of the kidney in radiotherapy. In: *Progress in Radiation Therapy*, Vol. II. F. Buschke, Ed, Grune & Stratton, New York, 1962, chapter 2.
19. KUNKLER, P., FARR, R., and LUXTON, R. The limit of renal tolerance to x-rays: An investigation into renal damage occurring following the treatment of tumors of the testis by abdominal baths. *Brit J Radiol*, 25:190–201, 1952.
20. LAMPE, I. Radiation tolerance of the central nervous system. In: *Progress in Radiation Therapy*, Vol. I. F. Buschke, Ed, Grune & Stratton, New York, 1958, chapter 10.
21. LEDERMAN, M. Place of radiotherapy in treatment of cancer of larynx, *Brit Med J*, 1:1639–1646, 1961.
22. LUXTON, R. The clinical and pathological effects of renal irradiation. In: *Progress in Radiation Therapy*, Vol. II. F. Buschke, Ed, Grune & Stratton, New York, 1962, chapter 1.
23. MACKAY, N. Tolerance of bladder to intracavitary irradiation. *J Urol*, 76:396–400, 1956.
24. PARKER, R. G. Tolerance of cartilage and bone in clinical radiation therapy. In: *Progress in Radiation Therapy*, Vol. II. F. Buschke, Ed, Grune & Stratton, New York, 1962, chapter 3.
25. PARKER, R. G., and WILDERMUTH, O. Radiation therapy of lesions overlying cartilage. I. Carcinoma of the pinna. *Cancer*, 15:57–65, 1962.
26. PARKER, R. G., BURNETT, L., WOOTTON, P., and MCINTYRE, D. Radiation cataract in clinical therapeutic radiology. *Radiology*, 82:794–799, 1964.
27. PHILLIPS, T. L., and BUSCHKE, F. Radiation tolerance of the thoracic spinal cord. *Amer J Roentgen*, 105:659–664, March 1969.
28. STEWART, J. R., and FAJARDO, L. F. Dose response in human and experimental radiation—induced heart disease. Radiology, 99, May 1971, pp. 403–408.
29. VAETH, J. Radiation induced myelitis. In: *Progress in Radiation Therapy*, Vol. III. F. Buschke, Ed, Grune & Stratton, New York, 1965, chapter 1.
30. VAETH, J., and BUSCHKE, F. Radiation therapy of carcinoma of the vocal cord without mucosal reaction. *Amer J Roentg*, 97:931–932, 1966.
31. VAETH, J., FEIGENBAUM, L., and MERRILL, M. Effects of intensive radiation on the human heart. *Radiology*, 76:755–762, 1961.
32. ZUELZER, W., PALMER, H., *and* NEWTON, W., JR. Unusual glomerulonephritis in young children, probably radiation nephritis; report of three cases. *Amer J Path*, 26:1019–1031, 1950.

SELECTION OF PATIENTS

The selection of patients for radiation therapy is beyond the capabilities of the referring physician regardless of competence in his chosen medical specialty. Thus, the selection of patients for radiation therapy must be made by the therapeutic radiologist just as the selection of patients for surgery must be the decision of the surgeon.

Radical radiation therapy has an objective of permanent control of tumor ("cure") as contrasted with *palliative radiation therapy*, which has an objective of patient comfort through relief of tumor-produced symptoms and signs. The surgeon recognizes similar indications for radical or palliative surgery. Radical radiation therapy differs from palliative radiation therapy in indications, techniques, and acceptable risks. Intermediate between these two forms of radiation therapy there is a type—used mainly in the treatment of some patients with lymphoma—which may be neither "curative" nor "palliative." This, for want of a better word, may be called "suppressive" therapy.

The selection of patients for radical radiation therapy is guided by certain criteria: (1) type of tumor, (2) primary site, (3) extent of tumor, and (4) general condition of the patient.

Type and Primary Site of Tumor

The degree of tumor radiovulnerability in relation to the radiovulnerability of the adjacent normal structures determines whether a tumor can be treated effectively by radiation methods. There is a wide spectrum of inherent "radiosensitivity" of malignant tumors. Although clinical observation has shown that for tumors of a particular histologic type an average degree of radiovulnerability can be expected, the radiation response of any individual tumor in such a group may differ considerably in either direction from the average. This deviation can be determined only by an actual therapeutic test. Tumors which, because of their relatively low degree of "radiosensitivity," usually cannot be controlled by irradiation alone may still respond sufficiently to make radiation therapy a useful procedure, either in conjunction with surgery or for palliation.

At one end of the spectrum of radiosensitivity, tumors are classified as "radio-resistant." These include soft tissue sarcomas, chondrosarcoma, neurogenic sarcoma, osteosarcoma, and melanoma. These tumors belong in the realm of surgery as long as there is a chance of complete removal. However, some of these tumors respond sufficiently for radiation therapy to be considered in selected situations.[3-7] There have been infrequent instances of unexpectedly long control of melanomas, although it is impossible to predict the response of a particular melanoma. Some liposarcomas are sufficiently radiovulnerable to encourage irradiation with curative intent in surgically hopeless situations. Some fibrosarcomas have been significantly radio-responsive so that palliative or postoperative radiation may be useful if removal is incomplete. A possible reason for incurability of partially radioresponsive mesenchymal tumors is that the diagnosis often is established only when the tumor is large and contains foci of poor vascularity and decreased tumor cell oxygenation. A correlation between tumor type and radiation response is hindered because of difficulty in specifically identifying these neoplasms. For example, all tumors designated as fibrosarcomas may not be the same distinct biological entity.

In the treatment of large or rapidly growing tumors, preoperative irradiation may reduce the incidence of marginal persistence of tumor, may decrease the chance of spread of tumor at the time of surgery, may mechanically facilitate surgery, and occasionally may permit the reduction of functional or cosmetic surgical damage by reducing the necessary extent of resection.[1,2]

At the other extreme are the highly "radiosensitive" tumors such as lymphosarcoma, lymphoepithelioma, and anaplastic carcinoma. These belong in the realm of radiation therapy. Their tendency to early and widespread extension through the regional lymphatics and blood vessels makes these tumors poor objects for surgical removal, even if removal may be anatomically tempting, as for example in patients with carcinoma of the tonsil.

Between these two extremes are the majority of clinical cancers which originate from skin, mucosa, mucocutaneous junctions, and ductal epithelium. These tumors may be only slightly more radiovulnerable than the adjacent normal structures. However, compared with the very radiovulnerable tumors, this group is less likely to have spread at the time of diagnosis, making the likelihood of permanent control greater.

Radiosensitivity and radiocurability are not synonymous and may even be mutually exclusive. *Epidermoid carcinomas are the most favorable objects for radiation therapy.* These tumors are sufficiently vulnerable for destruction by irradiation, but have minimal tendency to rapidly spread from the primary site. A decision whether surgery or irradiation is the best treatment of these tumors of moderate radiovulnerability does not depend entirely on the biological characteristics of the tumor, but partially on secondary considerations, such as location (surgical or radiological accessibility), functional or cosmetic end results, primary risk of surgery or irradiation, and availability of surgical or radiological competence. These decisions will be discussed in detail under specific tumors.

The concept that adenocarcinoma is not suitable for radiation therapy because of insufficient response is incorrect. Some glandular carcinomas, such as those of the endometrium and breast, and even certain gastrointestinal adenocarcinomas, may respond well to radiation therapy. Nevertheless, most of these carcinomas are primarily surgical lesions, partly because of their size when recognized and partly because of some associated anatomical peculiarity. The dose necessary for the destruction of these moderately radiovulnerable tumors is tolerated only if the irradiated tissue volume is small. A carcinoma of the larynx, pharynx, or esophagus, even if clinically advanced, is still small in volume compared with most cancers of the stomach at the time of diagnosis. In addition, tumors in a mobile organ, such as the gastrointestinal tract, are impossible to treat in a relatively limited tissue volume.

It is important to realize that the preference for surgery for most patients with adenocarcinomas results from such secondary considerations and not from lack of inherent tumor radiovulnerability, because in situations in which resection is not possible (such as some obstructing carcinomas of the gastric cardia and some carcinomas of the rectum and of the endometrium), radiation therapy may be useful for temporary retardation of tumor or palliation of specific problems. Under certain circumstances, as in patients with uterine adenocarcinoma, permanent control may be attained. Radiation therapy is very important in the treatment of patients with carcinoma of the breast, and has been used with increasing frequency as an adjunct to surgery in some other adenocarcinomas, such as those arising in the endometrium or rectum.

Extent of Tumor

A careful appraisal of the extent of tumor is essential in planning treatment. The major absolute contraindication for radical radiation therapy of a radiovulnerable tumor is demonstrable distant metastases. However, in some patients with very radioresponsive tumors (i.e., Wilm's tumor, Ewing's tumor) "curative" therapy may be considered even in the presence of pulmonary and other metastases. In their absence, the local tumor extent and the involvement of regional lymphatics must be determined as accurately as may be permitted by available clinical and laboratory procedures. In addition, biologically predictable—but as yet clinically undetectable —tumor extension must be related to the estimated radiovulnerability of a specific tumor and its adjacent normal tissues. Thus, patients with highly sensitive anaplastic carcinomas of the tonsil still may have a fair chance of cure in the presence of large regional lymph adenopathy, whereas the control of a differentiated carcinoma of the tongue or floor of the mouth and its much smaller regional adenopathy is less likely. A large carcinoma of the epiglottis may be more easily controlled than a much smaller tumor originating in the vocal cord. Tumor invasion of bone, cartilage, and muscle makes control by irradiation less likely, and usually makes surgery preferable. Radiation therapy infrequently controls lymph node metastases secondary to differentiated carcinomas, thus making resection preferable. However, node metastases of similar extent secondary to poorly differentiated carcinomas frequently may be controlled by radiation.

Condition of the Patient

The importance of the general condition of the patient frequently is underestimated. Patients may be referred for radiation therapy because their general condition is not good enough to tolerate major surgery. Only infrequently should the patient's general condition be decisive in the choice between surgery and irradiation. *A major radiotherapeutic procedure may be more demanding physiologically than surgery.* It is as important to prepare the patient prior to the institution of radical radiation therapy as it is prior to radical surgery. Certain specific contraindications to surgery, such as cardiovascular or metabolic disease, may not restrict radiation therapy. Surgical contraindications of this type have become less important with improved general medical care and anesthesia.

Indications for use of palliative radiation therapy will be discussed in a separate chapter.

REVIEW QUESTIONS

1. Can you describe any difference in principle between the surgeon being responsible for the selection of patients for surgery and the radiation therapist being responsible for the selection of patients for irradiation? What has been your experience?

2. What is the objective of radical radiation therapy? How does this differ from palliative radiation therapy? Can you think of some clinical situations which are not clearly defined? How would you resolve them?

3. What are the criteria for selection of patients for radical radiation therapy? Does this vary from criteria for selection for radical surgery?

4. Is tumor type a useful guide in selection of patients for irradiation? What are the limitations?

5. Name several tumor types you consider "radioresistant." Do they ever respond enough to make treatment worthwhile? If so, how would you select patients for a therapeutic trial?

6. What tumors are the most favorable for radiation therapy? Why? Does this surprise you? Why aren't highly radiosensitive tumors the most favorable type for treatment?

7. Distinguish between radiosensitivity and radiocurability of tumors. Must a tumor be very radiosensitive to be radiocurable?

8. What secondary considerations may determine whether a tumor which is radiocurable should be irradiated or removed surgically?

9. Based on preservation of normal anatomy, function, and cosmetics, is radical surgery or radical irradiation the more conservative treatment method? If the incidence of tumor control is comparable for several treatment methods, what are the advantages of the more conservative treatment?

10. Which adenocarcinomas may be controlled by irradiation? What limits radical irradiation in most patients with adenocarcinomas?

11. Do you think tumor type or tumor extent can be more closely related to prognosis? Give some examples.

12. Have you seen a patient referred for radiation therapy because he isn't "a candidate for surgery"? Is this a rational basis for selection? Why not?

BIBLIOGRAPHY

1. BLOEDORN, F. Radiation and surgery. In: *Progress in Radiation Therapy*, Vol. II. F. Buschke, Ed, Grune & Stratton, New York, 1967.
2. BUSCHKE, F., and GALANTE, M. Radical preoperative roentgen therapy in primarily inoperable advanced cancers of the head and neck. *Radiology*, 73:845–848, 1959.
3. DECHAUME, M., BACLESSE, F., CHAVANNE, G., and PAYEN, J. La rontgentherapie des ameloblastomes et des épitheliomas adamantis du maxillaire inférieur. *Presse Med*, 64:2177–2180, 1956.
4. DEL REGATO, J. A. Radiotherapy of soft tissue sarcomas. *JAMA*, 185:216–218, 1963.
5. WINDEYER, B. W. Chordoma. *Proc Roy Soc Med*, 52:1088–1100, 1959.
6. WINDEYER, B. W., DISCHE, S., and MANSFIELD, C. M. The place of radiotherapy in the management of fibrosarcoma of the soft tissues. *Clin Radiol*, 17:32–40, 1966.
7. ZUPPINGER, A., and RENFER, H. Zur Rontgen-Therapie der osteogenen Sarkome. *Radiol Clin* (Basel), 26:312–318, 1957.

4

SURGERY
AND RADIATION THERAPY

The major advance in clinical cancer management in the past decade has been the development of cooperation between surgeon and radiotherapist, with consequent improved selective and combined use of both treatment modalities. Until the development of this cooperation, each eyed the other suspiciously, competing for the opportunity to apply his method first, even though doomed to failure in a majority of patients, and anxious to blame the other for difficulties often inherent in the nature of the disease.

OBJECTIVE OF COMBINED TREATMENT

Combined treatment with surgery and irradiation should be used with an objective of improving the control of cancer, locally and ultimately systemically, beyond that possible by the best use of either modality alone. This requires close cooperation between surgeon and therapeutic radiologist, so that the combined treatment can be planned and systematic. Often in the past, use of the second modality was a move of desperation triggered by impending failure of the first. If use of the two modalities is separated by an interval longer than three months, it is unlikely that combined treatment was planned.[1]

INDICATIONS

Combined treatment is indicated[1,4,6] (1) when either method alone is unlikely to result in local tumor control and the tumor may be radioresponsive; (2) when there appears to be a high incidence of tumor dissemination following surgery; (3) when locally "complete" surgery is unlikely unless radiation therapy can favorably alter the tumor; and (4) when surgical mutilation can be avoided or reduced without a reduction in the possibility of local tumor control and "cure" of the patient.

50

NEED FOR DATA

Inasmuch as a voluminous past experience has been haphazard and unproductive of data necessary to judge the value of combined treatment, careful studies are in order. These require[1] (1) consistent, close cooperation between surgeon and therapeutic radiologist, (2) unrestricted use of both modalities, and (3) an "optimal" interval between use of each. By current standards the radiation therapy should be with supervoltage equipment, with delivery in a single continuous series (including planned "split-dose" techniques) to a patient in the best possible physiological state.

CLASSIFICATION OF COMBINED TREATMENT

Combined treatment includes programs in which (1) each modality may be directed to separate components of the tumor; or (2) both irradiation and surgery may be directed to the same tissue volume, bearing both the primary tumor and regional lymph nodes. The radiation therapy usually precedes or follows the surgery. However, on occasion, the radiation therapy may be interrupted for the surgery and then completed postoperatively.

1. Radiation treatment of the primary lesion and surgical treatment of the regional metastases have been used for patients with cancers of the head and neck, particularly when the tumor arises in the oral tongue. The potential advantage of this combination is that, whereas the control of the primary lesion is comparable by either method, irradiation is anatomically more conservative, and surgery is more effective in controlling the regional adenopathy. Because each treatment modality is directed to different anatomic sites, each must be used radically. The primary tumor should be treated first so that the blood supply will be intact for optimal radiation response. If possible, a short delay prior to resection of the regional nodes may allow an estimate of the probability of control of the primary lesion. If the response of the primary tumor has been unsatisfactory, an *en bloc* resection of both primary tumor and regional nodes is preferable to two separate operations, i.e., an initial removal of nodes and a later resection of the uncontrolled primary tumor.

Surgical treatment of the primary tumor with irradiation of the regional nodes may be used when local tumor control is more likely with resection, but regional adenopathy cannot be resected, but may be radioresponsive. Examples are carcinomas of the breast and testis.

2. Radiation therapy and surgery, in varying sequence, may be directed to the same tissue volume bearing both the primary tumor and the regional lymph nodes.

Preoperative radiation therapy should include the whole tumor complex, with subsequent resection within the irradiated tissue volume. This resection may be as extensive as considered necessary even without the preoperative irradiation, or it may be lesser in extent, for various reasons, with dependence on the irradiation for "safe" margins. This plan has been used in the treatment of patients with carcinomas of the anterior tonsillar pillar-retromolar trigone, floor of mouth, gingiva, maxillary sinus, uterine corpus, ovary, esophagus, bladder, kidney, and lung.

Postoperative radiation therapy of the whole tumor complex may be planned, as in McWhirter's[3] technique for patients with carcinoma of the breast. However, such treatment is likely to be unplanned or circumstantial.

In recent years, a few have advocated interruption of preoperative irradiation for resection with the intention of completing treatment postoperatively. This method, prompted by a concern about radical surgery in heavily irradiated tissue, has been championed by surgeons not concerned with possible violations of radiobiological fundamentals, i.e., disruption of the tumor bed and prolongation of the dose-time relationship, and who are unconvinced of improvements in radiotherapeutic techniques which result in improved tissue tolerance.

Regardless of the sequence, when radiation therapy and surgery are directed to the same tumor-bearing tissue volume, the principles[1] are the same: (1) Surgery controls only accessible localized tumors; and (2) radiation therapy often fails centrally while being effective at the tumor periphery.

Preoperative Radiation Therapy

The theoretical advantages of preoperative irradiation are[1, 4-6]: (1) The radiation effect will be the best possible biologically because the blood supply is intact; (2) the radiation therapy can control the tumor margins and even the regional adenopathy; (3) devitalization of tumor cells will reduce the incidence of local tumor persistence and distant metastases following surgery; and (4) reduction of the size of the tumor may facilitate surgery. The function of surgery in this program is the removal of tumor in situations in which local control by irradiation is of low order or when there is high risk of necrosis.

Patients likely to profit from this program have (1) locally advanced cancers, (2) cancers with a high likelihood of regional lymphatic metastases or blood vessel invasion, or (3) cancers with a high incidence of postoperative persistence.

Many radiotherapists have championed the potential biological advantages of preoperative irradiation, and enough surgeons have joined them to provide data showing that radical surgery can be performed in heavily irradiated tissue without morbidity in excess of that attributable to the surgery alone, if the procedure is planned, the irradiation is of high quality, the interval between irradiation and surgery is "optimal," and the surgeon uses meticulous technique.

Postoperative Radiation Therapy

Postoperative radiation therapy to the same tumor-bearing volume usually is dependent on modes of patient management.[1] The irradiation may be planned after surgery, which is necessary to determine tumor extent, i.e., for patients with brain tumors or breast carcinoma. More often such postoperative irradiation is unplanned and circumstantial, remembered only because resection was incomplete. The purpose of such treatment would be: (1) control of residual neoplasm at the margins of resection, (2) lessening of a high probability of tumor regrowth in the operative site, or (3) control of regional node metastases which were not resectable.

The likelihood of accomplishment is questionable because of disruption of the tumor bed and unexpected extensiveness of the tumor.

Interval between Radiation Therapy and Surgery

There is no concensus as to an optimal interval between irradiation and resection. This optimal interval may vary with radiation dose, extent of resection, anatomic site, and whether the radiation therapy is pre- or postoperative.

Patients and surgeons may become impatient after preoperative radiation therapy. However, if the radiation therapy favorably influences tumor, a supposition basic in planned combined treatment, then the interval does not increase the risk to the patient from tumor and is essential to minimize complications. Bloedorn[1] emphasized that the interval between irradiation and surgery must allow for the "full action of irradiation" on the tumor and the return of irradiated normal tissues to their best possible physiological condition, but must not exceed the period of tumor inactivation. The best time for surgery is after the acute radiation reaction has subsided, but before the onset of late changes, i.e., endarteritis. This interval after high dose irradiation usually is two to three months, although there may be considerable variation.

Radiation Dosage

Although theoretically the optimal radiation dosage for combined treatment might be related to (1) the number of tumor cells in the irradiated tissue volume not removed surgically, (2) the number of residual cells necessary to start tumor reactivation, (3) the radiovulnerability of the residual tumor cells, and (4) the radiovulnerability of the normal structures vital to postoperative healing,[6] lack of applicability of such considerations clinically makes it reasonable to use doses which are limited only by the tolerance of the normal tissues for the proposed surgery, whether the irradiation is preoperative or postoperative. Thus, even postoperatively when a smaller dose might be considered for "seeding" rather than for gross residual tumor,[2] dosage usually has been extended to the estimated limits of normal tissue tolerance. Thomlinson[7] has submitted laboratory data consistent with the long-standing clinical observation that the favorable influence of irradiation on tumor, even when combined with resection, is directly proportional to dose.

Surgery in Preparation for Radiation Therapy

Tolerance of radical radiation therapy requires that tissues and organs in the volume to be irradiated be in the best possible physiological condition. Often surgery can aid in this preparation, even though not a part of the definitive tumor treatment. Examples are: relief of bladder-neck obstruction by transurethral resection in patients with carcinoma of the bladder; tracheostomy when tumors obstruct the proximal airway; decompression of the brain when there is increased intracranial pressure incident to a brain tumor; decompression of the spinal canal when there is rapid loss of neurologic function secondary to tumor.

REVIEW QUESTIONS

1. What is the objective of combined surgery and radiation therapy?

2. What are the indications for combined treatment?

3. Give examples of combined treatment in which surgery and radiation therapy are directed to separate tumor components; to the same tumor-bearing volume. What determines this choice of application?

4. Why may combined treatment of the same tumor-bearing volume be more effective than either surgery or radiation therapy alone?

5. What are the theoretical advantages of preoperative radiation therapy? In which clinical situations may such treatment be advantageous?

6. When is postoperative radiation therapy likely to be planned?

7. When is the best time for planned surgery after radiation therapy? Why?

8. Compare the possible advantages and disadvantages of high-dose and lower-dose preoperative radiation therapy.

BIBLIOGRAPHY

1. BLOEDORN, F. G. Radiation and Surgery. In: *Progress in Radiation Therapy*, Vol. II. F. Buschke, Ed, Grune & Stratton, New York, 1962.
2. BLOEDORN, F. G. Radiation and surgery. In: *Textbook of Radiotherapy*. G. F. Fletcher, Ed, Lea & Febiger, Philadelphia, 1966.
3. MCWHIRTER, R. Simple mastectomy and radiotherapy in the treatment of breast cancer. *Brit J Radiol*, 28:128–139, 1955.
4. NIAS, A. H. W. Radiobiologic aspects of preoperative irradiation. *Brit J Radiol*, 40:166–169, 1967.
5. NICKSON, J. J., and GLICKSMAN, A. S. Preoperative radiotherapy in cancer. *JAMA*, 195:922–926, 1966.
6. POWERS, W. E., and PALMER, L. A. Biologic basis of preoperative radiation treatment. *Amer J. Roentgen*, 102:176–192, 1968.
7. THOMLINSON, R. H. An experimental method for comparing treatments of intact malignant tumours in animals and its application to the use of oxygen in radiotherapy. *Brit J Cancer*, 14:555–576, 1960.

ADDITIONAL READING ON SPECIFIC CANCERS

Uterus

LAMPE, I. Endometrial carcinoma. *Amer J Roentgen*, 90:1011–1015, 1963.

Ovary

LONG, R. T. L., and SALA, J. M. Radical pelvic surgery combined with radiotherapy in the treatment of locally advanced ovarian carcinoma. *Surg Gynec Obstet*, 117:201–204, 1963.
VAETH, J. M., and BUSCHKE, F. J. The role of preoperative irradiation in the treatment of carcinoma of the ovary. *Amer J Roentgen*, 105:614–617, 1969.

Breast

ASH, C. L., PETERS, V., and DELARUE, N. C. The argument of preoperative radiation in the treatment of breast cancer. *Surg Gynec Obstet*, 96:509–521, 1953.

BACLESSE, F. A method of preoperative roentgentherapy by high doses, followed by radical operation for carcinoma of the breast (showing survivals up to 10 years). *J Fac Radiol*, 6:145–163, 1955.

BORGSTROM, S., and LINDGREN, M. Preoperative roentgen therapy of cancer of the breast. *Acta Radiol [Ther]*, 58:9–16, 1962.

WHITE, E. C., FLETCHER, G. H., and CLARK, R. L. Surgical experience with preoperative irradiation for carcinoma of the breast. *Ann Surg*, 115:948–956, 1962.

Head and Neck

BUSCHKE, F., and GALANTE, M. Radical preoperative roentgen therapy in primarily inoperable advanced cancers of the head and neck. *Radiology*, 73:845–848, 1959.

FLETCHER, G. H., and JESSE, R. H., JR. The contribution of supervoltage roentgentherapy to the integration of radiation and surgery in head and neck squamous cell carcinomas. *Cancer*, 15:566–577, 1962.

HENDRICKSON, F. R., and LIEBNER, E. Results of preoperative radiotherapy for supraglottic larynx cancer. *Ann Otol*, 77:222–229, 1968.

HENSCHKE, U. K., FRAZELL, E. L., HILARIS, B. S., NICKSON, J. J., TOLLEFSEN, H. R. and STRONG, E. W. Local recurrences after radical neck dissection with or without preoperative x-ray therapy. *Radiology*, 82:331–332, 1964.

LINDBERG, R., and JESSE, R. H. Treatment of cervical lymph node metastasis from primary lesions of oropharynx, supraglottic larynx and hypopharynx. *Amer J Roentgen*, 102:132–137, 1968.

Esophagus

CLIFFTON, E. E., GOODNER, J. T., and BRONSTEIN, E. Preoperative irradiation for cancer of the esophagus. *Cancer*, 13:37–45, 1960.

DOGGETT, R. L. S. Combined radiation therapy and surgical treatment of carcinoma of the esophagus. Presented at the Fifth Annual San Francisco Cancer Conference, October, 1969.

NAKAYAMA, K., ORIHATA, H., and YAMAGUCHI, K. Surgical treatment combined with preoperative concentrated irradiation for esophageal cancer. *Cancer*, 20:778–788, 1967.

Lung

BLOEDORN, F. G., COWLEY, R. A., CUCCIA, C. A., and MERCADO, R. M., JR. Combined therapy: Irradiation and surgery in the treatment of bronchogenic carcinoma. *Amer J Roentgen*, 85:875–885, 1961.

MALLAMS, J. R., PAULSON, D. L., COLLIER, R. E., and SHAW, R. R. Presurgical irradiation in bronchogenic carcinoma, superior sulcus type. *Radiology*, 82:1050–1054, 1964.

Bladder

BLOEDORN, F. G., WIZENBERG, M. J., SEYDEL, H. G., and LIGHT, J. P. Radiotherapy in treatment of cancer of bladder. *Southern Med J*, 60:539–544, 1967.

WHITMORE, W. F. Preoperative radiation therapy in carcinoma of the bladder. Presented at the Fifth Annual San Francisco Cancer Conference, October, 1969.

Kidney

LACY, S. S., COX, C. E., and BLAKE, D. Preoperative radiotherapy of renal cell carcinoma: Feasibility study. *Amer Surg*, 33:943–948, 1967.

NG. E., and LOW-BEER, B. V. A. The treatment of Wilm's tumor. *J. Pediat*, 48:763–769, 1956.

RICHES, E. W. The place of irradiation. (Cancer of the urogenital tract: kidney.) *JAMA*, 204: 230–231, 1968.

Colon and Rectum

ALLEN, C. V. High-dose preoperative radiation therapy in carcinoma of the rectosigmoid colon. Presented at the Fifth Annual San Francisco Cancer Conference, October, 1969.

LEAMING, R. H., STEARNS, M. W., and DEDDISH, M. R. Preoperative irradiation in rectal carcinoma. *Radiology*, 77:257–263, 1961.

QUAN, S. H. Preoperative radiation for carcinoma of rectum. *New York J Med*, 66:2243–2247, 1966.

Bone

FRANCIS, K. C., PHILLIPS, R., NICKSON, J. J. WOODARD, H. Q., HIGINBOTHAM, N. L., and COLEY, B. L. Massive preoperative irradiation in the treatment of osteogenic sarcoma in children. *Amer J Roentgen*, 72:813–818, 1954.

LEE, E. S. The treatment of bone malignancy in children. Presented at Second Annual Children's Cancer Seminar, Seattle, 1967.

5

CHEMICAL MODIFICATION
OF RADIATION EFFECT

Inasmuch as the effects of ionizing radiation are mediated through chemical changes, it is logical and even enticing to attempt to alter radiation effect favorably by the use of chemicals. This attempt is as old as the use of ionizing radiation itself, although the recent increased intensity of interest may for the first time have some radiochemical basis.

Possible mechanisms for chemically altering the radiation response are: (1) changing the target, i.e., incorporation of purine or pyrimidine analogues into DNA; (2) modifying the ionization environment, i.e., by oxygen enhancement or depletion; and (3) selectively interfering with the repair of radiation damage.[3]

Clinical usefulness depends on improvement of the therapeutic ratio. This could be accomplished by a selective potentiation of the radiation effect on the tumor or by a selective decrease of radiation effect on normal tissues in the critical volume. Thus, chemicals which potentiate both tumor and normal tissue responses (i.e., actinomycin D) do not necessarily generate a clinical advantage. Also, many chemicals, although promising in the laboratory (i.e., BUdR), have proved highly toxic for the human.

In evaluating those chemical agents recently advocated for combined use with radiation therapy, criteria suggested by Kligerman[25] are valid: "The ultimate goal is to find drugs which when combined with irradiation cause an effect which is greater than simple addition of the two effects separately and where the increased effect on the tumor is disproportionately greater than any increased effect that the combination may have on the normal tissues" (Figure 5-1).

OXYGEN

The presence of oxygen at the time of irradiation influences the response of many biological and chemical systems. The amount of ionizing radiation needed to produce a specific change may be two to three times as great at anoxia as in the presence of oxygen. "Local oxygen tension in irradiated tissues has been manipulated, consciously or otherwise, almost since the inauguration of radiation therapy."[56] Although the oxygen effect in radiotherapy was noted by Schwartz in 1909[46] and confirmed by many (Mottram, 1924,[38] Crabtree and Cramer, 1933,[12] Lacassagne,

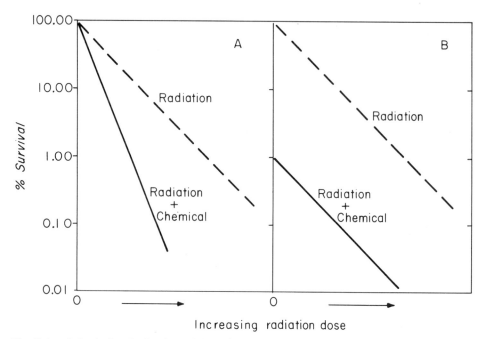

Fig. 5-1.   Criteria for Evaluation of Chemical Adjuvants for Radiation Therapy.   A.   The chemical adjuvant has amplified the response to radiation. The slope of the dose survival curve is steeper, indicative of an increased response per unit dose.   B.   The chemical adjuvant has not amplified the radiation response, but has introduced an independent additive effect.

1942[30]), the work of L. H. Gray and his colleagues dating to 1953,[21] stimulated the clinical application of methods aimed to increase oxygenation of tumor.[11,35,52,55]

Experimental data provide abundant stimuli for a trial of oxygen as a clinical radiotherapeutic adjuvant. Thorough reviews by Wootton,[56] Thomlinson,[50] Patt,[42] and Gray[22] provide the source of the following brief summation.

1.   The oxygen effect is real.

2.   Many, but not all, radiation effects are oxygen-dependent.

3.   The mechanism of the oxygen effect is not known. None of many theories covers all observations.

4.   Oxygen must be present at the time of irradiation if it is to influence effect.

5.   Other gases, i.e., nitric oxide, may be equally effective in producing the oxygen effect.

6.   The magnitude of the oxygen effect varies with the amount of oxygen available. There is a rapid increase of effect from anoxia to 10 percent of normal oxygen tension with a rapid plateau of effect beyond an oxygen tension of 20 mm Hg at 37°C (Figure 5-2). The variation of radiation effect from anoxia to normal physiological oxygen tension is approximately threefold.

7.   The oxygen effect varies with radiation quality, being maximum for x and gamma radiation (low ionization density) and practically absent for alpha particle radiation (intense ionization density).

8.   Many tumors have hypoxic foci, which are relatively poorly responsive to ionizing radiation. Although these hypoxic cells may constitute only 1 percent

of a tumor,[43,51] regeneration from these unresponsive hypoxic foci might result if destruction of adjacent well-oxygenated tumor was followed by better vascularization of the hypoxic cells.

9. Oxygen supplies tissues (and tumors) by diffusion. Therefore, an increased concentration of oxygen in the vascular supply to a tumor might lead to better oxygenation of hypoxic tumor foci. Such an increased availability of oxygen would not alter those tissues and tumor already at normal physiological tension, and thus would not increase their response to radiation. Therefore, such selective change in tissue and tumor oxygenation would be clinically favorable because the therapeutic ratio would be improved.

Clinical adversities related to the oxygen effect might be overcome by (1) increasing the blood flow to the tumor (although no direct method to achieve this is known, eventual improvement of the vascularity to hypoxic tumor foci may result from fractionation of radiation dose); (2) using high linear energy transfer (L.E.T.) radiations, which are less dependent on the presence of oxygen; (3) improving tumor oxygenation by increasing the oxygen in the blood; and (4) by depriving the entire tumor and critical normal tissue volume of oxygen and raising the radiation dose.

The most frequently used method of increasing oxygen in the blood has been through patient breathing of pure oxygen at 3–4 atm (30–45 pounds per square inch). Churchill-Davidson,[11] van den Brenk,[52] and Wildermuth[55] have claimed an increase in local tumor control using this method. Lack of patient controls and alteration of standard doses and patterns of application have made these impressions difficult to substantiate. Although it has been established that the early difficulties of convulsions, serious ear problems, and claustrophobia have been overcome and that patients can tolerate the 30–40 consecutive daily pressurization cycles necessary for irradiation with standard fractionation,[39] it has not been established that this pattern of application is optimal. If such a crude method of improving tumor oxygenation provides any benefit, it probably will be restricted to tumors that frequently are not controlled locally (or regionally), but remain localized for substantial periods (epidermoid carcinomas of the cervix, oral cavity, and hypopharynx).

Mallams, Finney, and Balla[35] developed a method of raising oxygen tension in tumors by regional arterial profusion of hydrogen peroxide (0.12–0.24 percent H_2O_2 in 5 percent dextrose solution). This method has the shortcomings and difficulties inherent in prolonged arterial catheterization, i.e., vessel spasm, placement and retention of a catheter in a major vessel.

Reduction of the adverse oxygen tension differential by deprivation of the entire tumor and adjacent normal tissues of oxygen has limited clinical application. Suit[48] has successfully treated malignant tumors of the extremities with high radiation doses (12,000 rads in 36 days) using a tourniquet technique.

ALKYLATING AGENTS

These heterogenous chemical agents, containing alkyl radicals which attach to proteins, nucleic acids, and amino acids, have been the most frequently used in cancer chemotherapy. Clinically useful agents include the nitrogen mustards, which contain the bis-amine groups (mechlorethamine hydrochloride—"Mustargen,"

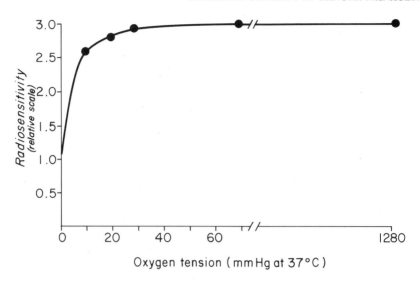

**Fig. 5-2. Relationship of Radiosensitivity (in Arbitrary Units) to Environ-
mental Oxygen Tension.** Note that return to full sensitivity occurs rapidly
with slight increase in oxygen tension.

chlorambucil—"Leukeran," cyclophosphamide—"Cytoxan," melphalan—"Alke-
ran," uracil mustard), the ethylenimines (triethylenethiophosphoramide—
"ThioTEPA," triethylenemelamine—"TEM") and the alkyl sulfonates (busulfan
—"Myleran"). Although the precise mechanism of action is unknown, the major
effect is the blockage of the synthesis of DNA by the combination of the alkyl radical
with the purine base, guanine.[9] Inasmuch as DNA is a likely radiation target,
enhancement of radiation effect seems possible.[15] Like ionizing radiation, alkylating
agents are mutagenic and carcinogenic, inhibit mitosis, produce nuclear pyknosis and
chromosome fragmentation,[26] thus gaining the misnomer "radiominetic."

Many clinical studies using nitrogen mustard and irradiation (carcinoma of the
bronchus—Krant et al.,[28] Chalmers,[10] localized Hodgkin's disease—Paterson[40, 41])
have failed to document any potentiation of radiation effect.

A seemingly specific effect has been claimed for the use of TEM with radiation
therapy for patients with retinoblastoma.[29, 44] However, a review of these data casts
doubt on any such optimism.[25, 49] Indeed, modern radiotherapeutic methods alone
have proved at least as successful.[4]

Alkylating agents, particularly Mustargen, have been used with radiation in a
few specific clinical situations, although no claim for synergism or potentiation has
been made. When rapidly growing tumors, usually anaplastic bronchial carcinomas
or lymphomas, compress the superior vena cava, trachea, or spinal cord, preirradiation administration of nitrogen mustard is supposed to avoid problems attributed to
radiation-produced edema. However, there is ample evidence to relieve this anxiety
and establish that radiation therapy alone, even in substantial dosage, is at least as
effective, without producing either local complications or the systemic morbidity
inherent with nitrogen mustard.[8, 15, 45]

ANALOGUE INHIBITORS

These agents may prevent the formation of nucleic acid bases (methotrexate or amethopterin and 5-fluorouracil) or interfere with the utilization of preformed bases (6-mercaptopurine).[9]

Methotrexate is a folic acid antagonist which interferes with the nucleic acid metabolism of growing cells and consequently prevents cell replication. It has been useful in the treatment of acute leukemia in children, reticulum cell sarcoma, and squamous cell carcinoma of the head and neck. Females with choriocarcinoma have been kept free of tumor for many years. Berry[7] proposed that methotrexate might sensitize radiation by interfering with repair of sublethal radiation damage. Friedman and Daly,[19] Kramer,[27] and Doggett et al.[14] suggested that the substantial methotrexate-induced reduction of volume of epidermoid carcinomas of the head and neck was merely additive to the radiation effect.

Fluorinated pyrimidines (5-FU and FUdR) interfere with DNA synthesis by inhibiting the enzyme, thymidylate synthetase.[15] 5-Fluorouracil is particularly active against adenocarcinomas arising in the gastrointestinal tract and breast. Although laboratory data have suggested a radiation potentiating effect of 5-FU,[2,7,53] data from clinical trials have been equivocal.[20,31,54]

Other halogenated pyrimidines with labeling by chlorine, bromine, and iodine (BUdR, CUdR, IUdR) are incorporated into DNA in place of thymine or thymidine.[15] These agents are radiosensitizers in vitro,[6,36] but no clinically useful augmentation of radiation effect has been demonstrated.

The purine analogues, 6-mercaptopurine and 6-thioguanine, interfere with purine synthesis, and both are incorporated into DNA and RNA. Laboratory evidence of increased radiosensitivity[24] has not been followed by demonstration of clinical usefulness.

ANTITUMOR ANTIBIOTICS

Actinomycin D, derived from the Streptomyces mold, selectively inhibits DNA-dependent RNA synthesis, especially nucleolar RNA synthesis.[9] Useful tumorocidal effects occur in Wilm's tumor, Ewing's tumor, embryonal rhabdomyosarcoma, neuroblastoma, and testicular tumors. Radiosensitization by actinomycin D has been reported in mammalian cell cultures[5] and in animal experiments.[33] Interference with postradiation cell recovery has been documented in the laboratory.[17] While under the systemic influence of actinomycin D, patients may have increased reactions in skin and other normal tissues within the irradiated volume. *Radiation reactions may be reactivated after long intervals by systemic actinomycin D.* However, evidence for a favorable alteration of the radiation therapeutic ratio is lacking. Many[15,25,32] consider the effects of systemic actinomycin D and ionizing radiation to be additive. "The case for the therapeutic synergism has not been made."[25] Although there is accumulating evidence that therapeutic regimens incorporating actinomycin D with surgery and radiation therapy have improved the outlook for patients with Wilm's tumor,[13,18,23,34] there is no evidence that local tumor control can be increased or local radiation-produced complications reduced by the combination of drug and smaller radiation dose as compared to adequate irradiation alone. Indeed the postirradiation aggrevation of radiation effects by actinomycin D can result in unwelcome developments avoidable only by routine "underdosing" by radiotherapists. Therefore, the combined use of actinomycin D and radiation therapy requires continuing close cooperation between pediatrician and radiation therapist.

ALKALOIDS

Vinblastine (Velban) and vincristine (Oncovin) are extracts of the periwinkle plant. They produce metaphase arrest and interfere with mitosis, with cell changes related to abnormal spindle development.[9] Acute leukemia in children, lymphomas, and choriocarcinoma have been usefully responsive.

The colchicine derivative demecolcin has had limited clinical trial.

No evidence is currently available that these alkaloids influence radiation response.

VITAMINS

Synkavit, a synthetic vitamin K, has been proposed as a radiation modifier by Mitchell,[37] based on an observation that this agent inhibited the mitosis of chick fibroblasts. In a randomized study of 18 patients with carcinoma of the bronchus, Deely[16] suggested that there might be a slight alteration in the shape of the intervening survival curve, although the incidence of survival at 12 months after irradiation was not increased.

CHEMICAL PROTECTIVE AGENTS

A wide spectrum of chemical compounds is known to protect cells irradiated in vitro and laboratory animals receiving total body irradiation. The best known are "radical scavengers" such as the sulfhydryl-containing cysteine, cysteamine, aminoethyl-thiouronium (AET), and 2-mercapto-ethylguanidine (MEG). This subject has been reviewed recently by Bacq.[1] However, selective protection of normal tissues adjacent to tumor has not been accomplished, and so there has been no clinical application.

At the present time, modification of the effects of ionizing radiation by chemicals is of little clinical value. However, the understanding of chemical modification of radiation effect ultimately should result in an increased understanding of radiation mechanisms and an improved clinical application. To date, as noted by Stein,[47] the efforts have resulted in a better understanding of the cancer problem and better cooperation between the radiotherapist and clinicians in other fields interested in the cancer patient.

REVIEW QUESTIONS

1. What is the basic objective of chemical modification of radiation effect if it is to be used clinically? How might this be accomplished?

2. Are any modifiers of radiation effect useful clinically?

3. What is the difference between synergism and additive effect? Which is preferable as an objective for modifiers of radiation effect? Why?

4. What are the possible mechanisms of chemical alteration of radiation effect? Give an example for each.

5. What is the theoretical basis for the use of oxygen at elevated pressure as a radiation adjuvant? Has this been tried clinically? Has it worked? In what tumors is the oxygen effect likely to be operative?

6. Have you seen alkylating agents used with radiation? In what situations? What was the rationale? Was such usage judged successful? Are there disadvantages in such usage?

7. Have you seen actinomycin D used as a radiation potentiator? Did it improve the therapeutic ratio?

8. Why are some alkylating agents called "radiomimetic"? Is this accurate? Why?

BIBLIOGRAPHY

1. BACQ, Z. M. *Chemical Protection Against Ionizing Radiation.* Charles C Thomas, Springfield, Ill., 1965.
2. BAGSHAW, M. A. Some experimental evidence for clinical enhancement of radiation response in vitro. In: *Research in Radiotherapy: Approaches to Chemical Sensitization.* R. F. Kallman, Ed, National Academy of Sciences, National Research Council, No. 35, Pub. 888, Washington, D.C., 1961, pp. 138–149.
3. BAGSHAW, M. A. Approaches for combined radiation and chemotherapy. *Laval Med,* 34: 124–133, 1963.
4. BAGSHAW, M. A., and KAPLAN, H. S. Supervoltage linear accelerator radiation therapy. VIII. Retinoblastoma. *Radiology,* 86:242–246, 1966.
5. BASES, R. E. Modification of radiation response determined by single-cell technics: Actinomycin D. *Cancer Res,* 19:1223–1229, 1959.
6. BERRY, R. J., and ANDREWS, J. R. Modification of the radiation effect on the reproductive capacity of tumor cells in vivo with pharmacologic agents. *Radiat Res,* 16:82–88, 1962.
7. BERRY, R. J. Modification of radiation effects. *Radiol Clin N Amer,* 3:249–258, 1965.
8. BOLAND, J. Personal communication.
9. BUSCH, H., and LANE, M. *Chemotherapy: An Introductory Text.* Year Book, Chicago, 1967.
10. CHALMERS, T. C. Combination of radiotherapy and chemotherapy in the treatment of carcinoma of the lung. *Cancer Chemother Rep,* 16:463–466, 1962.
11. CHURCHILL-DAVIDSON, I., SANGER, C., and THOMLINSON, R. H. High-pressure oxygen and radiotherapy. *Lancet,* 1:1091–1095, 1955.
12. CRABTREE, H. G., and CRAMER, N. The action of radium on cancer cells. II. Some factors determining the susceptibility of cancer cells to radium. In: *Eleventh Scientific Report on Investigations of the Imperial Cancer Research Fund.* Taylor and Francis, London, 1934, pp. 89–101.

13. D'ANGIO, G. J. Clinical and biological studies of Actinomycin D and roentgen irradiation. *Amer J Roentgen*, 87:106–109, 1962.

14. DOGGETT, R. L. S., BAGSHAW, M. A., KAPLAN, H. S., and NELSEN, T. S. Combination intra-arterial antimetabolite and radiation therapy of advanced head and neck cancer. Quoted in: *Modern Trends in Radiotherapy*. T. J. Deeley and C. A. P. Wood, Eds, Appleton-Century-Crofts, New York, 1967.

15. DOGGETT, R. L. S., BAGSHAW, M. A. and KAPLAN, H. S. Combined therapy using chemotherapeutic agents and radiotherapy. In: *Modern Trends in Radiotherapy*. T. J. Deeley and C A. P. Wood, Eds, Appleton-Century-Crofts, New York, 1967, pp. 107–131.

16. DEELEY, T. J. A clinical trial of synkavit in the treatment of carcinoma of the bronchus. *Brit J Cancer*, 16:387–389, 1962.

17. ELKIND, M. M., WHITMORE, G. F., and ALESCIO, T. Actinomycin D: Suppression of recovery in x-irradiated mammalian cells. *Science*, 143:1454–1457, 1964.

18. FERNBACH, D. J., and MARTYN, D. T. Role of Dactinomycin in improved survival of children with Wilm's tumor. *JAMA*, 195:1005–1009, 1966.

19. FRIEDMAN, M., and DALY, J. F. Combined irradiation and chemotherapy in treatment of squamous cell carcinoma of the head and neck. *Amer J Roentgen*, 90:246–260, 1963.

20. GOLLIN, F. F., ANSFIELD, F. J., CURRERI, A. R., HEIDELBERGER, C., and VERMUND, H. Combined chemotherapy and irradiation in inoperable bronchogenic carcinoma. *Cancer*, 15:1209–1217, 1962.

21. GRAY, L. H., CONGER, A. D., EBERT, M., HORNSEY, S., and SCOTT, O. C. A. Concentration of oxygen dissolved in tissues at time of irradiation as factor in radiotherapy. *Brit J Radiol*, 26:638–648, 1953.

22. GRAY, L. H. The influence of oxygen on the response of cells and tissues to ionizing radiation. *Lectures on the Scientific Basis of Medicine, VII*, pp. 314–374, 1957–1958.

23. HOWARD, R. Actinomycin D in Wilm's tumor: Treatment of lung metastases. *Arch Dis Child*, 40:200–202, 1965.

24. KAPLAN, H. S., EARLE, J. D., and HOWSDEN, F. L. The role of purine and pyrimidine bases and their analogues in radiation sensitivity. *J Cell Physiol*, 64:69–89, 1964.

25. KLIGERMAN, M. M. Present status of combined radiation therapy and chemotherapy. In: *Progress in Radiation Therapy*, Vol. III. F. Buschke, Ed, Grune & Stratton, New York, 1965, pp. 183–199.

26. KNOCK, F. E. *Anticancer Agents*. Charles C Thomas, Springfield, Ill., 1967.

27. KRAMER, S. Combined chemotherapy and radiation therapy in the management of regional Cancer; in Cancer Chemotherapy, I. Brodsky and S. B. Kahn, Eds, Grune & Stratton, New York, 1967, pp. 319–330.

28. KRANT, M. J., CHALMERS, T. C., DEDERICK, M. M., HALL, T. C., LEVENE, M. B., MUENCH, H., SHNIDER, B. I., GOLD, G. L., HUNTER, C., BERSAK, S. R., OWENS, A. H., JR., DE LEON, N., DICKSON, R. J. BUNDLEY, C., BRACE, K. C., FREI, E., GEHAN, E., and SAVIN, L. Comparative trial of chemotherapy and radiotherapy in patients with non-resectable cancer of the lung. *Amer J Med*, 35:363–737, 1963.

29. KREMENTZ, E. T., SCHLOSSER, J. F., and PUMAGE, J. P. Treatment of retinoblastoma by fractional intra-arterial T.E.M. and x-ray therapy. *Southern Med J*, 56:1023–1025, 1963.

30. LACASSAGNE, A. Chute de la sensibilité aux rayons X chez la souris nouveau—neé en état d' asphyxie. *C R Acta Sci*, 215–232, 1942.

31. LATOURETTE, H. B., and LAWTON, R. L. Combined radiation and chemotherapy: Concomitant use for advanced malignant neoplasms. *JAMA*, 186:1057–1060, 1963.

32. LIEBNER, E. J. Actinomycin D and radiation therapy. *Amer. J Roentgen*, 87:94–105, 1962.

33. MADDOCK, C. L., BROWN, B., and D'ANGIO, G. J. Abstract 159. The enhanced response of Ridgway osteogenic sarcoma to x-radiation combined with Actinomycin-D. *Proc Amer Ass Cancer Res*, 2:131, 1960.

34. MAIER, J. G., and HARSHAW, W. G. Treatment and prognosis in Wilm's tumor: Study of 51 cases with special reference to role of Actinomycin D. *Cancer*, 20:96–102, 1967.

35. MALLAMS, J. T., FINNEY, J. W., and BALLA, G. A. The use of hydrogen peroxide as a source of oxygen in a regional intra-arterial infusion system. *Southern Med J*, 55:230–232, 1962.

36. MARUYAMA, Y., SILINI, G., and KAPLAN, H. S. Studies of the LSA ascites lymphoma of C57B1 mice. II. Radiosensitization in vivo with 5-bromo-deoxycytidine and combined 5-fluorodeoxyuridine and 5-bromodeoxycytidine. *Int J Radiat Biol*, 7:453–484, 1963.

37. MITCHELL, J. S. *Studies in Radiotherapeutics.* Blackwell, Oxford, 1960.
38. MOTTRAM, J. C. *Brit J Radiol,* May, 1924. Quoted in: Alteration in the sensitivity of cells. *Brit J Radiol* 8:32–39, 1935.
39. PARKER, R. G., and WOOTTON, P. Physiological evaluation of patients subjected to hyperbaric radiation therapy. In: *Proceedings of the First Annual San Francisco Cancer Symposium: Hyperbaric Oxygen and Radiation Therapy of Cancer,* November, 1967. Jerome M. Vaeth, Ed, S. Karger, Basel, 1967.
40. PATERSON, E. Evaluation of chemotherapeutic compounds in the reticuloses. *Brit J Cancer,* 12:332–341, 1958.
41. PATERSON, E. Evaluation of chemotherapeutic compounds in the reticuloses. *Acta Un Int Cancer,* 16:518–521, 1960.
42. PATT, H. M. The modification of radiation effects by chemical means. In: *Progress in Radiation Therapy,* Vol. I. F. Buschke, Ed, Grune & Stratton, New York, 1958, pp. 115–127.
43. POWERS, W. E., and TOLMACK, L. J. A multicomponent x-ray survival curve for mouse lymphosarcoma cells irradiated in vivo. *Nature,* 197:710–711, 1963.
44. REESE, A. B., and ELLSWORTH, R. M. The evaluation and current concept of retinoblastoma therapy. *Trans Amer Acad Ophthal Otolaryng,* 67:164–172, 1963.
45. RUBIN, P., GREEN, J., HOLZWASSER, G., and GERLE, P. Superior vena caval syndrome: Slow low-dose versus rapid high-dose schedules. *Radiology,* 81:388–401, 1963.
46. SCHWARTZ, G. Uber dosensensibilisenung gegen Röntgen und Radiumstrahlen. *München Med. Wschr.* 56:1217–1218, 1909.
47. STEIN, J. J. The question of chemical potentiators in radiation therapy. *Amer J Roentgen,* 88:989–992, 1962.
48. SUIT, H. D. Radiation therapy given under conditions of local tissue hypoxia for bone and soft tissue sarcoma. In: *Tumors of Bone and Soft Tissue, Eighth Annual Clinical Conference on Cancer.* Year Book, Chicago, 1963, pp. 143–163.
49. TAPLEY, N. DU V. Clinical results in the treatment of retinoblastoma with T.E.M. and radiation. In: *Research in Radiotherapy.* R. F. Kallman, Ed, Washington, National Academy of Science, National Research Council, 1961, and personal communication, 1969, pp. 199–200.
50. THOMLINSON, R. H. Oxygen therapy—Biological considerations. In: *Modern Trends in Radiotherapy.* T. J. Deeley and C. A. P. Wood, Eds, Appleton-Century-Crofts, New York, 1967, pp. 52–72.
51. THOMLINSON, R. H. A comparison of fast neutrons and x-rays in relation to the "oxygen effect" in experimental tumours in rats. *Brit J Radiol,* 36:89–91, 1963.
52. VAN DEN BRENK, H. A. S., MADIGAN, J. P., and KERR, R. C. Experience with megavoltage irradiation of advanced malignant disease using high pressure oxygen. Pp. 144–160 in: *Clinical Application of Hyperbaric Oxygen.* I. Boersma, Ed, Elsevier, Amsterdam, 1964.
53. VERMUND, H., HODGETT, J., and ANSFIELD, F. J. Effects of combined roentgen irradiation and chemotherapy on transplanted tumors in mice. *Amer J Roentgen,* 85:559–567, 1961.
54. VON ESSEN, C. F., KLIGERMAN, M. M., and CALABRESI, P. Radiation and 5-fluorouracil: A controlled clinical study. *Radiology,* 81:1018–1027, 1963.
55. WILDERMUTH, O. Hybaroxic radiation therapy in cancer management. *Radiology,* 82:767–776, 1964.
56. WOOTTON, P. Oxygen as a radiotherapeutic adjuvant. *Progress in Radiation Therapy,* Vol. II. F. Buschke, Ed, Grune & Stratton, New York, 1962, pp. 94–113.

6

CANCER OF THE SKIN
AND MUCOCUTANEOUS
JUNCTIONS

Malignant tumors of the skin and mucocutaneous junctions include basal cell and squamous cell carcinoma, adenocarcinoma arising in sweat or sebaceous glands, melanoma, mycosis fungoides, Kaposi's disease, lymphomatous infiltrations, and metastases from other sites.

BASAL AND SQUAMOUS CELL CARCINOMA

These visible lesions should be detected soon after their appearance and, because of infrequent and late occurring metastases, should be controlled in nearly all instances.

They constitute one of the most frequent forms of cancer in the human (40 percent of all malignancies at the Ellis Fischel State Cancer Hospital).[11]

Etiology

There is an association with long-term exposure to actinic rays, thermal or radiation damage, certain chemicals (arsenicals, nitrates, petroleum products), and infected chronic draining sinuses. The apparent common denominator is severe degenerative change with a long latent period (more than 15 years).

Therefore, it is predictable that most carcinomas of the skin will arise in chronically exposed sites (face, neck, dorsum of the hands), in certain groups (farmers and fishermen), and in the older population (median age 72 years and infrequently in those under 40 years).[1]

Pathology

Basal or squamous cell carcinomas of the skin may be nodular and superficial, flat with spread parallel to the surface, or deeply infiltrative with destruction of bone, cartilage, or soft tissues. Such gross appearances are usually distinctive, thus allowing a high order of accuracy in clinical diagnosis even as to histological type (accuracy of tumor type—90 percent of 2,000 cases).[17] However, even with expert judgment, about 15 percent of lesions clinically diagnosed as benign will be malignant.[17]

Except in extenuating circumstances (i.e., multiple, typical facial lesions, when one or more have been proved), lesions in question need to be biopsied. A good biopsy specimen obtained through the junction with normal skin with adequate depth facilitates diagnosis which is necessary license for institution of treatment.

Metastasis from a basal cell carcinoma is so rare as to merit reporting. Squamous cell carcinomas metastasize infrequently (5 percent of facial lesions,[1] 20 percent of lesions of the extremities[3]) and late in their clinical course. Such metastases with rare exception are to regional lymph nodes, and their incidence increases with longer duration, larger size, and lesser histological differentiation of the primary tumor and failure of previous treatment.

Basal cell carcinomas are about twice as frequent as squamous cell carcinomas. They have a distinctive, although varied, histological pattern, and may contain melanin, a finding which may give rise to some clinical confusion with melanomas. This confusion may be compounded by a few malignant melanomas which are without pigment (amelanotic melanoma).

Squamous cell carcinomas usually are well or partially differentiated.[10]

Clinical Presentation

Nearly all basal cell carcinomas are on the face and neck, with special affinity for the eyelids, nose, cheeks, forehead, skin of upper and lower lips, and chin (T-zone—Figure 6-1). They may be of slow evolution, histories of 10 years' duration not being rare.

Most squamous cell carcinomas also occur on the face and neck with an affinity for the scalp, ears, temples, cheeks, and vermilion surfaces of the lips. Lesions of the hands, feet, extremities, and trunk are likely to be squamous cell carcinomas. These lesions, often associated with hyperkeratoses, also may have a long history, although shorter than for basal cell carcinoma.

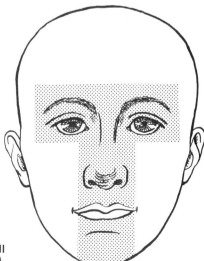

Fig. 6-1. T-zone of high incidence for basal cell carcinoma. (exclusive of vermilion surface of lips).

Treatment

Basal cell and squamous cell carcinomas of the skin have been treated by many means: surgery, irradiation, cautery, escharotic pastes, and dry ice. Excision and irradiation are the methods of merit based on control of the primary lesion and its metastases, good functional and cosmetic results, and flexibility of treatment application.

For many lesions, adequate surgery or radiation therapy would produce comparable results. However, surgery and radiation therapy are not optimally used in the same situations. Routine use of either modality to the exclusion of the other will not result in the best performance possible. The choice of treatment should not be based on the bias of an uninformed clinician. To merit use in any instance, surgery or radiation therapy must be done with competence. Even the *combination of both modalities used poorly will add up to poor treatment.*

Preference for resection or irradiation will depend on (1) site, size, and extent of the primary lesion; (2) presence of metastases; (3) condition of the surrounding tissue; (4) presence of other lesions; (5) previous treatment; (6) function of the part involved; (7) desire for cosmetic result; (8) expediency; and (9) cost (time and money).

Therefore, surgery might be preferable for small lesions of the head and neck where simple excision provides adequate margins (Figure 6-2), does not alter function, and should result in a good cosmetic result; for lesions of the trunk and extremities where ample skin allows effective simple excision with good cosmetic result; when there is advantage in simultaneous treatment of regional metastases; when the adjacent tissue is compromised, i.e., with burn scars; in the presence of other adjacent lesions, i.e., lupus, keratoses; when previous treatment at the site has failed and the recurrence is in scar tissue; and when speed of treatment is of great importance.

Inherent advantages of radiation therapy are that it can be adapted to nearly all clinical situations and can result in an unexcelled functional and cosmetic result. Therefore, radiation therapy has advantage when resection requires sizable repair, i.e., lesions of the eyelid, canthus, nose, ear, and lip (Figure 6-3). If resection is of such magnitude as to require hospitalization, radiation therapy on an outpatient basis should be less costly and more expeditious. Radiation therapy also can be used to advantage for some extensive lesions when resection is not applicable. The only

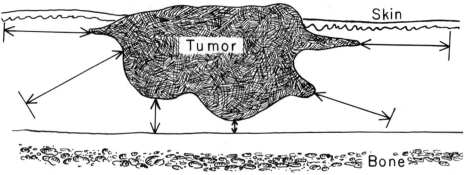

Fig. 6-2. Adequacy of margins of excision. Note that deep margins may be compromised by underlying structure. Adequate margins must be three-dimensional.

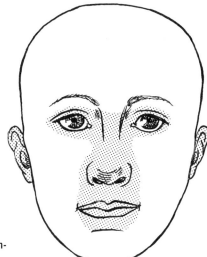

Fig. 6-3. Sites where radiation therapy has advantage over surgery for treatment of skin cancer.

major contraindications to irradiation are compromise of the adjacent tissue, i.e., scar or radiation damage, such that cancerocidal doses are not tolerated; extensive invasion of underlying bone; lack of available professional competence; or in a patient with other problems which make the skin cancer inconsequential.

Radiation Therapy Techniques

Skin cancers can be irradiated adequately by roentgen rays of various qualities or by radium or other isotopes in various contact applicators.

Flexibility, ease, and safety of application make roentgen rays the best physical choice. As with surgery, the skill of the physician outweighs the equipment used.

Inasmuch as the inherent advantages of irradiation include preservation of adjacent structures, radiation techniques maximizing normal tissue tolerance should be used. Thus, the most frequent technique consists of filtered x-rays (i.e., HVL 3.0 mm Al—2.0 mm Cu) applied in multiple increments (usually daily) for two to five weeks. Necessary increases in dose correlated with lengthening overall treatment periods have been documented by Strandquist,[17] Andrews,[2] and von Essen[19] (Figure 6-4). Structures such as the eye and teeth should be protected by custom-fitted shields of lead whenever such protection does not risk inadequate treatment of the tumor (Figures 6-5, 6-6).

Biological Response of Skin to Irradiation

The response of skin to ionizing radiation has been more exhaustively studied than has the response of any other tissue or organ. This has been a natural result of the application of a treatment modality which, in nearly all instances, needs to be introduced through the skin. Skin responses, often unwelcomed, have guided and limited nearly all technical application until the use of supervoltage radiation.

Radiation reactions of skin may be of a broad spectrum of intensity and appear in predictable sequence. These reactions are related to (1) radiation quality (less

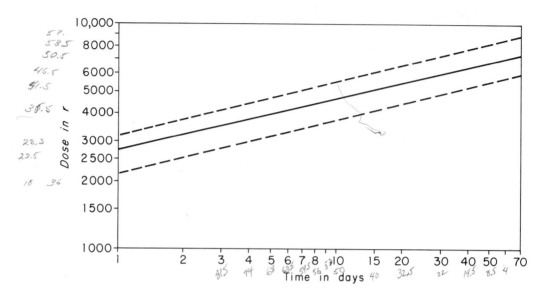

Fig. 6-4. Time-dose relationship for destruction of small epidermoid carcinomas of skin with optimum (and 20 percent variations) regression line. (after Andrews and Moody[2]).

intense with better filtered, more penetrating radiation); (2) total dosage; (3) over-all time of application (less intense with same dose administered over a longer period); (4) area of application (more intense with same dose when larger is area irradiated); (5) anatomic site (axillary or perineal skin less tolerant than skin of face, neck, back, and extremities); (6) poorly defined constitutional factors (skin of fair complexion responds more vigorously than pigmented skin; (7) pre-existing alteration of the skin and adjacent tissue (scar, surgical graft); and perhaps (8) coexistent administration of drugs (actinomycin D).

Changes detectable within hours to several weeks after irradiation may range from a barely detectable, transitory erythema through a brisk, persistent erythema

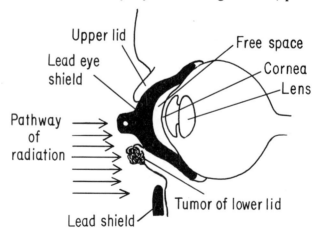

Fig. 6-5.   Protection of eye with lead shield.   (sagittal view).
Note lack of contact between shield and cornea.

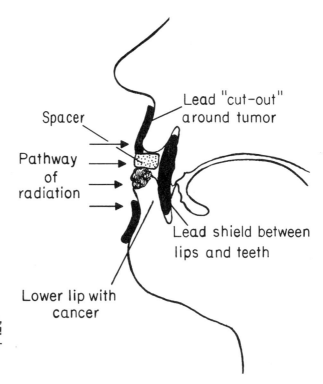

Fig. 6-6. Protection of teeth, gingiva, mandible, and oral structures when treating cancer of lip. (sagittal view).

and epilation, to gross loss of the epidermis (exudative radiodermatitis), or even necrosis of the dermis. These acute changes (except necrosis) are reversible and usually are followed by minimal sequelae. Acceptable changes occurring weeks to years after irradiation (chronic) may include atrophy, epilation, telangiectasia, and pigmentation. The severe changes of nonhealing ulceration or necrosis usually follow violation of sound principles of the therapeutic application of radiation. Squamous cell carcinomas on rare occasions may develop in this badly damaged skin many years later. *No irradiated skin, even if grossly normal, is unaltered.* Therefore, such skin will not tolerate the insults of trauma or infection as well as the normal. However, such altered skin in most instances has served the host well without loss of function, and may be superior to grafted skin or excision scar.

Sequelae and complications of radiation therapy depend on many factors: (1) size and extent of the lesion, especially with reference to destruction of normal tissue; (2) condition of tumor bed; (3) later trauma (i.e., excessive exposure) or infection, but depend most on (4) technique of treatment. Treatment with adequately filtered x-rays with cancerocidal but not excessive dosage delivered over a period of time (protraction) rarely should be followed by the undesirable sequelae of marked atrophy with telangiectasia, marked subepidermal atrophy and fibrosis, ulceration, or necrosis. (Necrosis with lesions less than 2 cm, about 3 percent).[18] Even when ulceration or necrosis occurs, conservative management usually results in healing. There has been much unwarranted concern about irradiation of lesions overlying cartilage or bone.[13] Intact, healthy cartilage and bone will tolerate necessary doses of radiation. If cartilage or bone has been invaded by tumor or is infected, localized sequestration usually will occur. Even in these instances, primary healing can follow.

Results

The prognosis of basal and squamous cell carcinomas of the skin is the best of all forms of cancer. However, unnecessary failure continues to be too frequent. Most of these failures are based on inadequate initial treatment. Survival rates are inaccurate as a measure of therapeutic performance because of the high number of deaths from intercurrent disease in an elderly population. Local control, especially in basal cell carcinoma, is an adequate measure of success, but such local control need be correlated with preservation of function and cosmetic appearance. Comparison of the reported results of surgery and radiation therapy is not valid, for the lesions treated in various series are not comparable. Following irradiation, less than 5 percent of previously untreated lesions will recur, although about 20 percent of previously recurrent lesions will recur again.[18] Recurrences will be most frequent in larger lesions, and 85 percent will be manifest within three years, with a majority within one year.[18]

Lower five-year survival rates of patients with squamous cell carcinoma compared with those with basal cell carcinoma may be a manifestation of metastases in the former.

MALIGNANT MELANOMA

Malignant melanoma may arise from many sites (skin, mucous membranes, retina, conjunctiva). In the past, all melanomas have been considered collectively and have been considered extremely malignant and nonresponsive to radiation therapy. It has become almost dogma to consider malignant melanoma to be outside the influence of radiation therapy.

It is now recognized that melanomas originating in different tissues differ in biological behavior, response to radiation therapy, and prognosis. Melanoma arising in ocular structures, such as the limbus or conjunctiva, is different biologically from melanoma arising in the skin. The former is radioresponsive and curable by radiation therapy.[7]

Melanoma of the skin is a distinct clinical entity. Radical surgery, when feasible, is the treatment of choice. However, some melanomas of the skin are responsive to radiation therapy. Gratifying, long-term palliation may be associated with complete disappearance of the irradiated lesion during the patient's lifetime. Inasmuch as it is impossible to predict responsiveness in the individual patient, radiation therapy for palliation is justified if the patient's general condition is good, and if a large, ulcerated tumor or lymph node mass causes significant clinical discomfort.

The prognosis for melanoma is not as hopeless as stated in many textbooks. Review of the material treated at the University of California has shown that the overall five-year salvage is better than for patients with carcinoma of the breast.[6]

CARCINOMA ARISING IN SWEAT OR SEBACEOUS GLANDS

These infrequent lesions, usually well-differentiated adenocarcinomas, usually have been managed by resection.

MYCOSIS FUNGOIDES, KAPOSI'S DISEASE, LYMPHOMATOUS INFILTRATIONS

These infrequent lesions are usefully radiation responsive and, therefore, in most instances irradiation is the treatment of choice for the local lesions.

METASTASES TO SKIN

Treatment should be based on the local problem and its relationship to overall management of the patient. Predictions of responsiveness to irradiation relate to the primary lesion as well as to the tumor bed. The most frequent lesions, those from the breast and lung, should be usefully responsive. The response of others, i.e., from stomach, uterus, kidney, whether present through biologic or iatrogenic means, will be problematical.

SPECIAL ANATOMIC SITES

Although most (numerically) skin cancers are best treated by excision, the inherent advantages of radiation therapy should be exploited when certain sites are involved. These are sites where excision is difficult, thus compromising adequate margins, where function and cosmetics following surgery would compare unfavorably with results of radiotherapy, and where surgical repair would be a major effort. These special sites are: eyelids, skin of the medial canthus, skin of the nose and nasolabial fold, skin of the pinna and immediate pre- and postauricular regions, and vermilion surface of the lip (Figure 6-3).

Carcinoma of the eyelid represents about 2.5 percent of all skin cancer, usually affects males beyond "middle age," and most frequently involves the lower lid and medial canthus.[15] Most are basal cell carcinomas (82 percent basal cell, 14.5 percent squamous cell carcinoma).[15] Although very small tumors in freely movable skin can be excised expeditiously, and massive lesions with invasion of the orbit and destruction of the eye may be treated best by orbital exenteration, most of these tumors are best treated by radiation methods. Failures of radiation therapy can be controlled by excision. Thus, Wildermuth and Evans[19] controlled 94.4 percent of 67 patients by primary irradiation and salvaged another 3 percent by postirradiation excision. With good technique, inclusive of protection of the anterior surface of the globe (Figure 6-5), mild transitory treatment-related complications (conjunctivitis, corneal ulcer, epiphora, and skin necrosis) are very infrequent, and serious late complications (i.e., cataract, corneal change) are very rare.[9, 19]

Selection of the best treatment for a specific patient requires cooperation between ophthalmologist, dermatologist, plastic surgeon, and therapeutic radiologist, any of whom may initially see the patient for primary treatment.

Other special anatomic sites, nose and pinna, have been the subject of a myth that radiation methods cannot be used because of the underlying cartilage. Long-standing evidence documents that not only can local irradiation be used, but that it is the treatment of choice in most skin cancers involving these structures.[1,4,5,8,12,14]

Our material[14] includes control of 29 of 34 skin cancers of the pinna and of over 100 of 110 skin cancers of the nose for more than three years or until death from intercurrent disease. Although mild atrophy and telangiectasia of the skin were frequent, rare cartilage problems (less than 2 percent) occurred only with uncontrolled tumor or when cartilage had been destroyed and infected prior to irradiation.

PREMALIGNANT SKIN CONDITIONS

Senile Keratoses

Squamous cell carcinomas may develop in association with these rough, granular, plaquelike lesions with overlying keratin, usually involving the skin of the upper face, ears, or dorsal surfaces of the hands of the elderly.

"Occupational" Keratoses

These lesions are like senile keratoses, but can be related to a specific etiologic agent, i.e., on the fingers of early radiation workers.

Bowen's Disease

Bowen described a solitary, slightly raised, occasionally ulcerated/crusted, erythematous, chronic lesion of the skin which should be considered a carcinoma-in-situ, which occasionally may become an invasive epidermoid carcinoma.

Xeroderma Pigmentosum

This rare, familial disease starts in infancy with photosensitive, irregularly atrophic and hyperpigmented skin which soon hosts multiple epidermoid carcinomas.

Erythroplasia of Queyrat

These rare, well-defined, erythematous, velvety lesions, which involve the prepuce, glans penis, vulva, and oral mucous membrane, may become epidermoid carcinomas.

REVIEW QUESTIONS

1. List six malignant tumors of the skin.

2. What are some etiological associations important in the management of patients with carcinomas arising in the skin?

3. What are the margins of error in the clinical diagnosis of skin cancer? How does this influence your decision to substantiate a skin lesion by biopsy?

4. What is the most important difference in the behavior of basal and squamous cell carcinomas of the skin? How does this affect clinical patient management?

5. What are the advantages of surgery in the treatment of skin cancer? the disadvantages?

6. What are the advantages of radiation therapy in the treatment of skin cancer? the disadvantages?

7. When would you recommend surgery? radiation therapy?

8. What factors influence the skin's reaction to radiation?

9. What is the incidence of local tumor control of previously untreated basal cell carcinoma and squamous cell carcinoma of the skin by radiation therapy? How does previous treatment failure influence this control?

10. What is a reasonable time interval after treatment to assess local tumor control?

11. In what circumstances can radiotherapy be of value for patients with malignant melanoma?

12. In what special anatomic sites involved by skin cancer has radiation therapy an advantage over other treatment methods?

BIBLIOGRAPHY

1. ACKERMAN, L. V., and DEL REGATO, J. A. *Cancer*, 4th Ed, Mosby, St. Louis, 1970.
2. ANDREWS, J. R., and MOODY, J. M. The dose-time relationship in radiotherapy. *Amer J Roentgen*, 75:590–596, 1956.
3. BROWNE, H. J., COVENTRY, M. B., and MCDONALD, J. R. Squamous carcinoma of the extremities. *Mayo Clin Proc*, 28:590–598, 1953.
4. DOWDY, A. H. Roentgen ray therapy of skin cancer overlying cartilage and bone. *New York J Med*, 40:620–626, 1940.
5. DRIVER, J. R., and COLE, H. N. Treatment of epithelioma of the skin of the ear. *Amer J Roentgen*, 48:66–73, 1942.
6. GALANTE, M. Personal communication.
7. LEDERMAN, M. Radiotherapy of malignant melanomas of the eye. *Brit J Radiol*, 34:21–42, 1961.
8. LEVI, W. The roentgen ray treatment of cutaneous carcinoma involving cartilage. *Amer J Roentgen*, 61:380–386, 1949.
9. LEVITT, S. H., BOGARDUS, C. R., JR., and BRANDT, E. N., JR. Complications and late changes following radiation therapy for carcinoma of the eyelid and canthi. *Radiology*, 87:340–347, 1966.
10. LUND, H. Z. Tumors of the skin. *Atlas of Tumor Pathology*, Sect. 1, Fasc. 2, Washington, D.C. Armed Forces Institute of Pathology, 1957.
11. MOSS, W. T. *Therapeutic Radiology*, 3rd Ed, Mosby, St. Louis, 1969.
12. MURPHY, W. T. *Radiation Therapy*, 2nd Ed, Saunders, Philadelphia, 1967.
13. PARKER, R. G. Tolerance of cartilage and bone in clinical radiation therapy. In: *Progress in Radiation Therapy*, Vol. II, F. Buschke Ed, Grune & Stratton, New York, 1962.
14. PARKER, R. G., and WILDERMUTH, O. Radiation therapy of lesions overlying cartilage. Carcinoma of the pinna. *Cancer*, 15:57–65, 1962.

15. STETSON, C. G., and SCHULTZ, M.D. Carcinoma of the eyelid. Analysis of 301 cases and review of the literature. *New Eng J Med*, 241:725–732, 1949.
16. STRANDQUIST, M. Studien uber die kumulative Wirkung der Rontgenstrahlen bei Fraktionierung. *Acta Radiol (Suppl. 55)*, 1944.
17. TORREY, F. A., and LEVIN, É. A. Comparison of clinical and pathologic diagnosis of malignant conditions of the skin. *Arch Derm Syph*, 43:532–535, 1941.
18. VON ESSEN, C. F. Roentgen therapy of skin and lip carcinoma: Factors influencing success and failure. *Amer J Roentgen*, 83:556–570, 1960.
19. WILDERMUTH, O., and EVANS, J. C. The special problem of cancer of the eyelid. *Cancer*, 9:837–841, 1956.

THE SPECIAL PROBLEM OF KERATOACANTHOMA
(Molluscum sebaceum, Self-healing Primary Squamous Carcinoma of Skin)

A curious lesion, often confused with basal and squamous cell carcinomas arising in the skin, was named keratoacanthoma by Rook and Whimster in 1950,[5] was described as molluscum sebaceum by MacCormack and Scarff in 1936,[4] and probably was recognized as a clinical entity as early as 1888 by Hutchinson.[1] The usual site of involvement is the skin of the face and neck of adults. Diagnosis can be based on a characteristic appearance of a hemispherical mass with rolled edges and thin atrophic margins and a central keratin core, a characteristic short history (four to six weeks) and a typical histologic appearance. Although these lesions will spontaneously subside in a few months, often leaving an atrophic scar with a crenated margin,[3] concern for the rapidly enlarging lesion on the face usually leads to treatment. Inasmuch as nearly any treatment is effective in this self-limiting lesion, many regimens have been advocated. Thus, Kunkler and Raines (radiotherapist and surgeon)[3] state: "Except to establish the diagnosis, surgery has little part to play, the earliest lesions can be removed with a sharp spoon and the largest most simply treated by radiation;" whereas Jackson (plastic surgeon)[2] recommends: "A reasonable management regime would be excision biopsy in all cases unless the lesion is already in the phase of involution, when shaving is undoubtedly the most satisfactory form of treatment. . . . This scheme of treatment precludes radiotherapy."

On the basis of four cases, Jackson[2] emphasizes the danger that squamous cell carcinomas, often highly malignant, may be misdiagnosed as keratoacanthoma, and consequently inadequately treated.

BIBLIOGRAPHY

1. HUTCHINSON, J. A., quoted by I. T. Jackson in: *Small Atlas of Illustrations of Clinical Surgery*, Vol. II, Plate 92, Philadelphia, 1888.
2. JACKSON, I. T. Diagnostic problem of keratoacanthoma. *Lancet*, 490–492, 1969.
3. KUNKLER, P. B., and RAINS, A. J. H. *Treatment of Cancer in Clinical Practice*. Livingstone, Edinburgh, 1959.

4. MACCORMACK, H., and SCARFF, R. W. Molluscum sebaceum. *Brit J Derm*, 48:624–626, 1936.
5. ROOK, A. J., and WHIMSTER, I. W. Le kérato-acanthoma. *Arch Belg Derm Syph*, 6:137–146, 1950.

CARCINOMA OF THE LIP

Carcinoma of the vermilion surface of the lip is a clinical entity distinct from carcinoma of the skin. When this tumor is included with oral cancers it comprises 25 percent of the entire group. The lower vermilion surface is involved ten times more frequently than is the upper vermilion surface.[1] One-half of the carcinomas arise lateral to the middle third, but exclusive of the lateral commissure, whereas one-third arise from the middle third just external to the line of contact[3] (Figure 6-7). One-third of the patients are between 60 and 69 years, but patients under 40 years are infrequent.[3] Nearly all cancers of the lower lip occur in men, whereas the proportion of females may be slightly higher in cancer of the upper lip.[1] There is an association with leukoplakia and long exposure to actinic rays, but only rare coexistence of syphilis, historically associated with some intraoral cancers.

Pathology

Nearly all lips cancers are well-differentiated squamous cell carcinomas. These tumors may be exophytic, superficial, or deeply infiltrating.

Metastases usually are orderly and progressive to ipsilateral submental, submaxillary, upper deep cervical and lower deep cervical lymph nodes without skipping node stations (Figures 6-8, 6-9). Occasional contralateral adenopathy usually is associated with midline primary tumors. The reported incidence of cervical adenopathy on initial examination has varied from 6.2 percent[10] to 28.7 percent[6] (average 10 percent), whereas adenopathy has been recognized after treatment of the primary tumor in 4.9 percent[8] to 8.6 percent[6] (average 7.4 percent) of patients. The incidence of regional adenopathy varies with the size of the primary tumor, the histologic grade of tumor, and previous treatment failure (Table 6-1).

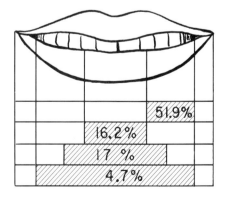

Fig. 6-7. Cancer of the lip. Incidence of Site of Involvement (after Gladstone and Kerr[3]).

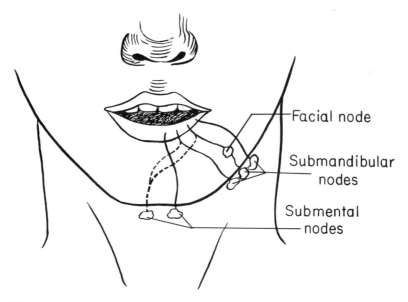

Fig. 6-8. Primary lymphatic drainage of lower vermilion. (precedes drainage to deep cervical nodes)

Distant metastases are rare (1 in 519 patients[3]). If metastases are to appear in relationship to a controlled primary tumor, they will be grossly detectable within two years of treatment.

Treatment

Comparable primary lip cancers can be controlled with equal frequency by radiation treatment or surgery.[5,10] Therefore, the choice of treatment method should be based on considerations other than local tumor control. If the tumor is small, good control, good preservation of function, and good cosmetic appearance

Table 6-1. Cancer of the Lip
Factors in Cervical Adenopathy

Total No. Patients	Previous Treatment	Size of Primary Tumor	Histologic Grade	Metastases On Admission	Later
	129 (none)	119 < 3.0 cm	105 gr. I	1	6
			14 gr. II	2	1
		10 > 3.0 cm	3 gr. I	0	1
161			7 gr. II	2	2
	32 (failure)	22 < 3.0 cm	17 gr. I	2	0
			5 gr. II	3	0
		10 > 3.0 cm	8 gr. I	3	1
			2 gr. II	2	0

After Modlin.[7]

can be accomplished by either treatment method, but surgery may be more expeditious. If the lesion is more extensive, but there is minimal destruction of normal tissue, radiation therapy has great advantage over a complicated resection. If the tumor is extensive with associated destruction of normal tissue, in itself requiring plastic repair, then surgery may be preferable although satisfactory results have followed irradiation.[5] Surgery is the choice (1) if there is coexistent widespread change, i.e., atrophy, leukoplakia; (2) if there is likely to be further prolonged exposure, i.e., in farmers; (3) if the tumor is recurrent in scar following either excision or irradiation; (4) if an immediately adjacent site, which would be in the treatment volume, previously has been vigorously irradiated; (5) if proved regional metastatic adenopathy coexists and treatment of the primary can be done expeditiously at the same time; and (6) if there is extension of tumor to bone.

The preferable treatment of regional metastatic adenopathy is radical neck dissection.[10] Clinical appraisal of cervical adenopathy may be in error, especially if the nodes are small (less than 2.0 cm), probably because of frequent ulceration and infection at the primary site. Spread of tumor follows a highly predictable pattern with consecutive involvement of nodes without "skipped" stations (Figures 6-8, 6-9). Thus, with therapeutic neck dissection, Modlin[7] found a single node involved in 57.7 percent, two nodes involved in 26.9 percent, and multiple nodes involved in only 15.3 percent. This low incidence and orderly progression of cervical adenopathy makes "prophylactic" neck dissection unprofitable in this group of elderly patients. Judd and Beahrs[4] did 322 "prophylactic" neck dissections to find 74 patients (23.0 percent) with tumor-bearing nodes, and Modlin[7] with

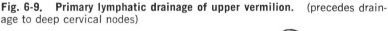

Fig. 6-9.   Primary lymphatic drainage of upper vermilion.   (precedes drainage to deep cervical nodes)

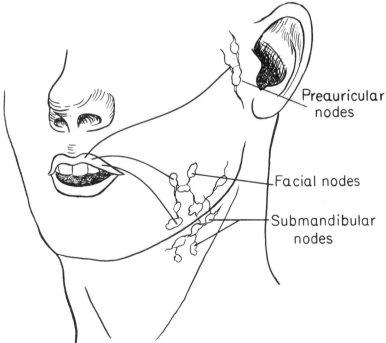

Preauricular nodes

Facial nodes

Submandibular nodes

"therapeutic" neck dissections found 25 of 30 patients (83 percent) to have tumor-bearing nodes. However, the five-year tumor-free survival for those with positive nodes was similar in both series (33 of 74 patients—46.0 percent[4]; 13 of 25 patients—52 percent[7]). Therefore, patient salvage is not compromised by restraining therapy pending clinical detection of adenopathy, and a large number of unnecessary operations is avoided.

Sequelae and Complications

The previously untreated lip is a good tumor bed with high radiation tolerance. Sequelae are comparable to those described for the treatment of skin cancer.

Prognosis

Tumor control varies with the site, extent, and histological grade of the primary lesion, the presence of metastases, and previous treatment failure. Thus, direct unqualified comparisons between reported series are prone to error. For example, 75 percent of our series had primary tumors less than 2.0 cm and only 10 percent had tumors larger than 3.0 cm in contrast to the material of Gladstone and Kerr[3] in which only 50 percent had tumors less than 2.0 cm but one-third had tumors larger than 3.0 cm.

Often the very small and the extensive tumors are resected, whereas the moderate-sized tumors are irradiated, thus negating unqualified comparison between the treatment methods.

Tumor control is related to tumor size in Table 6-2. The similar effectiveness of radiation therapy and surgery for comparable tumors has been documented by del Regato and Sala[10] (Table 6-3).

Tumors of the vermilion of upper lip and those involving the commissure and buccal mucosa may be more difficult to control, the former because of a higher incidence of adenopathy, the latter because of frequent extensive tumor with invasion of muscle as well as a higher incidence of regional adenopathy.

The presence of regional adenopathy reduces the likelihood of cure to about 50 percent whether the neck dissection is "prophylactic"[4] or "therapeutic."[7]

Poorly differentiated squamous cell carcinomas occasionally arise from the mucosa of the lip. The few observed have been biologically aggressive, with metastases to regional lymph nodes and via the bloodstream to distant sites. These lesions can be locally controlled by irradiation.

Table 6-2.   Cancer of the Lip
Treatment Effectiveness Related to Tumor Size

Size (cm)	Rate of Local Treatment Failure
0–1.4	2.6–4.7%
1.5–2.4	7.1–7.3%
3.5–4.4	13.3%
Over 4.5	40–50%
Total	5.5–7.2%

Swartz and Lesser[11]

Table 6-3.   Cancer of the Lip
Treatment Effectiveness Related to Tumor Size

Size (cm)	Treatment Method	Local Recurrence	Later Metastases	D/O	3-Year Survival Rate
0–2	Surgery	7/210	14	35	81%
	Radiation therapy	0/62	0	11	82%
2–12	Surgery	5/45	1	10	73%
	Radiation therapy	12/129	19	21	76%

del Regato and Sala[10]

REVIEW QUESTIONS

1. What is the anatomical definition of lip as used in clinical oncology? How does this differ from cancer of the skin of the lip?

2. Should carcinoma arising from the vermilion surface be included with cancer of the oral cavity or cancer of the skin? Why?

3. What is the usual histologic type of cancer arising from the vermilion surface? Does this differ from carcinomas arising from the mucosa of the oral cavity? from skin of the face?

4. Do you have any ideas why epidermoid carcinoma of the vermilion surface usually involves the lower lip of men?

5. Compare the metastatic cervical adenopathy of carcinoma of the lower lip with carcinoma of the oral tongue as to: (1) incidence, (2) pattern, (3) predictability. How does this influence treatment and prognosis?

6. Have you seen claims that either radiation therapy or surgery is more effective for lip cancer? What are the usual bases for such claims?

7. Why not combine radiation therapy and surgery for patients with carcinoma of the lip?

8. In the treatment of carcinoma of the lower lip, what are the advantages and disadvantages of radiation therapy? of surgery? If frequency of control of the primary tumor is comparable with either method, why not base selection on these advantages or disadvantages?

9. What is the preferable treatment of cervical adenopathy from carcinoma of the lip? Should this be done in anticipation ("prophylactic") of adenopathy or after adenopathy has become palpable ("therapeutic")? Why?

10. If your patient is a 67-year-old male with a lesion restricted to the lower vermilion and measuring 1.0 cm in greatest dimension, what is the probability of local tumor control with adequate treatment?

BIBLIOGRAPHY

1. ACKERMAN, L. V., and DEL REGATO, J. A. *Cancer*, 4th Ed, Mosby, St. Louis, 1970.
2. BACKUS, L. H., and DE FELICE, C. A. Five-year end results in epidermoid carcinoma of the lip with indications for neck dissection. *Plast Reconstr Surg*, 17:58–63, 1956.
3. GLADSTONE, W. S., and KERR, H. D. Epidermoid carcinoma of the lower lip: Results of radiation therapy of the local lesion. *Amer J Roentgen*, 79:101–113, 1958.
4. JUDD, E. S., and BEAHRS, O. H. Epithelioma of the lower lip. *Arch Surg (Chicago)*, 59:442–432, 1949.
5. LAMPE, I. The place of radiation therapy in the treatment of carcinoma of the lower lip. *Plast Reconstr Surg*, 24:34–44, 1959.
6. MARTIN, H. E., MACCOMB, W. S., and BLADY, J. V. Cancer of the lip. *Ann Surg*, 114:226–242; 341–368, 1941.
7. MODLIN, J. Neck dissections in cancer of the lower lip. *Surgery*, 28:404–412, 1958.
8. MOSS, W. T. *Therapeutic Radiology*, 3rd Ed, Mosby, St. Louis, 1969.
9. MURPHY, W. T. *Radiation Therapy*, 2nd Ed, Saunders, Philadelphia, 1967.
10. DEL REGATO, J. A., and SALA, J. M. The treatment of carcinoma of the lower lip. *Radiology*, 73:839–844, 1959.
11. SCHWARZ, H., and LESSER, J. C. Cancer of lip; control of primary lesion. *Missouri Med*, 51:355–359, 1954.

CARCINOMA OF THE ANUS AND ANAL CANAL

Carcinomas arising in the anus and anal canal are infrequent, comprising about 0.1 percent of all cancer[1] and about 1.8 percent of tumors of the large intestine.[9] Understanding of the behavior of these tumors and ultimately the management and prognosis of its victims must be based on a knowledge of the anatomy (Figure 6-10).

The anal canal extends 1–1.5 in. from the level of the puborectalis part of the levator ani muscles to the anal orifice. The proximal epithelium is simple columnar with glands, and the distal epithelium varies from stratified columnar to squamous. Blood is supplied by the inferior hemorrhoidal and middle sacral arteries, whereas the venous drainage forms the hemorrhoidal plexus, part of which goes to the portal system (hepatic metastases 3.5[3]–12.0 percent[7]). The major lymphatic pathway follows the inferior hemorrhoidal vessels to hemorrhoidal, sacral, and lumbar nodes. Drainage to lateral pelvic, abdominal, and inguinal (retrograde along the external iliac nodes) nodes is less frequent.

The anal orifice or margin commences at the level of the anal valves (embryologic junction of postallantoic gut and proctodeal membrane) and extends 1.0–1.5 cm to include immediate perianal skin. The lining is simple squamous epithelium. The blood is supplied by the inferior hemorrhoidal vessels with drainage into the inferior vena cava. The lymphatics join the cutaneous vessels and cross the perineum and thigh to the inguinal nodes.

These anatomic differences explain why cancers of the anal canal may spread to the liver (3.5[3]–12.0 percent[7]) and lateral pelvic nodes (47 percent[7]), and hemorrhoidal nodes (43 percent[9]), while cancers limited to the anal margin are unlikely to do so. Cancers from either site may spread to inguinal nodes by different routes (canal tumors, 36 percent and margin tumors, 40 percent[9]).

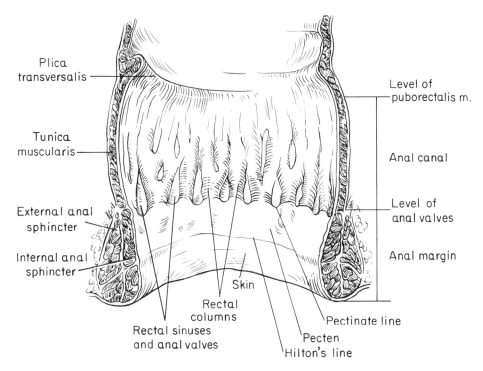

Plica transversalis

Level of puborectalis m.

Tunica muscularis

Anal canal

External anal sphincter

Level of anal valves

Internal anal sphincter

Anal margin

Skin

Rectal columns

Pectinate line

Rectal sinuses and anal valves

Pecten

Hilton's line

Fig. 6-10. Anatomy of anal canal and anal margin.

Loss of sphincter function, whether incident to tumor or treatment, is a major morbidity. The internal sphincter is a complete smooth muscle ring, 2.0–3.0 mm thick, encircling the proximal anal canal. The external sphincter is a tripartate voluntary muscle encircling the anal canal and margin with attachments to the coccygeus and perineal central tendon.

Anal canal cancers are slightly more frequent in females, but anal margin cancers are more frequent in males.[9] The average age of patients is 60 years. There is frequent association with long-standing fistulas in addition to those fistulas of short duration which develop with the neoplasm. Condylomas, leukoplakia, or pruritis ani are not predisposing conditions.[2]

Pathology

The primary lesion may have raised, indurated borders; it may be nodular or proliferative; or it may be flat and diffusely spreading. Ulceration is common. Two-thirds of the primary lesions will be larger than 3 cm in greatest dimension when diagnosed.[6]

Inasmuch as most lesions arise from an unstable transitional zone of epithelium adjacent to the anal valves, the histology is variable.[5] Tumors of the margin are more often differentiated epidermoid carcinoma (keratin formation in 84.2 percent[5]) than their counterpart in the canal (keratin formation in 45.1 percent[5]).

The primary lesion may spread by direct extension, frequently to the sphincter muscles and perianal tissues and proximally to the rectum; but infrequently to the neighboring viscera, i.e., vagina, prostate, and bladder[3]; infrequently by the blood stream and by regional lymphatics, where lesions of the canal metastasize to perirectal and mesocolic nodes (28 percent of those operated on[3]), and later to the inguinal glands (36 percent[8]), whereas lesions of the margin rarely spread to intrapelvic glands, but may involve inguinal glands (8.2[3]–40 percent[9]).

Treatment

Choice of treatment should be based on anatomical site, size, extent, and the histology of the primary lesion, the presence of metastases, and the condition of the patient.

Tumors of the anal canal are most effectively treated by abdomino-perineal resection. If the intrapelvic nodes are positive, radical dissection may be attempted with modest chance of success. Vigorous pelvic irradiation of the adenopathy, once deemed futile because of technical as well as biological reasons, should be considered, especially if the primary lesion is undifferentiated, now that technical limitations can be avoided with modern equipment.

Many tumors of the anal margin can be treated effectively by local excision, inasmuch as intrapelvic node metastases are rare. If such an excision will result in sphincter incompetence, radium implantation may be justified, inasmuch as the primary site control will be comparable.[8] The possible complications of radium implantation (fibrosis, necrosis with resultant pain), considered overwhelming and unavoidable in the surgical literature, can be related to technique[1] and can be minimal (8–16 percent[8,9]).

Carcinomas of the anal margin, when superficial, also can be treated effectively by external irradiation with minimal morbidity. Extension across the pectinate line and deep invasion are associated with an increased likelihood of pelvic adenopathy and so may be better treated surgically.

Inguinal adenopathy may be the only metastases from cancers of the anal margin. Block dissection, either unilateral or bilateral, is the treatment of choice despite a substantial complication incidence of edema of the lower limb. Use of "therapeutic" rather than "prophylactic" dissection apparently does not lessen the prognosis. Inguinal adenopathy associated with anal canal cancers probably is accompanied by pelvic adenopathy, making the use of groin dissection of doubtful value. Radiation therapy may be used as a palliative measure.

Prognosis

Anal canal tumors are more dangerous than similar lesions of the anal margin. This is manifest by reported "corrected" five-year clinically tumor-free survival rates of 48.7 percent for canal lesions and 60.8 percent for margin lesions.[5] In this series, major reliance was placed on surgery, with operability rates of 85.9 percent for canal lesions and 78.4 percent for margin lesions. Local excision was applicable in 69 percent of the margin lesions, but in only 7 percent of the lesions of the canal. The prognosis is poorer for anaplastic lesions of comparable clinical extent.[2,6]

Radiation therapy has been relegated to palliative treatment of patients with far-advanced tumors, in most series. However, with selection of cases, control of the primary site can be comparable to resection.[1] Watson[8] locally controlled all six anal carcinomas treated by radium implantation. Only one of these patients developed regional adenopathy. Williams[9] reported control of 12 of 32 patients (37.5 percent) for over five years by use of radiation therapy. The influence of irradiation of pelvic adenopathy exclusive of, or in conjunction with, resection is unknown.

REVIEW QUESTIONS

1. Compare the anal canal and anal margin as to boundaries, epithelium, lymphatic and venous drainage. What is the clinical significance of these differences for patients with cancers in these sites?

2. What is the significance of inguinal adenopathy in patients with cancers in these two sites?

3. Although surgery is the mainstay of treatment for patients with these cancers, how might radiation therapy be used to the patient's advantage?

BIBLIOGRAPHY

1. BOND, W. H. Discussion on squamous cell carcinoma of the anus and anal canal. *Proc Roy Soc Med,* 53:411–414, 1960.
2. GABRIEL, W. B. Discussion on squamous cell carcinoma of the anus and anal canal. *Proc Roy Soc Med,* 53:403–409, 1960.
3. GRINNELL, R. S. An analysis of forty-nine cases of squamous cell carcinoma of the anus. *Surg Gynec Obstet,* 98:29–39, 1954.
4. MORGAN, C. N. (1960) Quoted by I. G. Williams (ref. 6).
5. MORSON, B. C. The pathology and results of treatment of squamous cell carcinoma of the anal canal and anal margin. *Proc Roy Soc Med,* 53:416–420, 1960.
6. RAMSEY, G. S. Discussion on squamous cell carcinoma of the anus and anal canal. *Proc Roy Soc Med,* 53:414–416, 1960.
7. STEARNS, M. W., JR. Epidermoid carcinoma of the anal region. *Surg Gynec Obstet,* 106:92–96, 1958.
8. WATSON, T. A. Treatment of cancer of the anus. *Radiology,* 77:783–787, 1961.
9. WILLIAMS, I. G. Carcinoma of the anus and the anal canal. *Clin Radiol,* 13:30–34, 1962.

7

CANCER
IN CHILDREN

GENERAL CONSIDERATIONS

Cancer causes about 20 percent of the deaths of children under 15 years, being second only to accidents in this age group.[11,12] During the past few years, cancer has become an increasingly important pediatric problem because prevention and effective treatment have reduced the threat of infection. Also, it appears that there has been an absolute increase of cancer in children.[6]

Types of cancer and their biological behavior are different in the child than in the adult. For example, the bizarre biological behavior of neuroblastoma and the innocuous behavior of ominous-appearing, melanin-pigmented skin neoplasms have no counterparts in the adult.

Tumors of hematopoietic tissues, including leukemias, account for more than one-third, and tumors of the nervous system, particularly astrocytoma, medulloblastoma, and neuroblastoma, account for about one-fifth of malignant neoplasms in children; the remainder includes a great variety.[20]

Specific cancers which kill children under 15 years in order of decreasing frequency (mortality rates per million) are:[12] leukemia, 34.6; central nervous system tumors, 11.4; lymphoma, 5.4; neuroblastoma, 5.1; Wilms' tumor, 3.9; bone tumors, 2.9; rhabdomyosarcoma, 1.6; liver tumors, 0.87; and retinoblastoma, 0.59.

Tumor types vary with age. Those tumors predominant in infancy and early childhood are embryonic and include Wilms' tumor, retinoblastoma, medulloblastoma, neuroblastoma, embryonic sarcomas, and rare tumors of the liver and testis. Many teratomas involving the ovary, testis, mediastinal and retroperitoneal structures, are present at birth, but become clinically manifest in later childhood. Gliomas and hematopoietic tumors have no peak age incidence. Most sarcomas, bone tumors, and carcinomas occur in later childhood.[20]

The management of children with cancer differs from the care of adults, and the problems vary with age.[4,17] These problems include: variations in awareness and understanding of the illness by the child; participation of the parents; effect on the siblings and the family unit; impact on the child's development.

If the child potentially is curable, the long-term effects of the tumor and any treatment must be assessed in the perspective of survival for 50 to 70 years. Thus, tissue damage, disability, gonadal effects, and carcinogenesis are of greater concern than in the adult.

Any effective cancer treatment can cause undesired, serious side effects. The risk of these complications must be considered in the perspective of survival. What is an acceptable "price" for life? Often amputation or colostomy are accepted with relative tranquility, although, mild nonsymptomatic, radiation-produced scoliosis may be condemned. The deleterious effects of ionizing radiation on gonads, bone marrow, growth centers, and other structures have been studied, are reasonably well known, and should be avoided or minimized whenever possible. That long-term effects of cytotoxic agents are less well known should not license their indiscriminate use.

Specific Effects of Radiation in Children

Ionizing radiation, in doses used for cancer treatment, can interfere with growth. This interference varies with radiation dosage, pattern of radiation application, the part irradiated, and the age of the child. Although good technique may minimize this effect, possible interference with growth always must be evaluated and often properly prompts use of another form of treatment.

Bone growth may be affected by irradiation of epiphyses. Effects vary with the specific site, the child's development at the time of irradiation, and the dose. Although doses used for the treatment of cancers, such as Wilms' tumor (i.e., over 2,000 rads in two to four weeks in a single course with daily fractionation), usually cause detectable change, the resultant deformity, i.e., scoliosis, may be of little clinical importance.[18,19] Youngsters have tolerated calculated doses of 1,500–2,000 rads without grossly measurable effect.[13] The need for irradiation over growing long bones or facial bones in a possible survivor is rare.

Significant changes in skin and soft tisues, often the undesired, but unavoidable results of orthovoltage x-ray techniques should be rare with modern techniques. However, unexpected, violent responses may be correlated with the administration of actinomycin. Unfortunately, this accentuation of radiation effect on normal tissues may occur after the use of radiation, making the child a potential victim of poor communication between pediatric oncologist and radiotherapist.

This danger is maximal when the lungs have been irradiated as they might be in patients with Wilms' tumor or Ewing's tumor. Margolis and Phillips[10] documented that, when the equivalent of one entire lung is irradiated, normal tissue tolerance is significantly reduced by systemic actinomycin D, whether administered before, during, or after the radiation therapy (limits 1,100 rads in 10 fractions with actinomycin D compared with 1,800 rads in 10 fractions without the drug).*

The hematopoietic system of children is more labile than that of the adult.[2] Both response and recovery may be more rapid. Because of a more widespread distribution of functioning marrow, hematopoietic depression may follow irradiation of parts rarely of importance in the adult. In contrast irradiation of the entire vertebral column, such as in the treatment of medulloblastoma in children and testicular

---

*We prefer somewhat smaller daily fractions with a somewhat higher total dose, and our present technique consists of 1,500 rads in 15 fractions with actinomycin D (100 rads per day or 500 rads per week, 19 days), and 2,500 rads in 20 fractions without the drug (125 rads per day or 625 rads per week, 26 days).

tumors in adults, may be better tolerated by children because of a more widespread, functioning marrow with better reserve. This greater spectrum of hematopoietic response to irradiation in the child is accentuated by the frequent use of chemotherapeutic agents.

Gonads of the child must be protected, if possible, in any potential survivor. Thus, undescended testes and ovaries outside the true pelvis may cause unexpected problems. If the gonads inadevertently are irradiated in an ultimate survivor, the dose must be measured and recorded, and the radiotherapist must assume the responsibility of advising the parents, and later the patient, of current scientific knowledge of the somatic and genetic effects.

Long-term changes in the thyroid will be discussed later. The effects of irradiation of other endocrine organs are less well known.

Knowledge of the limits of renal tolerance to radiation is increasing.[7,9] It is likely that the limits in the growing child are lower than those tolerated by the adult ($\pm$2,500 rads in 2½–3½ weeks to include all the renal parenchyma).

Central nervous system tolerance is of importance inasmuch as 20 percent of malignant tumors of children arise from this tissue, and some tumors such as medulloblastoma, ependymoma, and pinealoma are radiocurable. Although long-term changes in the brain related to technique have been reported,[8] specific complications, i.e., radiation myelitis, are much less frequent than in the adult.[14] This may, in part, result from use of lower doses.

Induction of Tumors

Radiation carcinogenesis has been a concern to those responsible for the treatment of children. This potential hazard is maximized by the long life expectancy of the surviving, treated child. Malignant tumors arising in skin, bone,[1,5] and thyroid[3,15,16] are well documented.

Those rare malignant tumors arising in irradiated skin and bone have originated in tissue badly damaged by high doses of poor quality radiation delivered in a poor time distribution and, therefore, should be eliminated by modern treatment techniques.

Cancer arising many years later in thyroids irradiated in infancy has been reported by several.[3,15,16] It is likely that radiation was a contributing rather than a sole factor in this relationship.[15] Inasmuch as the major contributor, irradiation of the thymus in infants, justifiably has been abandoned, this threat has been eliminated.

It is important for the welfare of all patients that the remote possibility of radiation carcinogenesis be kept in perspective. With proper selection of patients for treatment and use of modern techniques, this risk is much less than that accepted for use of anesthesia and surgery.

Although the benefits of radiation therapy in the care of children with cancer have been well documented for many years, actual use has been restricted by a shortage of qualified radiotherapists and by a lack of understanding of the method by physicians primarily involved in the care of these children. Radiation therapy occasionally should be the primary and only initial definitive treatment (i.e., in limited Hodgkin's disease, medulloblastoma). Often it is combined with surgery and chemotherapy. "It is important for the radiotherapist to see the patient as early as possible and to arrive at a cooperative decision with the others concerned as to the plan of treatment. Such a plan may have to be altered as circumstances arise, but the initial timing and amount of the various forms of therapy should be organized and not merely conform to expediency. Unfortunately, more often than not, the radiotherapist is faced with a patient in whom all the decisions have been made and the treatment already carried out, or instituted".[2]

REVIEW QUESTIONS

1. What is the scope of the problem for children that is created by cancer? Does the frequency of cancer in children surprise you? Is this problem likely to decrease in the foreseeable future?

2. What tissues are most often affected, and which cancers are most frequent in children? How does this compare with cancer in adults?

3. Can you relate specific cancers to pediatric age groups?

4. List five significant potentially adverse responses to irradiation which must be considered in the treatment of a child with cancer. How can these be minimized or eliminated? How do these risks compare with other risks in the treatment of the child with cancer?

5. Why is radiation carcinogenesis of greater concern in the child than in the adult? How great is this risk?

6. Does your critical evaluation of the use of radiation therapy for benign tumors in children differ from use for cancer? Why?

7. What are the major deterrents to the effective use of radiation therapy for children with cancer? How can this situation be improved?

BIBLIOGRAPHY

1. CAHAN, W. B., WOODWARD, H. Q., HIGINBOTHAM, N. L., STEWART, F. W., and COLEY, B. L. Sarcoma arising in irradiated bone. *Cancer*, 1:3–28, 1948.
2. DARTE, J. M. Radiation therapy in childhood. In: *Progress in Radiation Therapy*, Vol. III, F. Buschke, Ed, Grune & Stratton, New York, 1965.
3. DUFFY, B. J., JR., and FITZGERALD, P. J. Thyroid cancer in childhood and adolescence: A report of 28 cases. *Cancer*, 3:1018–1032, 1950.
4. EVANS, A. E. If a child must die. *New Eng J Med*, 278:138–142, 1968.
5. FOREST, A. W. Tumors following radiation about the eye. *Trans Amer Acad Ophthal Otolaryng*, 65:694–717, 1961.
6. GRANT, R. N. The challenge of childhood cancer. *CA*, 18:35–39, 1968.
7. KUNKLER, P. B. The significance of radiosensitivity of the kidney in radiotherapy. In: *Progress in Radiation Therapy*, Vol. II, F. Buschke, Ed, Grune & Stratton, New York, 1962.
8. LAMPE, I. Radiation tolerance of the central nervous system. In: *Progress in Radiation Therapy*, I. F. Buschke, Ed, Grune & Stratton, New York, 1958.
9. LUXTON, R. W. The clinical and pathological effects of renal irradiation. In: *Progress in Radiation Therapy*, II, F. Buschke, Ed, Grune & Stratton, New York, 1962.

10. MARGOLIS, L. W., and PHILLIPS, T. L. Whole lung irradiation for metastatic tumor. *Radiology*, 93:1173–1179, 1969.

11. Metropolitan Life Insurance Co.: Statistical Bulletin, 37:3, 1956.

12. MILLER, R. W. Fifty-two forms of childhood cancer: United States mortality experience, 1960-1966. *J Pediat*, 75:685–689, 1969.

13. PARKER, R. G. Tolerance of cartilage and bone in clinical radiation therapy. In: *Progress in Radiation Therapy*, II, F. Buschke, Ed, Grune & Stratton, New York, 1962.

14. PATERSON, E. Malignant tumors of childhood. *J Fac Radiol*, 9:170–174, 1958.

15. SAENGER, E. L., SILVERMAN, F. N., STERLING, T. D., and TURNER, M. E. Neoplasia following therapeutic irradiation for benign conditions in childhood. *Radiology*, 74:889–904, 1960.

16. SIMPSON, C. L., HEMPELMANN, L. H., and FULLER, L. M. Neoplasia in children treated with x-rays in infancy for htymic enlargement. *Radiology* 64:840–845, 1955.

17. TOCH, R. Management of the child with a fatal disease. *Clin Pediat*, (Phila), 3:418–427, 1964.

18. VAETH, J. M., LEVITT, S. H., JONES, M. D., and HOLTFRETER, C. Effects of radiation therapy in survivors of Wilms' tumor. *Radiology*, 79:560–568, 1962.

19. WHITEHOUSE, W. M., and LAMPE, I. Osseous damage in irradiation of renal tumors in infancy and childhood. *Amer J Roentgen*, 70:721–729, 1953.

20. WILLIS, R. A. *The Pathology of the Tumours of Children*. Charles C Thomas, Springfield, Ill., 1962.

NONCANCEROUS CONDITIONS IN CHILDREN

Concern about undesired long-term sequelae of irradiation, effectiveness of other treatments, and frequency of self-limiting disease restrict the use of radiation therapy for noncancerous conditions in children. However, in a few specific circumstances local irradiation in small doses still may be optimal treatment.

Nonlipid reticuloendotheliosis (Histiocytosis X) includes the three syndromes of Letterer-Siwe disease, Hand-Schüller-Christian disease, and eosinophilic granuloma. Variations in the bony and soft tissue lesions and in the histology make strict categorization of specific patients difficult. However, recognition of these syndromes may have useful therapeutic and prognostic function for specific patients.

Eosinophilic granuloma of bone, described by Lichtenstein and Jaffe in 1940,[4] is a benign, often self-limited lesion (may be multiple) affecting nearly any bone.

Symptoms are tenderness, pain, swelling, and occasionally disability. The well-circumscribed osteolytic defects are granulomas, with histiocytes, eosinophils, and giant cells, which do not incite osseous regeneration.[1]

Hand-Schüller-Christian disease is an uncommon chronic involvement of the reticuloendothelial system with osteolytic lesions usually involving membranous bones, particularly the skull; diabetes insipidus; and exophthalmos. The youngsters may have fever, malaise, anorexia, malnutrition, pallor, hepatosplenomegaly, adenopathy, and tender tumefactions.[1]

Letterer-Siwe disease was described in 1924 by Letterer[3] as a fatal syndrome of infants and included an eczematous hemorrhagic rash, widespread adenopathy, hepatosplenomegaly, fever, anemia, and osteolytic lesions. It now can be considered as a rare subclassification of "acute reticuloendotheliosis," generally disseminated, usually affecting infants, and having a grave but not invariably fatal course.[1]

Darte[2] emphasized the necessity for physicians to be aware that, with careful management, a large proportion of these patients can enjoy long clinical remissions and cure. At the Hospital for Sick Children in Toronto, between 1958–1964, only 1 of 23 patients with nonlipid reticuloendotheliosis died. Even in patients dating to 1921, only 15 of 77 patients (27 diagnosed as having eosinophilic granuloma) died, all before their third birthdays.

Lesions in bone may respond to curettage or small doses of radiation, or may be self-limiting. If lesions are causing pain or threaten the structural integrity of bone and are not easily curetted, small doses of radiation can be effective. When persistent otitis media is associated with destruction of the mastoid, radiation therapy often is necessary.

Other sites of involvement, i.e., skin and lymph nodes, occasionally may profit from local irradiation.

Irradiation of the pituitary of patients with diabets insipidus and of the orbit of patients with exophthalmos has been disappointing.[2]

BIBLIOGRAPHY

1. DARGEON, H. W. *Tumors of Childhood.* Hoeber-Harper, New York, 1960.
2. DARTE, J. M. Radiation therapy in childood. In: *Progress in Radiation Therapy,* Vol. III, F. Buschke, Ed, Grune & Stratton, New York, 1965.
3. LETTERER, E. Aleukämische Retikulose (Ein Beitrag zu den proliferativen Erkrankungen des Retikuloendothelial apparates). *Frankfurt Ztschr Path,* 30:377–394, 1924.
4. LICHTENSTEIN, L., and JAFFE, H. L. Eosinophilic granuloma of bone; with report of a case. *Amer J Path,* 16:595–604, 1940.

Hemangioma

Lister's[4] documentation that most strawberry nevi in infants spontaneously involute established a basis for conservative management. Such a policy depends on identification of those lesions likely to conform to this biological pattern. Lampe and Latourette[3] have noted that any lesion likely to involute spontaneously will actively enlarge in the first few months of the infant's life. In their series of 471 "hemangiomas of the involuting type," 61 percent were present at birth, 86 percent were detectable by the age of one month, and early growth was noted in 86 percent. The typical growth pattern described by Lister[4] is: appearance at or shortly following birth; enlargement for the first few months of life; cessation of growth, usually after 6 to 8 months and always by 12 months; regression complete by the fifth year, characterized by initial lessening of the redness with replacement by central grayness, followed by generalized color loss and ultimate loss of bulk.

Of the three most frequent types of hemangiomas, cavernous and simple hemangiomas may spontaneously involute, although nevus flammeus (port wine stain) and the many infrequent types do not.[1] These latter lesions are recognizable by their gross appearance and their nonconformity with a pattern of early growth.[3]

The objective of any management is disappearance of the hemangioma and replacement with residual normal tissue. Accomplishment of this objective is most likely with correct identification of the lesion which will involute, and no treatment. Of all treatment methods used—irradiation, excision, cautery, injecting of sclerosing solutions—local irradiation to low doses is least likely to produce sequelae. However, Lampe and Latourette[3] question the concept that involuting hemangiomas are highly sensitive to ionizing radiation, implying that reported good results may be the result of biological behavior rather than small doses of radiation.

Apparent advisability of a conservative policy of observation rather than treatment is based on several reported series[2,5] in which the results were no better with treatment. However, in such series, treatment is likely to be used for the unfavorable lesions.

Andrews et al.[1] emphasized the disturbing potentials of continued growth, ulceration, and infection with an ultimate compromise of cosmetic result. Indeed, in their group of 1,113 patients, 37 percent of the simple hemangiomas (strawberry mark) and 84 percent of the cavernous hemangiomas did not completely involute by five years of age.

In those patients with hemangiomas partially obstructing the upper airway or interfering with eating, interfering with vision, or causing problems from ulceration and infection, treatment is indicated. Treatment with a few, small (200–400 R) doses of ionizing radiation is more widely applicable, at least equally effective, and less morbid than other currently used treatment methods. Extensive experience has documented that such usage can be beneficial and even life-saving.

REVIEW QUESTIONS

1. Why should therapeutic use of ionizing radiation be minimized for children with noncancerous diseases? Are there possible exceptions? What is your opinion?

2. How does your experience with children with nonlipid reticuloendothelioses compare with those discussed?

3. What is the optimal treatment of a strawberry nevus? When might irradiation be useful? Why is local irradiation with small doses preferable to other treatment methods?

BIBLIOGRAPHY

1. ANDREWS, G. C., DOMONKOS, A. N., TORRES-RODRIGUEZ, V. M., and BEMBENISTA, J. K. Hemangiomas—Treated and untreated. *JAMA*, 165:114–1117, 1957.
2 BRAIN, R. T., and CALNAN, C. D. Vascular naevi and their treatment. *Brit J Derm*, 64:147–163, 1952.
3. LAMPE, I., and LATOURETTE, H. B. Management of hemangiomas in infants. *Pediat Clin N Amer*, 6:511–528, 1959.

4. LISTER, W. A. Natural history of strawberry naevi. *Lancet,* 1:1429–1434, 1938.
5. WALTER, J. Treatment of cavernous hemangioma with special reference to spontaneous regression. *J Fac Radiol,* 5:134–140, 1953.

LEUKEMIA IN CHILDREN

Leukemia is by far the most frequent cancer of children, affecting more youngsters under 15 years of age than tumors of the central nervous system, lymphomas, neuroblastoma, Wilms' tumor, and bone tumors combined.[6] In nearly all instances leukemia in children is in the acute form, and often the specific cell type cannot be identified. The highest incidence is in males 2 to 4 years of age.[2] An apparent rising incidence[2] may be based on better diagnosis of the leukemias and less mortality from infectious disease.

Improvement in the management of these youngsters has been a documentary in the development of chemotherapeutic methods and ancillary care. Complete clinical remissions have become more frequent and more long-lasting with the development of new chemotherapeutic regimens. Concurrently, special problems such as infections, hyperuricemia and nephropathy, and leukemic infiltrations of particular organs have become more important.

Radiation therapy's very restricted value for these patients is in the treatment of some of these special problems.

Hyman et al.,[3] reported that 26 percent of the children with leukemia in their study developed CNS involvement of some form—infiltration of the meninges, brain substance, or cranial or spinal nerve roots. With adequate treatment there was no adverse effect on mean survival. Although both intrathecal drugs, i.e., methotrexate,[4] and small doses of irradiation can control meningeal involvement, irradiation is necessary for involvement of CNS tissue deep to the surface. Sullivan[7] reported that symptomatic control of meningeal leukemia lasted three to four months following doses of "400–2,000 R", although 43 percent of the children developed recurrences, which occasionally were multiple.

Leukemic infiltrations of the kidneys range from the insidious to those producing massive bilateral enlargement. In Sullivan's report,[7] 60 percent of 124 children dying with acute leukemia had some degree of renal enlargement at autopsy. These infiltrations, at least initially, are predominantly cortical.[7] Clinical renal function tests may be normal even with extensive infiltration.[7] Radiation therapy has been used in treatment regimens in an attempt to destroy subclinical deposits in renal "sanctuaries." No advantage from this attempt has been documented. Of 9 children receiving irradiation of *enlarged* kidneys, renal function improved in 4, and the kidneys decreased in size in 5.[7]

The superior mediastinal syndrome, although rare in children, may be caused by lymphomatous masses.[1] These rapidly enlarging tumors are sensitive to small doses of radiation, with consequent rapid, lasting relief. We have seen a large mediastinal mass in a youngster with leukemia completely resolve radiographically within 24 hours following a dose of less than 200 rads. In such circumstances, use of a xanthine oxydase inhibitor (Allopurinol) is advisable to prevent hyperuricemia.[5]

Local cellular infiltrates may cause discomfort disproportionate to their size. Thus, a retro-orbital chloroma may cause proptosis, diplopia, and blindness. A nasopharyngeal mass may cause airway obstruction and epistaxis. A gingival mass may interfere with eating. A skin nodule may be irritated by clothing. A bony lesion may cause pain. Often these lesions develop while the patient is on systemic treatment, and the quickest, most certain resolution follows small doses of local irradiation.

REVIEW QUESTIONS

1. By what margin is leukemia the most frequent cancer of children? Is the incidence of leukemia changing? Why?

2. What are the uses of radiation therapy for children with leukemia? Have you seen such usage?

1. D'ANGIO, G. J., MITUS, A., and EVANS, A. E. Superior mediastinal syndrome in children with cancer. *Amer J Roentgen*, 93:537–544, 1965.
2. DARGEON, H. W. *Tumors of Childhood*. Hoeber–Harper, New York, 1960.
3. HYMAN, C. B., BOGLE, J. M., BRUBAKER, C. A., WILLIAMS, K., and HAMMOND, D. Central nervous system involvement by leukemia in children. I. Relationship to systemic leukemia and description of clinical and laboratory manifestations. Blood, 25:1–12, 1965.
4. HYMAN, C. B., BOGLE, J. M., BRUBAKER, C. A., WILLIAMS, K., and HAMMOND, D. Central nervous system involvement by leukemia in children. II. Therapy with intrathecal methotrexate. Blood, 25:13–22, 1965.
5. KRAKOFF, I. H., and MEYER, R. L. Prevention of hyperuricemia in leukemia and lymphoma: Use of Allopurinol, a xanthine oxidase inhibitor. *JAMA*, 193:1–6, 1965.
6. MILLER, R. W. Fifty-two forms of childhood cancer: U.S. mortality experience, 1960–1966. *J Pediat*, 75:685–689, 1969.
7. SULLIVAN, M. P. Complications in the treatment for acute leukemia. In: *Neoplasia in Childhood*, Year Book, Chicago, 1967.

LYMPHOMA IN CHILDREN

General principles of clinical and histopathological recognition, evaluation of tumor extent, treatment, and prognosis are discussed in Chapter 11. Variations peculiar to children will be emphasized here.

Lymphomas are biologically different in children than in adults in that they are more aggressive; are associated with leukemia twice as often; present more frequently in extranodal sites; and more frequently involve the mediastinum, retroperitoneum, and abdomen,[12] although primary gastric involvement is rare.[14] These differences are reflected in a shorter survival.

Lymphomas comprise about 6 percent of childhood cancer,[14] afflicting children about one-sixth as frequently as leukemia and about one-half as often as primary CNS malignant tumors, but exceeding both neuroblastoma and Wilms' tumor in incidence.[10] Males are involved two to three times as often as females.[14]

Diagnostic delay averaging four months can be attributed to both parent and physician.[14]

Lymphomas in children may be classified as they are in adults, although the incidence of follicular lymphoma may be less and that of lymphosarcoma greater in children than in the adult.[14] The incidence of associated leukemia is far greater in children.[12-14]

Hodgkin's disease increases in frequency to the arbitrary upper age of childhood, thus possibly representing but a segment of the general incidence curve.[7] In Butler's report[1] the clinical findings were similar to those in the adult, peripheral adenopathy being the presenting complaint in 90 percent. In 47 patients diagnosed as having Stage I–II disease, adenopathy was initially noted in the left neck in 32, in the right neck in 21, and in the mediastinum in 20.[7]

The prognosis for children as compared with that for adults with Hodgkin's disease has been reported as better (Kelly[9]), worse (Evans and Nyhan,[3] Pitcock, Bauer, and McGavran[11]), and the same (Jackson and Parker,[6] Jenkins, Peters, and Darte[7]).

Jenkins, Peters, and Darte[7] found the survival, as in adults, to be primarily correlated with tumor extent at the time of adequate treatment. The frequency of survival for patients with Stage I–II$_A$ tumor was 13 of 21 at 5 years, 6 of 12 at 10 years, 4 of 7 at 15 years, and 3 of 3 at 20 years. Butler found the prognosis to be worse for patients under 9 years of age and, as in the adult, worse for patients with more extensive tumor and for those with lymphocyte-depleted tumor.

Lymphosarcoma in many reports includes all lymphomas other than Hodgkin's disease. Thus, data in the literature may be more confusing than enlightening. Dargeon[2] reported that between 1926 and 1956 at Memorial Hospital, New York, only 41 (3.5 percent) of 1,248 children with malignant tumors had lymphosarcoma or reticulum cell sarcoma exclusive of a leukemic component. Most of these young patients were males. Jenkins and Sonley[8] noted that the primary clinical site was more often the gastrointestinal tract and retroperitoneum than it was in Hodgkin's disease. Neoplasm often involved the terminal ileum, cecum, appendix, or ascending colon or the retroperitoneum, with the diagnosis established at laparotomy.[8]

Acute leukemia developed in 20 of 121 patients (16.5 percent) with a special predilection for those with mediastinal involvement (12/26—46 percent). Sagerman et al.[13] noted that of the 9 of 30 patients thought to have "localized" lymphosarcoma or reticulum cell sarcoma prior to treatment, 7 died in less than eight months with disseminated tumor.

Treatment of localized (Stages I–II) lymphoma should be with local irradiation. Gellhorn[4] summarized the statistics from the End-Results Committee at the Third National Cancer Conference, and concluded that chemotherapy or surgery did not improve results beyond those possible with radiation therapy alone. Rosenberg[12] reviewed 613 patients with Stage I–II lymphosarcoma and noted that postirradiation survivors exceeded postsurgical ones by a 2:1 margin.

Although surgery occasionally still is advocated for localized, accessible adenopathy, its lesser applicability and effectiveness, as compared with radiation therapy, plus its direct mortality (perhaps as high as 6 percent[5]) should restrict use to selected problems, i.e., relief of tumor-caused intussusception and intestinal obstruction.

Although Dargeon[2] again raised the question of long-term radiation sequelae, Schneider[14] emphasized that (1) preservation of life must be the major criterion of the value of treatment; (2) the best survival for patients with localized tumor results from radiation therapy; and (3) there should be no serious sequelae after "proper administration of radiotherapy."

Youngsters, as well as adults, with widespread lymphoma are best treated by coordinated use of several modalities. Often chemotherapy is the mainstay of treatment for these patients, with local irradiation reserved for specific problems.

REVIEW QUESTIONS

1. How do lymphomas differ biologically in children as compared with those in adults? How does this affect prognosis? Has treatment been comparable?

2. What are the sequelae in children following radical radiation therapy for localized Hodgkin's disease? What are the sequelae of chemotherapy?

3. What is the place of surgery in the management of children with lymphomas?

BIBLIOGRAPHY

1. BUTLER, J. J. Hodgkin's disease in children. In: *Neoplasia in Childhood*, Year Book, Chicago, 1969.
2. DARGEON, H. W. *Tumors of Childhood*, Hoeber–Harper, New York, 1960.
3. EVANS, H. E., and NYHAN, W. L. Hodgkin's disease in children. *Johns Hopkins Med J*, 114:237–248, 1964.
4. GELLHORN, A. End-results in lymphosarcoma and Hodgkin's disease. *Proc Third National Cancer Conference*, 862–869, 1957.
5. HELLWIG, C. A. Malignant lymphoma: The value of radical surgery in selected cases. *Surg Gynec Obstet*, 84:950–958, 1947.
6. JACKSON, H. J., and PARKER, F., JR. Hodgkin's disease; pathology. *New Eng J Med*, 231:35–44, 1944.
7. JENKINS, R. D. T., PETERS, M. V., and DARTE, J. M. M. Hodgkin's disease in children. *Amer J Roentgen*, 100:222–226, 1967.
8. JENKINS, R. D. T., and SONLEY, M. J. The management of malignant lymphoma in childhood. In: *Neoplasia in Childhood*, Year Book, Chicago, 1969.
9. KELLY, F. Hodgkin's disease in children. *Amer J Roentgen*, 95:48–51, 1965.
10. MILLER, R. W. Fifty-two forms of childhood cancer: U.S. mortality experience, 1960–1966. *J Pediat*, 75:687–688, 1969.
11. PITCOCK, J. A., BAUER, W. C., and MCGAVRAN, M. H. Hodgkin's disease in children: A clinicopathological study of 46 cases. *Cancer*, 12:1043–1951, 1959.
12. ROSENBERG, S. A., DIAMOND, H. D., DARGEON, H. W., and CRAVER, L. F. Lymphosarcoma in childhood. *New Eng J Med*, 53:877–897, 1960.

13. SAGERMAN, R. H., WOLFF, J. A., SITARZ, A., and LUKE, K. H. Radiotherapy for lymphomas in childhood. *Radiology*, 86:1096–1099, 1966.
14. SCHNEIDER, M. Malignant lymphomas in children. In: *Progress in Radiation Therapy*, Vol. III, F. Bushke, Ed, Grune & Stratton, New York, 1965, pp. 172–182.

LYMPHOMA IN AFRICAN CHILDREN

In 1958, Burkitt[1] described a lymphoma considered to be the most frequent malignant tumor in children in a section of Africa, later defined as a geographic belt adjacent to the equator.[2] This tumor most frequently was found in those three to eight years of age, usually presented clinically with involvement of the facial bones or mandible (often multiple) or the abdominal vescera; it was rarely associated with leukemia, and without treatment resulted in the patient's death within a few months.[3] Although peripheral adenopathy has been an infrequent clinical finding, tumor-bearing nodes usually have been found at autopsy.[6]

Regardless of variations in anatomical distribution of tumor, there is marked cytological uniformity.[6] The predominant cell is a primitive lymphoreticular cell, whether lymphoblastic or histiocytic.[7] Numerous large phagocytic histiocytes account for the "starry sky" or "water pot" histological appearance.

Whether Burkitt's tumor is a distinct form of lymphoma in children[8] or is an unusual incidence phenomenon in a section of Africa[7] may depend on criteria of definition and whether the proponent is a "lumper" or a "splitter." O'Conor[6] notes that except for the unusual frequency of jaw and facial bone involvement (and probably the infrequency of associated leukemia), the anatomical distribution of tumor is not greatly different from that of lymphoma in children reported elsewhere. Indeed, cases have been reported from the midwestern United States[5] and the AFIP (Armed Forces Institute of Pathology).

This tumor was found to be very responsive to cytotoxic agents,[4] at least for limited observation periods. Radical surgery is inappropriate because of failure of local tumor control and frequency of widespread tumor. Radiation therapy has not been used, except sporadically,[3] for local control.*

BIBLIOGRAPHY

1. BURKETT, D. A sarcoma involving the jaws in African children. *Brit J Surg*, 46:218–223, 1958–1959.
2. BURKITT, D. A "Tumour Safari" in East and Central Africa. *Brit J Cancer*, 16:379–386, 1962.
3. BURKITT, D., and O'CONNOR, G. T. Malignant lymphoma in African children. I. A clinical syndrome. *Cancer*, 14:258–269, 1961.

*There is an on-going study directed by the faculty of the Radiumhemmet and Karolinska Institute, Stockholm, Sweden.

4. BURKITT, D., and WRIGHT, D. H. The African lymphoma. Preliminary observations on response to therapy. *Cancer*, 18:399–410, 1965.
5. DORFMAN, R. F. Childhood lymphosarcoma in St. Louis Missouri, clinically and histologically resembling Burkitt's tumor. *Cancer*, 18:418–430, 1965.
6. O'CONNOR, G. T. Malignant lymphoma in African children. II. A pathological entity. *Cancer*, 14:270–283, 1961.
7. O'CONNOR, G. T., RAPPAPORT, H., and SMITH, E. B. Childhood lymphoma resembling "Burkitt Tumor" in the United States. *Cancer*, 18:411–417, 1965.
8. WRIGHT, D. H. Burkitt's tumor and childhood lymphosarcoma. *Clin Pediat* (Phila), 6:116–123, 1967.

TUMORS OF THE CENTRAL NERVOUS SYSTEM IN CHILDREN

Intracranial tumors are second only to leukemia in incidence (12 percent[1]–23 percent[3]) among the cancers of children under 15 years. Several features distinguish brain tumors in children compared with those in adults: a higher percentage (52 percent[2]–75 percent[5]) arise in the posterior fossa; the incidence of gliomas is higher (60–80 percent in children compared with 40–60 percent in adults[5]); glioblastomas are less frequent, and when they occur 50 percent involve the brain stem[1]; astrocytomas have a predilection for the infratentorial region; the most frequent glioma is medulloblastoma followed by tumors of the midbrain and brain stem[1]; meningiomas acoustic neurinomas, pituitary adenomas,[5] and pinealomas[1] are infrequent.

Intracranial tumors are rare in the first year of life, but the incidence rises to a peak between six and ten years.[1] Males are afflicted slightly more often (3:2[6]). The presenting complaints in order of frequency are headache, ataxic gait, vomiting, extremity weakness, focal epilepsy, squint, failing vision, and dyplopia.[6]

Special Features of Management

Although there has been concern for the irradiated brain and endocrine structures of children, Bouchard,[1] Richmond,[6] Lampe,[4] and other have documented that heavily treated long-term survivors may have little or no measurable sequelae. Richmond[6] has advocated age-related dose reductions (1 year, 50 percent adult dose; 5 years, 75 percent adult dose; 12 years, full adult dose), and Bouchard has used doses of 4,500–5,000 rads in 45 to 50 days, which he considers 20 percent less than the adult dose. However, the validity of this dose reduction, which must be based on assumptions of normal tissue tolerance rather than tumoricidal dose, is far from certain.

General Considerations of Results

The overall incidence of long-term tumor control in children is gratifying. Bouchard[1] reported that 50 of 119 treated patients were clinically free of tumor more than five years following treatment, and Richmond[6] had nearly identical

Table 7-1.   Tumor Types in Children[1]

Gliomas
 Medulloblastoma −31 percent
 Brain-stem glioma−17 percent
 Astrocytoma   −14 percent
 Midbrain glioma −−12 percent
 Ependymoma   − 6 percent
 Unclassified   − 9 percent
Nongliomatous Tumors
 Sarcoma   −6 percent
 Craniopharyngioma −2 percent

success (53 percent of 32 patients). These general figures only emphasize that the treatment of brain tumors in children is far from hopeless and that radiation therapy should be a major contributor.

Specific Tumors

Each tumor type requires study as an entity. Those types encountered by Bouchard[1] are listed in Table 7-1 in the order of frequency and may be used to direct your attention to each in Chapter 9, Tumors of the Central Nervous System.

REVIEW QUESTIONS

1. What is the incidence of CNS tumors in children?

2. What is the most frequent site involved?

3. What is the most frequent glioma in children? Is it curable?

4. Which tumors should be objects of radiation therapy?

BIBLIOGRAPHY

1. BOUCHARD, J. *Radiation Therapy of Tumors and Diseases of the Nervous System.* Lea & Febiger, Philadelphia, 1966.
2. FRENCH, L. A. Some aspects of diagnosis and treatment of brain tumors in children. In: *The Biology and Treatment of Intracranial Tumors.* W. S. Fields and P. C. Sharkey, Eds. Charles C Thomas, Springfield, Ill., 1962, pp. 412–433.
3. GRANT, R. N. The challenge of childhood cancer. *CA,* 18:35–39, 1968.
4. LAMPE, I. Radiation tolerance of the central nervous system. In: *Progress in Radiation Therapy,* Vol. I. F. Buschke, Ed, Grune & Stratton, New York, 1958.

5. LIEBNER, E. J., PETRO, J. I., HOCKHAUSER, M., and KASSARABA, W. Tumors of the posterior fossa in childhood and adolescence. *Radiology*, 82:193–201, 1964.
6. RICHMOND, J. J. Radiotherapy of intracranial tumours in children. *J Fac Radiol*, 4:180–189, 1953.

MALIGNANT TUMORS OF BONE AND SOFT TISSUE IN CHILDREN

Malignant tumors of bone, whether primary or secondary, are an important and difficult group in children. The clinical onset usually is insidious and the diagnosis, difficult. Infectious diseases (i.e., osteomyelitis and tuberculosis), changes incident to trauma (i.e., subperiosteal hemorrhage, exuberant callus), reticuloendothelial lesions, and certain benign tumors have been mistaken for malignant tumors and treated inappropriately, with tragic consequences. The physician responsible for these young patients must carefully integrate the clinical, roentgenographic, pathologic, and laboratory findings in establishing the most likely diagnosis. Even then the uncertainties of roentgenographic and pathologic interpretation must be recognized. As noted by Caffey,[1] "Uncertainties in the radiographic interpretation of the micropathology are the rule rather than the exception."

Treatment, whether by surgery or irradiation, probably will result in sequelae disproportionately more severe in the child than in the adult. Irradiation of an epiphysis in a youngster will be followed by growth suppression, less in consequence with increasing age at the time of treatment. Whether this deformity is worse than amputation is doubtful.

Indeed primary radiation therapy is the treatment of choice for two frequent primary malignant bone tumors, Ewing's tumor and reticulum cell sarcoma, and for metastases to bone.

Primary malignant tumors of bone most important in children are:[2,3,6] Ewing's tumor, osteosarcoma, fibrosarcoma, and reticulum cell sarcoma.

Metastatic bone tumors usually are incident to neuroblástoma, retinoblastoma, Ewing's tumor, and occasionally Wilms' tumor.[2,3,6]

Infrequently, malignant tumors of soft tissues involve bone by extension.

Specific primary tumors of bone will be discussed separately in Chapter 17, Tumors of Bone.

Soft tissue tumors, of mesenchymal origin, are a numerous and complex group in children. Although those tumors of older children usually have counterparts in the adult, tumors of the infant usually do not.[4,6] The latter may be embryonic sarcomas with rhabdomyoblastic differentiation or myxomatous change.[6] These biologically aggressive neoplasms frequently involve the urogenital organs (vagina, urethra, bladder, prostate, spermatic cord) or structures about the head (mouth, palate, nose, pharynx, middle ear, eustachian tube, orbit).

Other mesenchymal tumors may be predominantly fibrous, lipoid, or may arise from smooth muscle or synovia.

Radiation therapy has been considered of little value in this group of tumors.[3,6] However, it now has been established that embryonal rhabdomyosarcomas, particularly about the head and neck, may be responsive to and controlled by irradiation.[5] The response of other tumors in this group is even less predictable and needs very careful study and documentation.

Specific soft tissue tumors will be discussed in Chapter 18.

REVIEW QUESTIONS

1. What is the incidence of malignant tumors of bone in children?

2. What are the three most frequent types of bone tumors in children?

3. What difficulties hinder the definitive diagnosis of malignant tumors of bone in youngsters?

4. What anatomic structures are frequently involved by embryonic sarcomas in the child?

5. Have you seen an embryonal rhabdomyosarcoma controlled by radiation therapy?

BIBLIOGRAPHY

1. CAFFEY, J. *Pediatric X-ray Diagnosis,* Year Book, Chicago, 5th ed., 1967.
2. DAHLIN, D. C., *Bone Tumors,* Charles C Thomas, Springfield, Ill., 2nd ed., 1967.
3. DARGEON, H. W., *Tumors of Childhood,* Hoeber–Harper, New York, 1960.
4. ENZINGER, F. M., Fibrous tumors of infancy in *Tumors of Bone and Soft Tissue,* Year Book, Chicago, 1965.
5. LINDBERG, R. D., Rhabdomyosarcoma in children: Treatment and results. In: *Neoplasia in childhood,* Year Book, Chicago, 1969.
6. WILLIS, R. A., *The Pathology of the Tumours of Children,* Charles C Thomas, Springfield, Ill., 1962.

WILMS' TUMOR (NEPHROBLASTOMA)

Wilms' tumor is a highly malignant neoplasm which arises from embryonic remnants within the renal parenchyma and contains epithelial structures and mesenchymal tissues of varying degrees of maturation. This varied cellular composition is reflected in the abundant descriptive terminology (nephroblastoma, renal embryoma, embryonal mixed tumor, adenomyosarcoma).[16]

The rarity of nephroblastoma, about two new cases per year per million population,[12] explains the small number of cases in most reported series and the consequent difficulty in reaching statistically valid answers as to the efficacy of various therapeutic approaches. Nevertheless, nephroblastoma represents 15 to 20 percent of solid cancers in childhood,[28] competes with neuroblastoma as the most common abdominal tumor in children,[28] and constitutes 60 percent of all renal cancers in children.[19] In about 7–10 percent of patients, the tumor is bilateral.[20,28] These tumors are most commonly found in children between the ages of two and five years,[6] but they may be initially detected in the newborn or in the adult.

Pathologic Findings

Nephroblastomas probably arise in the growth zones of the renal cortex[11] and usually remain well-defined with a connective tissue "capsule" until they become large. Hemorrhage and necrosis are frequent. The remaining renal parenchyma may become atrophic from pressure from the rapidly enlarging neoplasm.

More than half of the children with Wilms' tumor will have distant metastases at the time of diagnosis or will develop them.[24] Approximately 50 percent of all patients develop pulmonary metastases, usually bilateral.[20] [30] Wilms' tumor may invade the renal vein and inferior vena cava and may cause tumor thrombi. Hematogenous metastases are most frequent in the lungs and less frequent in the liver, bone, and other sites. The likelihood of invasion of the renal capsule, with consequent paracapsular extension, increases with larger tumors. Martin and Reyes[22] found tumor-bearing regional adenopathy in 7 of 20 patients undergoing retroperitoneal lymph node dissection. Inasmuch as the prognosis is influenced by the extent of tumor at the time of institution of therapy,[10,33] earlier clinical recognition may explain the better prognosis reported for children less than two years of age.[10,30,32]

Clinical Presentation

The most frequent initial clinical finding is a palpable mass in the abdomen or flank.[6,12] This is as likely to be discovered by the parent as by the physician.[12] Abdominal pain, nausea, vomiting, ileus or partial bowel obstruction also may be the clinical presentation. Microscopic hematuria, indicating extension into the renal pelvis, is found in about 50 percent of patients, but gross hematuria is much less frequent.[6] Fever and weight loss may be associated with large primary nephroblastomas or metastases. Pyelography usually is diagnostic with findings of an intrarenal mass, renal distortion, and/or nonfunction. Calcification may be radiographically demonstrable, but is much less frequent than in neuroblastoma.

Treatment

The availability of effective treatment makes the prognosis for the individual patient directly dependent on correct management. In contrast to the pessimistic outlook previously accepted, currently more than 50 percent of these children can be saved.[7,10,33]

An estimate of tumor extent is necessary for treatment planning and evaluation and as a prognostic guide. Schneider[28] suggested the following *clinical staging:*

Stage I

The enlarged kidney is not fixed (on physical examination and/or radiography in supine and erect positions). The longest axis of the involved kidney does not exceed 10 cm. There is no hematuria, or pain, or physical or radiographic evidence of metastasis.

Stage II

The involved kidney is larger than 10 cm in its longest axis, or is fixed to adjacent tissues, or is accompanied by pain or hematuria. No metastases are found on physical and radiographic examination.

Stage III

Metastatic lesions are found by physical and/or radiographic examinations.

Radiation Therapy

The radioresponsiveness of Wilms' tumor varies, probably in relationship to the heterogeneous cellularity of the neoplasm. Many of these tumors respond rapidly to moderate doses. Occasionally doses less than 1,000 rads have resulted in regressions so complete that tumor was not identified easily in the specimens. However, a dose of at least 3,000 rads in three to four weeks is reasonable because of a substantial chance of tumor effect with minimal chance of significant morbidity. How this dose should be altered in combination with chemotherapy, i.e., actinomycin D, is uncertain. Necessary reduction of radiation dose may be more closely related to the lessened tolerance of normal tissue (i.e., liver and lung) in the irradiated volume than to any increased tumor response.

Preoperative radiation therapy may facilitate the necessary surgery by reducing the tumor size, the blood loss, and the risk of rupture of the neoplasm. In addition, it may devitalize tumor cells and thus reduce the risk of surgical manipulation. The primary objection to preoperative irradiation is the lack of histologic proof of tumor prior to the institution of treatment.[30] This diagnostic error should be very small with good evaluation and thus not a serious deterrent, if preoperative irradiation is of biological advantage. For example, in a report covering 1936–1960,[35] there was no diagnostic error in 17 patients irradiated preoperatively. Such a criticism of lack of diagnosis prior to institution of treatment would be equally valid for preoperative chemotherapy.[31]

Radiation therapy usually has been used following nephrectomy when there has been evidence of direct extension of tumor into the renal bed or spread to regional lymph nodes in a patient without known distant metastases. Such local spread, which may be occult, has been estimated to occur in over 80 percent of these patients.[29]

Irradiation of the tumor bed has been divided into preoperative and postoperative courses of approximately equal dosage. The rationale for this approach must be that some of the benefits of preoperative irradiation may be obtained with lesser treatment-produced sequelae, although further treatment, when necessary, can be better directed after determination of regional tumor extension.

Local irradiation can control regional extensions of Wilms' tumor and thus can particularly benefit those patients not victimized by distant metastases. The inaccuracy of necessary determinations of tumor extent often has resulted in "routine" use of local irradiation as a surgical adjuvant, and improved survival rates have been attributed to such usage.[13,16,35] Also, it has been stated that in patients so treated "local recurrence is not common except as part of generalized disease."[30]

Pulmonary metastases often have responded to tolerable radiation doses, and on occasion have been controlled. Exclusive of the use of actinomycin D, both lungs irradiated consecutively or even simultaneously tolerate doses up to 2,500 rads (with correction for air transmision) at a rate of 750 rads per week. Margolis and Phillips[21] have suggested that when the equivalent of one entire lung is irradiated, adjuvant actinomycin D will decrease the tolerance to irradiation by 35–40 percent.

Sequelae of Radiation Therapy.   Although frequently emphasized, radiation effects in normal tissues do not constitute a valid objection to the use of radiation therapy for youngsters with Wilms' tumor.

The remaining kidney should not be damaged because it should not be irradiated unless the tumor is bilateral. Careful studies of long-term survivors have documented the normal function of the remaining kidney.[23,34]

Growing bone, vertebrae in particular, is damaged and roentgenographic change is demonstrable in all long-term survivors.[13,34,36] The degree of alteration increases with larger doses and decreases with greater age at the time of irradiation. The frequent resultant scoliosis usually is not clinically significant[36] and can be minimized by orthopedic care during the patient's growth.[34]

Hematopoietic changes, i.e., leukopenia and thrombocytopenia, are transitory and infrequently interrupt treatment.

Chemotherapy

Several chemicals have a profound effect on Wilms' tumor. Actinomycin D and Vincristine have been used most frequently clinically. Tumor masses, particularly in the lungs, have been controlled for several years by use of these drugs alone.[9,14,18,32] In addition to this antitumor effect, a claim for radiation potentiation has been made for actinomycin D.[3,4] This augmentation of effect occurs in normal tissues, i.e., skin, lung. However, clinical usefulness depends on a favorable alteration of the therapeutic ratio, and "the case for therapeutic synergism has not been made."[15]

Thus, limits of current knowledge encourage the use of actinomycin D as a specific antitumor agent in situations in which it is unlikely that tumor has been removed completely by surgery or destroyed by local irradiation. Such usage, even in the uncontrollable future of a patient, must be accounted for by the radiotherapist, for whether or not actinomycin D reduces the tumoricidal dose of radiation, it necessitates reduction of dosage because of dangerous reactions in normal tissues.

When actinomycin D is used in combination with surgery and radiation therapy to "prevent" metastases, the time of administration may be very important.[1] Variations in time of administration may partially account for apparent contradictions in reported results.[27]

Surgery

Removal of the tumor-bearing kidney is the optimal treatment of the primary neoplasm. Improvements in surgical technique, including use of the thoracico-abdominal approach and early ligation of the renal pedicle, have led to better tumor control, as exemplified by a 32 percent "cure rate" without operative mortality reported by Ladd and Gross[17] as early as the period 1931–1939.

For patients without demonstrable distant metastases, nephrectomy is the major treatment effort, and radiation therapy and chemotherapy remain ill-defined adjuvants.

For patients with demonstrable distant metastases, nephrectomy still may be reasonable to remove the primary neoplasm, a source of further metastases, hemorrhage, and discomfort.

Although the removal of regional lymph nodes can be considered standard procedure, retroperitoneal lymph node dissection, advocated by some,[22] has not been universally adopted.

Although hematogenous metastases imply surgical futility, occasional carefully considered resections of masses poorly responsive to chemotherapy or radiation therapy may benefit the patient.

When Wilms' tumor involves both kidneys, a unique therapeutic problem exists. If the tumor is more extensive in one kidney, particularly if there is little remaining functional parenchyma, nephrectomy and local irradiation are in order. If the tumor in the second kidney is small, partial nephrectomy and local irradiation to a tolerable dose (i.e., 1,200 rads in two weeks with actinomycin D) has resulted in long-term tumor control with preservation of life-sustaining renal function. The improving technology of renal transplantation offers an interesting possibility for these patients, particularly if the tumor is extensive in both kidneys.

Prognosis

Within the lifetime of many of today's practicing physicains, the prognosis for youngsters with Wilms' tumor has improved dramatically. This favorable change has been in part the result of better surgery, radiation therapy, and general medical care, but the major thrust has been based on development of effective chemotherapy and a now justifiable therapeutic aggressiveness.

Results can be related to extent of tumor as "mirrored" in clinical findings. Thus, the following factors have been considered prognostically unfavorable: tumor invasion of blood vessels; tumor in lymphatics or nodes; tumor extension to nonresectable structures; tumor invasion of the renal pelvis; rupture of the "capsule" of the tumor; tumor cells in the bone marrow; and other distant metastases.

Platt and Linden,[26] on the basis of a study of 83 patients, claimed that both a fixed two-year post-treatment survival rate and Collin's risk period[2] are comparably good measures of prognosis. Only 2 of their 83 patients died of tumor beyond these periods of risk.

In the report of Garcia et al.,[10] when Wilms' tumor was uncontrolled and considered the cause of death, 50 percent died within 6 months, 75 percent within 12 months, and 97 percent within 2 years of diagnosis.

In a recent report,[7] Farber has chronicled improvements in prognosis as related to the development of therapeutic regimens. In a group of 53 patients treated by actinomycin D starting at the time of surgery, nephrectomy, and local irradiation, 47 (89 percent) were alive without evidence of tumor from two to over nine years. Sixteen of these 53 patients developed demonstrable metastases after the initial treatment, and 10 of these 16 (53 percent) survived after further treatment. Eight of 15 patients who developed pulmonary metastases survived after treatment with actinomycin D and irradiation of both lungs. Farber attributes the improved results, compared with a previous treatment regimen of nephrectomy and local irradiation, to the addition of actinomycin D.

Likewise, Fernbach and Martyn[9] attributed an improved survival in a small group of patients to the addition of actinomycin D to a regimen of nephrectomy and local irradiation.

Stone and Williams[30] reported a two-year survival rate of 54 percent for 38 patients treated by nephrectomy, postoperative irradiation of the renal bed, and actinomycin D. Seventy-five percent of those without gross evidence of spread at the time of surgery survived. These authors stated that actinomycin D used concurrently with radiation therapy was of doubtful value in preventing metastases.

Maier and Harshaw[20] reported a two-year survival rate of 44 percent for 51 patients, and noted the importance of clinical staging in assessing treatment results. In comparing two consecutive groups of patients, the latter receiving actinomycin D in addition to nephrectomy and local irradiation, all 4 Stage I and 9 of 10 Stage II patients survived, whereas in Stage III only 2 of 13 patients without actinomycin D and 3 of 14 patients with actinomycin D survived. These authors concluded that when used concurrently with radiation therapy in the primary treatment program, survival was not influenced, but patients with known metastases lived longer when actinomycin D was added to the treatment regimen.

As noted earlier, the time and pattern of administration of actinomycin D may be important,[1] and variations in usage may partially account for contradictions in reported results.[27]

REVIEW QUESTIONS

1. List three synonyms for Wilms' tumor. What does the variety of names reflect?

2. What is the usual clinical presentation of a child with Wilms' tumor? What is the usual age range? Does age at diagnosis have prognostic significance? If so, what?

3. How radiation responsive is Wilms' tumor? How predictable is this response?

4. What are the advantages of preoperative irradiation? the disadvantages?

5. What is the most frequent cause of failure to control Wilms' tumor? How does this biological behavior influence the use of radiation therapy?

6. What are the sequelae of radiation therapy in youngsters with Wilms' tumors? How important are these sequelae? How can they be minimized?

7. In contrast to other malignant renal tumors, several chemotherapeutic agents are tumorocidal for cells of Wilms' tumors. How may this influence use of radiation therapy?

8. Even if actinomycin D augments the response of several tissues and tumor cells to radiation, what criterion must it fulfill to be a clinically useful radiation potentiator?

9. What is the incidence of salvage of patients with Wilms' tumor? Has this changed in recent years? Why? Using currently available treatment modalities, is survival likely to further improve? Why?

BIBLIOGRAPHY

1. BURGERT, E. O., JR., and GLIDEWELL, O. Dactinomycin in Wilms' tumor. *JAMA*, 199:464–468, 1967.

2. COLLINS, V. P. Wilms' tumor; its behavior and prognosis. *J Louisiana Med Soc*, 107:474–480, 1955.

3. D'ANGIO, G. J., FARBER, S., and MADDOCK, C. L. Potentiation of x-ray effects of actinomycin D. *Radiology*, 73:175–177, 1959.

4. D'ANGIO, G. J. Clinical and biologic studies of Actinomycin D and roentgen irradiation. *Amer J Roentgen*, 87:106–109, 1962.
5. D'ANGIO, G. J. Radiation therapy in Wilms' tumor. *JAMA*, 204:987–988, 1968.
6. DARGEON, H. W. *Tumors of Childhood*. Hoeber–Harper, New York, 1960.
7. FARBER, S. Chemotherapy in the treatment of leukemia and Wilms' tumor. *JAMA*, 198:826–836, 1966.
8. FARBER, S., D'ANGIO, G. J., EVANS, A., and MITUS, A. Clinical studies of Actinomycin D with special reference to Wilms' tumor in children. *Ann NY Acad Sci*, 89:421–425, 1960.
9. FERNBCH, D. J., and MARTYN, D. T. Role of Dactinomycin in improved survival of children with Wilms' tumor. *JAMA*, 195:1005–1009, 1966.
10. GARCIA, M., DOUGLASS, C., and SCHLOSSER, J. V. Classification and prognosis in Wilms' tumor. *Radiology*, 80:574–580, 1963.
11. GESCHICKTER, C. F., and WIDENHORN, H. Nephrogenic tumors. *Amer J Cancer*, 22:620–658, 1934.
12. GLENN, J. R., and RHAME, R. C. Wilms' tumor: Epidemolgical experience. *J Urol*, 85:911–918, 1961.
13. GROSS, R. E., and NEUHAUSER, E. Treatment of mixed tumors of the kidney in childhood. *Pediatrics*, 6:843–852, 1950.
14. HOWARD, R. Actinomycin D in Wilms' tumor: Treatment of lung metastases. *Arch Dis Child*, 40:200–202, 1965.
15. KLIGERMAN, M. M. Present status of combined radiation therapy and chemotherapy. In: *Progress in Radiation Therapy*, Vol. III, F. Buschke, Ed, Grune & Stratton, New York, 1965.
16. KLAPPROTH, H. J. Wilms' tumor: A report of 45 cases and an analysis of 1,351 cases reported in the world literature from 1940 to 1958. *J Urol*, 81:633–648, 1959.
17. LADD, W. E., and GROSS, K. E. In: *Abdominal Surgery of Infancy and Childhood*. Saunders, Philadelphia, 1941, pp. 411–426.
18. LIEBNER, E. J. Actinomycin D and radiation therapy. *Amer J Roentgen*, 87:94–105, 1962.
19. LUCKE, B., and SCHLUMBERGER, H. C. Tumors of the kidney, renal pelvis and ureter. Armed Forces Institute of Pathology, Fasc. 30, Section VIII.
20. MAIER, J. G., and HARSHAW, W. G. Treatment and prognosis in Wilms' tumor: Study of 51 cases with special reference to role of actinomycin D. *Cancer*, 20:96–102, 1967.
21. MARGOLIS, L. W., and PHILLIPS, T. L. Whole lung irradiation for metastatic tumor. *Radiology*, 93:1173–1179, 1969.
22. MARTIN, L. W., and REYES, P. M., JR. An evaluation of 10 years' experience with retroperitoneal lymph node dissection for Wilms' tumor. *J Pediat Surg*, 4:683–687, 1969.
23. MITUS, A., TEFFT, M., and FELLERS, F. X. Renal function in children after nephrectomy. *Pediatrics*, 44:912–921, 1969.
24. MOSS, W. T. *Therapeutic Radiolgy*, 3rd ed. Mosby, St. Louis, 1969.
25. NG, E., and LOW-BEER, B. V. A. Treatment of Wilms' tumor. *J Pediat*, 48:763–769, 1956.
26. PLATT, B. B., and LINDEN, G. Wilms' tumor: Comparison of two criteria for survival. *Cancer*, 17:1573–1578, 1964
27. RUBIN, P. Comment: The prevention of metastases. *JAMA*, 204:989–990, 1968.
28. SCHNEIDER, M. Renal embryoma. In: *Progress in Radiation Therapy*, Vol. I, F. Buschke, Ed, Grune & Stratton, New York, 1958.
29. SNYDER, W. H., JR. *Pediatric Surgery*. Year Book, Chicago, 1962.
30. STONE, J., and WILLIAMS, I. G. Treatment of Wilms' tumor with special reference to actinomycin D. *Clin Radiol*, 20:40–46, 1969.
31. SULLIVAN, M. P., SUTOW, W. W., CANGIR, A., and TAYLOR, G. Vincristine sulfate in management of Wilms' tumor. Replacement of preoperative irradiation by chemotherapy. *JAMA*, 202:381–384, 1967.
32. SUTOW, W. W., and SULLIVAN, M. P. Vincristine in primary treatment of Wilms' tumor. *Texas Med*, 61:794–799, 1965.
33. VAETH, J. M., and LEVITT, S. H. Five-year results in the treatment of Wilms' tumor of children. *J Urol*, 90:247–249, 1963.
34. VAETH, J. M., LEVITT, S. H., JONES, M. D., and HOLTFRETER, C. Effects of radiation therapy in survivors of Wilms' tumor. *Radiology*, 79:560–568, 1962.

35. WESTRA, P., KIEFFER, S. A., and MOSSER, D. G. Wilms' tumor: A summary of 25 years of experience before actinomycin D. *Amer J Roentgen*, 100:214–221, 1967.
36. WHITEHOUSE, W. W., and LAMPE, I. Osseous damage in irradiation of renal tumors in infancy and childhood. *Amer J Roentgen*, 70:721–729, 1953.

NEUROBLASTOMA

Neuroblastoma is the most frequently used term for malignant, embryonic, nonchromaffin tumors arising from sympathogonia. Other names include neurocytoma, sympathicoblastoma, sympathicogonioma, and sympathicocytoma.[12,22] Occasionally these tumors spontaneously mature to the benign, differentiated ganglioneuroma through intermediary mixed forms,[3,8,10,21] and there are well-recorded, apparent spontaneous "cures" of patients with widespread tumor.[6,7,9,11,22]

Neuroblastoma is one of the most common cancers of childhood, rivaling embryonic tumors of the kidney as the most frequent malignant abdominal neoplasm in children.[4,22] Twenty percent of those afflicted are less than one year old and 75 percent are less than four years of age.[4,10] These tumors can originate from any sympathetic nerve structure, but the frequent primary sites in descending order of incidence are[9]: adrenal (40 percent); intrathoracic, paravertebral (11 percent); pelvic; retroperitoneal; and in the neck. In about 25 percent the primary site cannot be determined. The predominance of adrenal origin is less pronounced in older patients.[16]

Pathologic Findings

Neuroblastomas are soft, friable, and highly vascular. Apparent encapsulation of small tumors is followed by extensive invasion of surrounding structures. Hemorrhage, necrosis, cystic change, and calcification are frequent. This calcification is important in the x-ray differential diagnosis from Wilms' tumors, which exhibit radiographically demonstrable calcification much less often.[15]

Histologically, these tumors may consist of sheets of small, round, deeply staining cells, indistinguishable from Ewing's tumor, or there may be evidence of increasing differentiation with rosettelike clusters of tumor cells around young nerve fibers with an ultimate appearance of ganglioneuroma.[22]

Neuroblastoma spreads rapidly and relentlessly by direct invasion of surrounding structures or by widespread hematogenous or lymphatic metastases. In a large series,[14] bone metastases were found on initial examination in 75 percent and gross liver involvement on laparotomy in 20 percent of patients.

Clinical Manifestations

In view of the multiplicity of possible primary sites, the frequency of metastases and the evolution from undifferentiated to more differentiated forms, it is not surprising that the clinical manifestations are protean. Neuroblastoma should be a primary consideration in any child with an abdominal or pelvic mass, especially if the mass contains calcium, or when there is periorbital ecchymosis, cervical or mediastinal adenopathy, hepatomegaly, or widespread bony metastases. The presenting clinical findings may be nonspecific, i.e., fever, anemia, loss of appetite, localized pain, or locomotor disturbance.[4]

Biochemistry

An important advance in the diagnosis and management of patients with neuroblastoma has resulted from measurement of catecholamines and metabolites excreted in the urine. These substances of greatest importance are VMA (from noradrenaline) and HVA (from dopamine and dopa).[2] Inasmuch as testing for a single catecholamine or metabolite is not absolutely reliable, testing for a combination raises the accuracy of the examination.[2] Thus, using a random urine sample, a diagnostic test of 95 percent accuracy can be completed within two hours. For example, Williams and Greer[20] found the HVA elevated in 74 percent and the VMA in 77 percent of patients, but if both were sought simultaneously, 95 percent of patients had elevations of one or both. These abnormal values have ranged to multiples of normal of 140 for total catecholamines, 380 for NMA; 58 for VMA.[2] Such accurate and sensitive tests should be useful, not only for diagnosing neuroblastoma, but in assaying response to treatment.

Treatment

Evaluation of the treatment of patients with this unpredictable cancer is difficult and precarious. Survival has been reported without any treatment[6,7,9,11,22] and following biopsy only.[4,10] Surgery, radiation therapy, and chemotherapy have been advocated in various combinations and sequences.

Surgery

Although "complete resection," by definition, would be admirable treatment, the possibility of accomplishment is small (14 percent in the series of Gross, Farber, and Martin[10]).

Removal of a large tumor mass may be indicated even in the presence of metastases, for the host-tumor relationship may be favorably altered.

Postoperative irradiation of the tumor bed is indicated if removal has been incomplete.

Radiation Therapy

Although the radiovulnerability of neuroblastomas may vary with differentiation and vascularity, most are sufficiently responsive to allow local tumor control. Such control has followed use of small doses (400 rads in 16 days[17]). However, except for transitory responses for palliation, optimal doses for tumor control are in the range of 2,500–3,000 rads delivered in three to four weeks.

A great advantage of radiation therapy is its flexibility of application, allowing effective treatment of tumor in nonresectable sites, i.e., liver, mediastinum, orbit, skull, long bones, and vertebrae.[19]

Table 7-2.   Neuroblastoma UC, SF 1944–1964
Total: 42 patients

Pt. No.	Name	Age Year	Primary	Metastases	Biopsy	Treatment	Result	Primary Removed
1	J.P.	F 10 mo 1950	R. adrenal	—	Primary	1070 R/16 days primary	1960 Gn. same site 1965 Nbl. same site	No
2	J.L.	M 3 yr 1955	L. adrenal	Bones, orbit	Primary: Nbl. Bone: Gn Cerv. n: Nbl.	3000 R/44 days primary	1960 Gn. bone (Vert.) 1966 Nbl. cerv. n.	Partial
3	D.E.	F 4 mo 1954	L. adrenal	Liver, supraclav. node	Primary, liver	6-mercapto. Primary 25 mg × 19	W 1967 (13 years)	No
4	D.S.	M 9 mo 1959	Posterior mediastinum	Left axillary node, left supraclavicular node	Primary	3000 R/65 days primary	W 1967 (8 years) with neurologic deficit	No
5	M.B.	M 3 mo 1963	L. adrenal	Liver, skin	Primary, liver, skin	Vit. B$_{12}$ 1½ years	W 1967 (4 years)	No
6	G.O.	F 6 yr 1960	Mediastinum	Bone, supraclav. node cervical n., liver	Bone, mediastinum	600 R/9 days cerv. and mediast. n. 345 R/5 days maxilla 700 R/12 days (skin) to liver	W 1967 (4 years)	No
7	M.J.	M 2 mo 1963	L. adrenal	Bone marrow, liver	Primary, liver	1000 R } 1500 R } primary Cytoxan 2 yrs. Vit. B$_{12}$ 2 yrs.	W 1967 (4 years)	Partial
8	G.C.	M 7 mo 1950	L. adrenal	Both femurs (1 yr postoperative)	Primary	—	W 1967 (17 years)	Yes

From Hinton[11]
Gn = ganglioneuroma
Nbl = neuroblastoma

Chemotherapy

Various direct cell toxins, antifolic acid compounds, steroids, and even vitamin B_{12} in massive doses have been used. Vincristine and cyclophosphamide have been effective in causing tumor regression.[18]

Spontaneous "cure" by maturation of the neoplasm has been frequent enough that such a possibility should be considered in clinical manage-[1, 6, 7, 9-11, 13, 14, 16, 21] ment. Everson[6, 7] recorded 28 well-documented cases. We[11] have observed spontaneous regression of neuroblastoma and apparent "cure" of 8 patients in whom widespread tumor would have indicated a hopeless prognosis with most cancers (Table 7-2). Seven of these 8 patients were from a total of 42 patients with neuroblastoma observed at the University of California Hospitals, San Francisco, between 1944 and 1964.[11] In these patients unexpectedly "cured," host-tumor balance seemed more important than the specific therapy used. Consequently, in patients with nonremovable tumor at the primary or secondary sites, local treatment of tumor in critical sites, i.e., mediastinum, may prevent serious complications and provide an opportunity for tumor maturation. Such a treatment policy, of not abandoning as "hopeless" those children with extensive neuroblastoma, requires careful, periodic re-evaluation of each patient. However, the uncertainty of "cure" must be emphasized. Two of our patients (Table 7-2, patients 1 and 2) were considered "cured" until five and six years following biopsy documentation of maturation to ganglioneuroma, when each succumbed to clinically reactivated neuroblastoma.

D'Angio et al.[4a] have called attention to a group of patients, aged one year or less, with disease involving liver, skin and bone marrow (but not bone) who recovered spontaneously. Twenty-one of 25 such patients (84 percent) survived for two years or longer. However, our group also included older children and those with bone involvement. It is important to recognize this in order to avoid—possibly harmful-overtreatment.

Results

Until the 1940 report of Farber,[8] neuroblastoma was considered nearly uniformly fatal. However, since then, many have reported patients surviving after various types of treatment (Table 7-3). The prognosis can be related to several factors:

1.   Extent of tumor at the time of treatment: Gross et al.[10] reported an 88 percent survival at two years after "complete excision" of tumor and a 44 percent survival at two years after partial excision of tumor. However, patients have survived with neuroblastoma involving the liver, lung, bone, or distant lymph nodes.

2.   Primary tumor site: Survival may be better with cervical, intrathoracic or intrapelvic primary sites and poorer for primary sites in the adrenal medulla and retroperitoneal sympathetic chain.[10] If real, this may reflect earlier diagnosis in the former sites.

3.   Histology: The prognosis is better with tumors having evidence of maturation.

4.   Age: Gross et al.[10] reported "cure" in 56 percent of those under 12 months compared to an overall survival of 37 percent. de Lorimier[5] has confirmed this in patients recorded in the California Tumor Registry.

Table 7-3. Collected Clinical Tumor-Free Survival Rates

Author	Years	Number of Cases	Type of Treatment	Post Rx Interval	Percent Survivors
Phillips[14]	1932–1949	58	Surgery Radiation Chemical	3 years	17
Wittenborg[23]	?–1949	73	Surgery Radiation Chemical	3 years	30
Gross, Farber, and Martin[10]	1940–1950	68	Surgery Radiation Chemical	2 years	22
Uhlmann and von Essen[19]	1940–1952	19	Radiation	3 years	31
Seaman and Eagleton[17]	1949–1955	19	Radiation	3 years	26
Gross, Farber, and Martin[10]	1950–1957	49	Surgery Radiation Chemical	2 years	37
Dargeon[4]	?–1958	135	Surgery Radiation Chemical	4-5 years	12

Of those patients with uncontrolled neuroblastoma, 90 percent will die within 12 months and 99 percent within 24 months of treatment without any periods of clinical freedom from tumor.[10] Therefore, two-year clinical tumor-free survivals would seem significant.

REVIEW QUESTIONS

1. What are the two most frequent intra-abdominal malignant tumors in children?

2. Have you been aware of "spontaneous cure" concurrent with maturation of neuro-blastoma? How would this affect your philosophy of treatment? your evaluation of treatment?

3. What are the frequent sites of origin of neuroblastoma? How does this variation influence diagnosis, treatment, and prognosis?

4. What is the x-ray differential between Wilms' tumor and neuroblastoma?

5. Is there a "typical" clinical presentation for patients with neuroblastoma? Why?

6. What biochemical substances can be measured in increased amounts in the urine of patients with neuroblastoma? How accurate is this measurement as a diagnostic test?

7. How often is "complete resection" possible for patients with neuroblastoma? Is partial resection recommended? Why?

8. When can radiation therapy be used to the advantage of these patients?

9. List four prognostic factors.

10. Why can the evaluation of the treatment of patients with neuroblastoma be accurate two years after treatment?

BIBLIOGRAPHY

1. ANDERSON, O. Neuroblastoma with skeletal metastases and apparent recovery. *Amer J Dis Child,* 83:782–787, 1952.
2. BELL, M. Neuroblastoma: Newer chemical diagnostic tests. *JAMA* 205:105–106, 1968.
3. CUSHING, H., and WOLBACH, S. Transformation of a malignant paravertebral sympathico-blastoma into a benign ganglioneuroma. *Amer J Path,* 3:203–216, 1927.
4a. D'ANGIO, G. J., EVANS, A. E., and KOOP, C. E. Special Pattern of Widespread Neuroblastoma with Favorable Prognosis. *Lancet,* May 22, 1971, pp. 1041–1049.
4. DARGEON, H. *Tumors of Childhood.* Hoeber–Harper, New York, 1960.
5. DE LORIMER, A. Neuroblastoma in childhood. *Amer J Dis Child,* 118:441—450, 1969.
6. EVERSON, T. Spontaneous regression of cancer. *Ann N Y Acad Sci,* 114:721–735, 1964.
7. EVERSON, T., and COLE, W. *Spontaneous Regression of Cancer.* Saunders, Philadelphia, 1966.
8. FARBER, S. Neuroblastoma. *Amer J Dis of Children,* 60:749—751, 1940.
9. GOLDRING, D. Neuroblastoma sympatheticum with metastases. *J Pediat,* 38:231–234, 1951.
10. GROSS, R., FARBER, S., and MARTIN, L. Neuroblastoma sympatheticum: Study and report of 217 cases. *Pediatrics,* 23:1179–1191, 1959.
11. HINTON, P., and BUSCHKE, F. Neuroblastoma in children, 42 cases. *Radiol Clin* (Basel), 37:19–28, 1968.
12. KARSNER, H. T. Tumors of the adrenal. Atlas of Tumor Pathology, Section VIII, Fascicle 29, 1950.
13. KING, R., STORAASLI, J., and BOLANDE, R. Neuroblastoma. Review of 28 cases and presentation of 2 cases with metastases and long survival. *Amer J Roentgen,* 85:733–747, 1961.
14. PHILLIPS, R. Neuroblastoma. *Ann Roy Coll Surg Eng,* 12:29–48, 1953.
15. PHILLIPS, T., CHIN, F., and PALUBINAKAS, A. Calcification in renal masses: An 11-year survey. *Radiology,* 80:786–794, 1963.
16. RUSSELL, D., and RUBENSTEIN, L. *The Pathology of Tumours of the Nervous System.* E. Arnold, London, 1959.
17. SEAMAN, W., and EAGLETON, M. Radiation therapy of neuroblastoma. *Radiology,* 68:1–8, 1957.
18. SINKS, L. F., and WOODRUFF, M. W. Chemotherapy of neuroblastoma. *JAMA,* 205:161–162, 1968.
19. UHLMANN, E., and VON ESSEN, C. Neuroblastoma (Neuroblastoma sympatheticum). *Pediatrics,* 15:402–412, 1955.
20. WILLIAMS, C. M., and GREER, M. Homovanillic acid and vanilmandelic acid in diagnosis of neuroblastoma. *JAMA,* 183:836–840, 1963.
21. WILLICH, E., and BUSCHMANN. *Amer J Dis of Children,* 60:749—751, 1940. Suppl. to Vol. 203, Karger, Basle, 1964.
22. WILLIS, R. *The Pathology of Tumours of Children.* Charles C Thomas, Springfield, Ill. 1962.
23. WITTENBORG, M. Roentgen therapy in neuroblastoma: Review of 73 cases. *Radiology,* 54:679–688, 1950.

RETINOBLASTOMA

Retinoblastoma is a radiosensitive tumor probably arising from the retinal glial cells most numerous in the inner nuclear layer.[12] Either sex is equally at risk, with diagnosis usually made within the first year of life and infrequently established after the third birthday.[21] There is a marked tendency for these tumors to be multiple, either in one or both eyes.[13] The overall incidence of bilateral involvement is at least 25 percent,[21] being most frequent in patients with a familial history of retino-blastoma (40 percent in sporadic cases and 100 percent in familial cases in Stallard's series[16]).

Retinoblastoma will appear as a result of spontaneous mutation about once in every 20,000 births.[7] This abnormal gene will be transferred to the children of a survivor as an "autosomal dominant" resulting in a 40–50 percent incidence of retinoblastoma.[5] The unaffected children of affected parents probably are carriers.[19] This influence of heredity was of little medical or social importance when all victims died. However, effective treatment with resulting survivors makes possible an ever-increasing population segment affected by this genetic abnormality.

The clinical findings of visual impairment, dilatation of the pupil, and abnormal reflection of light from the pupil (it appears white rather than black) are easily overlooked in the infant and small child.[4] If initial involvement is unilateral and treatment is successful, careful, periodic examination of the second eye is imperative, for the incidence of involvement exceds 25 percent, and this risk continus for several years.[20] One of our patients, initially treated when an infant, reached the age of 13 years before tumor was noted in the second eye.

Pathologic Findings

Many tumors are anaplastic, consisting of unarranged collections of small round cells. Distinctive rosettes are indicative of increasing differentiation. Necrosis may leave clusters of surviving tumor cells about blood vessels, and roentgenographically detectable calcification is frequent in these necrotic foci.[21] Spontaneous regression of tumor with survival has been reported.[17]

The principal route of tumor extension is via the optic nerve into the cranial cavity (beyond the lamina cribrosa in 27 percent of Reese's series[13]). This may be followed by widespread involvement of the intracranial and spinal meninges.[21]

Remote metastases are reported infrequently, but may involve bone, lymph nodes, or viscera.[3, 11]

Treatment

The low incidence of tumor in the general population and continuing failure to establish the diagnosis when tumor is of limited extent have hindered establishment of an optimal treatment regimen even though surgery, radiation therapy, and chemotherapy may be effective in specific circumstances.

Radiation therapy may control retinoblastoma with preservation of useful vision if the diagnosis is established before extensive tumor destroys vision. These limited tumors, except through fortuitous location, are unlikely to extend along the optic nerve into the cranial cavity.

Thus, radiation therapy, rather than enucleation, is optimal, primary treatment for patients with limited retinoblastoma that is not destroying vision. However, in reviewing his most recent experience, Ellsworth[6] found such a policy applicable in only 19 of 250 patients.

If extensive tumor has destroyed vision, the major advantage of radiotherapy over *surgery* no longer exists. Therefore, enucleation is preferable as a rapid, comparably effective treatment devoid of risk to the remaining eye. The full orbital segment of optic nerve should be studied, for evidence of tumor extension should prompt irradiation of the orbit and the immediate intracranial path of the optic nerve. Whether treatment should be extended to include the intracranial and spinal meninges, as recommended for medulloblastoma, is questionable.

Although there has been some risk of error in clinical diagnosis,[1] improved clinical diagnostic skill should eliminate the need for enucleation of the first eye to establish the diagnosis.

Chemotherapeutic agents, particularly the alkylating agents T.E.M. and cyclophosphamide, may produce useful tumor responses. However, there is no evidence that the combination of T.E.M. and radiation is synergistic, thus allowing subtumoricidal doses of radiation, or that the combination has improved results for patients with limited tumor beyond what is possible with radiation therapy alone.[2, 8, 18]

Complications reported in irradiated eyes include retinal exudates and hemorrhages and retinal detachment, all of which may be found in association with untreated tumor. Radiation-stimulated cataracts, which can be minimized by good treatment technique, develop many years after treatment and thus only afflict survivors. Such lens opacities can be managed surgically. Other complications reported in the literature also can be minimized or eliminated by careful, protracted megavoltage radiation therapy, as illustrated by Bagshaw and Kaplan.[2]

Results

Accomplishments of treatment must be related to tumor extent. The use of a classification suggested by Reese[13] and Ellsworth[6] allows comparison of various methods (Table 7-4).

Bagshaw and Kaplan[2] reported the primary treatment of 11 patients with linear accelerator irradiation and localizing techniques which can be considered optimal by current standards. Retrospectively, two of these patients were considered in Group III of the Reese-Ellsworth classification, although the others were in Groups I and II. Tumor was controlled in seven of 11 eyes (64 percent) by the first course of treatment. Of the four failures, two of three were controlled by re-irradiation for an overall incidence of success of 82 percent.

Bagshaw and Kaplan's overall experience[2] includes the radiation treatment of retinoblastoma in 15 eyes in 10 patients who have been followed for over six years. There have been no tumor-related deaths. All patients have "useful vision" except one who had enucleation, although such an evaluation is precluded in a second patient by his mental deficiency. At the University of California[10] between 1959 and 1969, 12 patients with retinoblastoma of the second eye have been treated with radiation methods. Eleven are alive without evidence of disease for more than two years. In 5, useful vision was preserved.

Table 7-3.   Classification of Intraocular Retinoblastoma[6]

Group I (very favorable prognosis)	Solitary or multiple tumors less than 4 dd* in size at or behind the equator
Group II (favorable prognosis)	Solitary or multiple tumors 4–10 dd at or behind the equator
Group III (doubtful prognosis)	Any tumor anterior to equator or solitary tumor larger than 10 dd behind equator
Group IV (unfavorable prognosis)	Any tumor anterior to ora serrata or multiple tumors, some larger than 10 dd
Group V (very unfavorable prognosis)	Tumors involving over half the retina or vitreous seeding

*dd—optic disc diameter

In a series of 118 patients using a surface applicator of ^{60}Co, Stallard[16] preserved useful vision in 65 percent of those patients with tumors occupying between 25–50 percent of the retina of one eye and in 91 percent of those patients with tumors occupying less than 25 percent of the retina.

Skeggs and Williams[14] treated 45 patients with "advanced" retinoblastoma with irradiation and cyclophosphamide. Of the 30 followed, three had uncontrolled tumor, but 21 of the survivors had at least some vision.

Krementz, Schlosser, and Rumage[9] treated 19 patients (17 with tumor confined to one eye) with x-ray plus intra-arterial (carotid) T.E.M., with seven survivors and 12 deaths attributed to tumor.

Reese and Ellsworth[6] treat those patients in Groups I, II, and III with radiation, those in Groups IV and V with radiation plus intra-arterial T.E.M., and those with residual orbital tumor with exenteration plus intra-arterial T.E.M. plus irradiation. Their results for 175 patients treated between 1958–1963 are:

Group	No. Patients	"Cure" Rate Averaging 5 Years
I	20	95%
II	29	83%
III	33	76%
IV	17	71%
V	59	32%

REVIEW QUESTIONS

1. In what age range is retinoblastoma most frequent? What other malignant tumors are frequent in this same group?

2. How often does retinoblastoma involve both eyes? How does this influence management of the patient?

3. How would you advise parents of a child afflicted by retinoblastoma regarding additional children if there was no family history of this tumor? if either parent or a grandparent had had retinoblastoma?

4. How is the clinical diagnosis made? How accurate is this?

5. What tumors may resemble anaplastic retinoblastoma histologically?

6. What is the common route of spread of retinoblastoma? How does this affect treatment? prognosis?

7. Why is radiotherapy the conservative method of treatment compared to surgery?

8. When should radiotherapy be used?

9. What is the role of chemotherapy?

10. How often can retinoblastoma be controlled with irradiation when tumor masses are less than 10 dd? How often is useful vision preserved?

11. How often can "useful vision" be retained when limited tumor is treated by irradiation?

BIBLIOGRAPHY

1. ACKERMAN, L. V., and REGATO, J. A. Cancer. Diagnosis, Treatment and Prognosis. Mosby, St. Louis, 1962.
2. BAGSHAW, M. A., and KAPLAN, H. S. Retinoblastoma, megavoltage therapy and unilateral disease. Trans Amer Acad Ophthal Otolaryng, 70:944–950, 1966.
3. CARBAJAL, U. M. Metastasis in retinoblastoma. Amer J Ophthal, 48:47–69, 1959.
4. DARGEON, H. W. Tumors of Childhood. Hoeber–Harper, 1960.
5. DUNPHY, E. B. The story of retinoblastoma. Amer J Ophthal, 58:539–552, 1964.
6. ELLSWORTH, R. M. Treatment of retinoblastoma. Amer J Ophthal, 66:49–51, 1968.
7. FALLS, H. F., and NEEL, J. V. Genetics of retinoblastoma. Arch Ophthal (Chicago), 46: 367–389, 1951.
8. KLIGERMAN, M. M. Present status of combined radiation therapy and chemotherapy. In: Progress in Radiation Therapy, Vol. III. F. Buschke, Ed, Grune & Stratton, New York, 1965, pp. 183–199.
9. KREMENTZ, E. T., SCHLOSSER, J. V., and RUMAGE, J. P. Combined radiation and regional chemotherapy in treatment of retinoblastoma. Amer J Roentgen, 96:141–146, 1966.
10. MARGOLIS, L., and HILL, D. Radiotherapy of retinoblastoma (in preparation).
11. MERRIAM, G. R., JR. Retinoblastoma. Analysis of seventeen autopsies. Arch Ophthal (Chicago), 44:71–108, 1950.
12. PARKHILL, E. M., and BENEDICT, W. L. Gliomas of the retina: A histopathologic study. Amer J Ophthal, 24:1354–1373, 1941.
13. REESE, A. Tumors of the eye and adnexa. Armed Forces Institute of Pathology, Fascicle #38, 1956.
14. SKEGGS, D. B. L., and WILLIAMS, I. G. Treatment of advanced retinoblastoma by means of external irradiation combined with chemotherapy. Clin Radiol, 17:169–172, 1966.
15. STALLARD, H. B. The irradiation of retinoblastoma. Trans Ophthal Soc UK, 80:589–595, 1960.
16. STALLARD, H. B. Retinoblastoma. St. Bartholomew's Hosp J, 68:1–8, 1964.
17. STEWARD, J. K., SMITH, J. L. S., and ARNOLD, E. L. Spontaneous regression of retinoblastoma. Brit J Ophthal, 40:449–461, 1956.

18. TAPLEY, N. DU V. Clinical results in the treatment of retinoblastoma with T.E.M. and radiation. Pp. 199-209 in: *Research in Radiotherapy*. R. F. Kallman, Ed, Washington National Academy of Science, National Research Council, 1961, and personal communication, 1969.

19. WELLER, C. V. The inheritance of retinoblastoma and its relationship to practical eugenics. *Cancer Res*, 1:517–535, 1941.

20. WILLIAMS, I. G. Radiation therapy in the treatment of retinoblastoma. *Amer J Roentgen*, 77:786–795, 1957.

21. WILLIS, R. A. *The Pathology of the Tumours of Children*. Charles C Thomas, Springfield, Ill., 1962.

8

CANCER OF THE HEAD AND NECK
(Excluding CNS, Skin, Orbit)

CANCER OF THE ORAL CAVITY

The upper digestive tract between the vermilion surfaces of the lips and the constrictor muscle at the entrance to the cervical esophagus is host to cancers of great clinical complexity. This mucosa-lined muscular tube contains two important structures, tongue and larynx, on its ventral surface and has direct communication with the upper airway. An understanding of the intricate anatomy is basic to an understanding of the behavior of tumors and consequent competence in their clinical management. Based on development, structure, and function, the proximal digestive tract can be divided into oral cavity, oropharynx, and hypopharynx.

The oral cavity extends from the vermilion surfaces of the lips to include the anterior faucial pillars which divide it from the oropharynx (Figures 8–1, 8–2). The oral portion of the tongue (anterior two-thirds, mobile) is divided from the pharyngeal tongue (posterior one-third, base of tongue) at the circumvallate papillae.

Malignant tumors originating in the mucosa of the oral cavity must be differentiated from those arising in the mucosa of the oropharynx, because these two groups of tumors differ biologically and, consequently, they differ as to treatment and prognosis. These biological differences include variations in histological differentiation, local tumor extension, and regional lymphatic spread. Examples are carcinomas of the oral tongue compared with those of the pharyngeal tongue and carcinomas of the anterior tonsillar pillar compared with malignant tumors of the tonsil and tonsillar fossa.

The epithelium of the oral cavity is thick with progressing differentiation toward the surface, whereas the submucosa is sparse and contains relatively small lymphatic spaces. In comparison, the epithelium of the oropharynx is less differentiated, and the underlying lymphatics are abundant. Carcinomas of the oral mucosa are more differentiated, more likely to invade adjacent structures, and less likely to spread to regional lymph nodes than are malignant tumors of the oropharyngeal mucosa. Adenopathies incident to oral mucosa carcinomas are more likely to be unilateral and discrete compared with those secondary to oropharyngeal tumors, which often are bilateral, massive, and confluent.

These biological variations, in addition to anatomical factors, often make

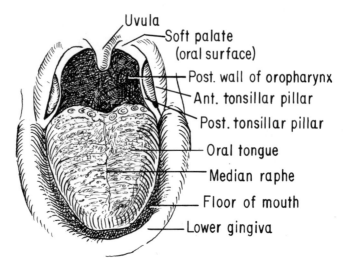

Fig. 8-1.   Oral cavity; anterior view.

surgery preferable to radiation therapy for carcinomas of the oral mucosa, although radiation therapy is the method of choice for malignant tumors of the oropharynx.

Structures of the oral cavity are involved by cancer in the following order of frequency: oral tongue, floor of mouth, buccal mucosa, lower gingiva, anterior faucial pillar (and retromolar trigone), soft palate, upper gingiva, and hard palate.[2, 10] Carcinomas of the vermilion surface of the lip, often included with oral cancers, will be discussed with cancers of the skin and mucocutaneous junctions,

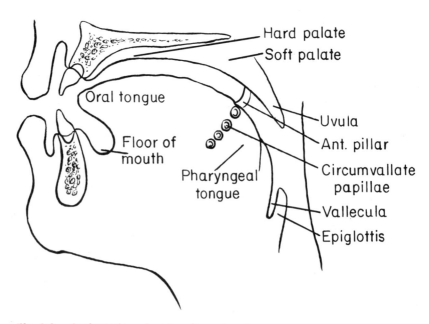

Fig. 8-2.   Sagittal view of oral cavity and orpharynx.

and cancers of the pharyngeal (base) tongue will be discussed with those of the oropharynx.

Correlation with Pathology

The majority of oral cavity cancers are epidermoid carcinomas. Those originating in the tongue, buccal mucosa, gingiva, and anterior pillar often are highly differentiated. Epidermoid carcinomas of the floor of the mouth usually are less differentiated. Infrequent histologic types are muco-epidermoid carcinomas which originate from glandular structures in the mucosa and aberrant salivary gland tumors. Muco-epidermoid carcinomas occur in any portion of the oral mucosa, and their histological differentiation from epidermoid carcinoma may be difficult because of epithelial metaplasia. However, this differentiation is of prognostic and therapeutic significance. Aberrant salivary gland tumors are similar in their clinical evolution to salivary gland tumors originating in the major salivary glands, although they may be more malignant. Both muco-epidermoid and aberrant salivary gland tumors usually grow slowly, invade locally, and spread "late" into the lymphatics. These two varieties are less radiovulnerable than epidermoid carcinomas. Complete removal by radical surgery is therefore preferable. Initial removal needs to be successful, for with clinical reactivation management becomes increasingly difficult.

A biologically indolent squamous cell carcinoma with little inclination to local invasion or spread to regional lymphatics (verrucous carcinoma) has been described by Ackerman.[1] This tumor usually involves the buccal mucosa or lower gingiva. With adequate excision it has an excellent prognosis. However, there are cases on record in which, after initial regression following radiation therapy, the tumor became anaplastic and rapidly fatal.[19]

Small foci of leukoplakia frequently are best excised. Large areas not easily removed surgically should be closely observed for the development of carcinomas and then excised as necessary. Radiation therapy usually is ineffective in the treatment of leukoplakia and may be less effective in the control of carcinomas arising in leukoplakic mucosa compared to those arising elsewhere.

A general estimate of radiation responsiveness of oral epidermoid carcinomas can be made by correlation with gross tumor appearance. Highly vascular, exophytic tumors usually are radiovulnerable, whereas deeply infiltrating, ulcerating lesions are difficult to control. However, variations in either direction make the prediction of response in any individual uncertain.

General Principles of Management

Victims of oral cancer are likely to be 45 to 75 years of age with associated vascular and degenerative diseases. There is frequent association with leukoplakia, poor oral hygiene, large alcohol intake, and heavy smoking. In the past, there was a frequent association between syphilis and cancer of the oral tongue. However, oral carcinomas occur in patients in whom none of these conditions prevail.

Evaluation for treatment must include assessment of the location, extent, histology, and gross characteristics (exophytic or infiltrating) of the primary lesion, involvement of regional nodes, and the condition of the patient.

The primary tumor and the regional adenopathy may be considered as separate parts of the same problem. In many situations, radiation therapy is preferable for the primary lesion because structures, and consequently function, may be preserved without compromise in tumor control.

Radical neck dissection is the treatment of choice for cervical adenopathy secondary to oral carcinomas. The potential contribution of preoperative irradiation is being studied.[16]

Four radiotherapeutic techniques for treatment of the primary tumor are available: external irradiation; peroral irradiation; a mold containing radioactive material, usually radium; and interstitial irradiation.

External irradiation alone rarely controls the highly differentiated squamous cell carcinomas, but may control the less well-differentiated carcinomas which arise in the floor of the mouth. Peroral irradiation through a cone is suitable for small tumors in favorable anatomic locations in cooperative patients.[9] Interstitial irradiation is the best procedure for many tumors of the oral tongue, floor of mouth, and buccal mucosa, but usually is not applicable and may be contraindicated when the tumor is immediately adjacent to or involves bone.

Great improvement in radical surgery during the past decade has prompted preference for initial surgery for many patients formerly treated by radium implantation. Improvement of radiotherapeutic techniques, such as use of higher radiation energies and longer protraction of application, has facilitated the combined use of preoperative radiation therapy and surgery.

Consequently, patients with oral cancers should be treated only after evaluation by surgeon and radiation therapist working together, each with an understanding of the accomplishments and limitations of their own and the other's methods.

Preliminary to any local treatment of the primary tumor, it is important to treat existing oral infection. This permits better evaluation of the true extent of the tumor, lessens complications during and following radiation therapy, and improves the radiation response and normal tissue tolerance.

Many patients with oral cancers eventually develop additional oral cancers. Therefore, in overall planning of a patient's management, an advantage of initial surgery is the reservation of radiation tolerance for the later treatment of a tumor not amenable to excision.

Management of the teeth in the heavily irradiated mandible has been a controversial problem. Heavily irradiated bone, particularly the mandible, is intolerant of infection or trauma. Therefore, even simple tooth extraction has been followed by the clinical disaster of extensive osteonecrosis. Fear of this uncommon result has prompted policies of preirradiation extraction of all teeth. Wildermuth and Cantril[22] have emphasized that careful tooth extraction from the irradiated mandible is possible without unnecessary risk. A rare, curious decay of teeth at the junction with the gingiva may be associated with suppression and quality change of saliva incident to heavy irradiation of the salivary glands. Decision regarding disposition of the teeth often is unnecessary because the population with oral cancer frequently is edentulous or has teeth beyond repair, which should be extracted for other reasons. If the patient is intelligent and reliable so that future dental care can be supervised, healthy teeth may be allowed to remain. Otherwise it may be prudent to extract those teeth which will be within the radiation beam and others in poor condition prior to starting treatment. Preirradiation tooth extraction must be accompanied by careful removal of the irregular bone between the sockets (radical

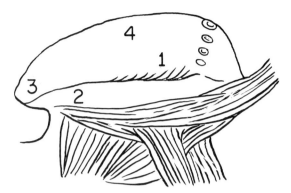

Fig. 8-3. Sites of primary cancers of oral tongue in order of frequency.

1 – Lateral margin
2 – Under surface
3 – Tip
4 – Dorsum

alveolectomy) and followed by an interval of seven to ten days to allow initial healing. Later use of dentures causing pressure on such heavily irradiated mucosa and bone is accompanied by substantial risk of nonhealing ulceration, infection, and eventual osteonecrosis.

Cancer of the Oral (Mobile, Anterior Two-Thirds) Tongue

Cancer of the oral tongue usually develops in males 45 to 75 years of age. Association with poor oral hygiene, leukoplakia of the oral mucosa, smoking, alcoholism, cirrhosis, or syphilis has been noted in a majority of these patients.

These epidermoid carcinomas, usually well-differentiated, most frequently arise from the lateral border of the oral tongue, although they may originate from the undersurface, tip, or dorsum, or they may be multiple (3.0 percent[7]) (Figure 8-3). The primary tumor may spread in the mucosa and submucosa to involve the floor of the mouth, lower alveolus, pharyngeal tongue, or anterior faucial pillar; may invade the extrinsic muscles of the oral tongue; and may metastasize to regional lymph nodes, usually the ipsilateral subdigastric or submandibular nodes, although there may be "clinical skipping" to lower ipsilateral cervical or contralateral cervical nodes (Figure 8-4).

Treatment

Treatment of the primary lesion of the oral tongue depends on the site and the extent of the tumor, the condition of the adjacent tissue (tumor bed), and the general condition of the patient. Thus, resection might be preferable for small tumors at the tip, multiple small tumors, tumors in a tongue with syphilitic endarteritis, in conjunction with a radical neck dissection for cervical adenopathy, or in an infirm patient when interstitial implantation of radium might be comparably more strenuous treatment.

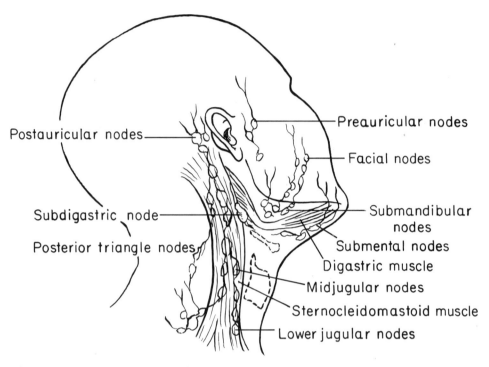

Fig. 8-4. Lymph nodes of the neck

Radiation therapy of the primary lesion has the advantage of preserving the anatomy and function of the tongue while controlling the tumor as effectively as does resection. Radiation techniques nearly always should be interstitial implantation, usually with radium needles (Figure 8-5) or x-ray through a peroral cone. Interstitial techniques are major operative procedures requiring general endotracheal anesthesia, followed by hospitalization, with careful nursing care for about seven

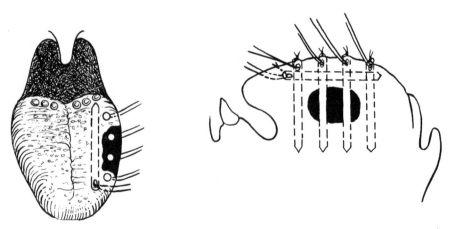

Fig. 8-5. Interstitial Application of Radium in Needles for Tongue Cancer.
1. Tumor within volume of high dose from row of needles. 2. "Crossing" needle at top improves distribution of dose. 3. Needles separated by ±1.0 cm. 4. Needles tied with two sutures, one fixed through the tongue, the other taped to the cheek.

days. Peroral x-ray has been useful in well-selected circumstances.[9] It is an out-patient clinic procedure, thus avoiding need for anesthesia or hospitalization.

Metastatic cervical adenopathy preferably is treated by radical neck dissection often in combination with resection of the primary lesion if untreated or uncontrolled after irradiation. Irradiation may suppress and infrequently sterilize cervical node metastases from oral tongue lesions and should be used only if resection is not possible or in controlled clinical studies as an adjuvant.[16]

Results

Control of the primary lesion of the oral tongue can be related to tumor site, size, and extent. With combined therapeutic management, reserving surgery for treatment of a few specific lesions and irradiation failures, Fletcher and MacComb[10] controlled 51 of 52 lesions less than 3 cm; 36 of 40 lesions 3–5 cm; 32 of 40 lesions over 5 cm, but involving less than half the oral tongue; and 15 of 25 lesions involving more than half the oral tongue. Ash[4] reported better local control of tumors of the tip (75 percent 5 YSR*) and lateral margin (57 percent 5 YSR) than for those of the dorsum (44 percent 5 YSR), although this in part may be related to tumor extent.

The prognosis is more closely related to failure of control of regional metastases than to lack of control of the primary tumor. The likelihood of metastases to cervical nodes increases with larger primary tumors and less histological differentiation of the tumor. Thirty-five to 40 percent of these patients will have palpable cervical adenopathy at the time of initial diagnosis, and another 20–30 percent will develop detectable cervical node metastases,[2,4] usually within 12 months. Radical neck dissection should control seven of ten "operable" necks.[8] Bilateral cervical adeno-pathy is infrequently controlled. The prognostic significance of clinically detectable adenopathy has been reported by Fletcher and MacComb[10]: never detected, 5 YSR = 78 percent; developing after treatment of the primary lesion, 5 YSR = 30 percent; present at time of initial diagnosis, 5 years = 14 percent.

This importance of cervical adenopathy has led some physicians to advocate radical neck dissection in anticipation of the development of clinically detectable abnormality ("prophylactic radical neck dissection"). Although from 35–40 per-cent of these patients with palpably "normal" necks will have histologically identi-fiable tumor in the cervical nodes,[2] the evidence remains inconclusive whether such "routine" application of radical surgery results in greater patient survival than a policy of withholding radical neck dissection pending discovery of clinical adeno-pathy, or use in certain situations of high risk, i.e., large primary tumors, undifferen-tiated tumors, in patients with necks difficult to examine, and in unreliable patients. This "individualized" management is licensed only by frequent, careful clinical exam-ination of the neck (every month by the same examiner for two years), but can show a profit of reduced patient morbidity.

Cancer of the Floor of the Mouth

The floor of the mouth is the inferior limiting structure of the oral cavity, being bound anteriorly and laterally by the inner surface of the mandible and posteriorly

*YSR = year survival rate.

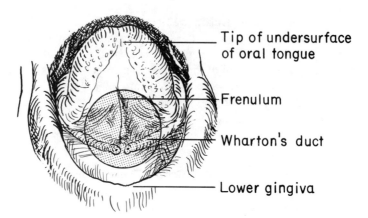

Fig. 8-6. Cancer of floor of mouth. Eighty percent arise anteriorly within shaded circle.

by the anterior faucial pillars (Figure 8-6). The centrally situated oral tongue divides the floor of the mouth into two symmetrical "alimentary grooves"[14] functionally continuous with the glossopharyngeal sulci and pyriform sinuses. Ducts of the submaxillary and major sublingual glands empty into the floor of the mouth through the sublingual caruncle and frequently are obstructed by tumor.

Carcinoma of the floor of the mouth constitutes about 15 percent of cancers of the oral cavity.[2] The vast majority of these tumors are epidermoid carcinomas, less differentiated than those of the oral tongue. They usually occur in males with a history of a large, prolonged alcohol intake. Most cancers originate in the anterior

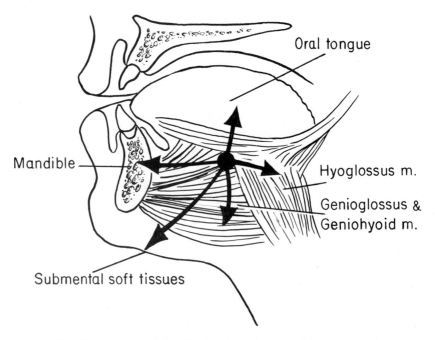

Fig. 8-7.   Routes of direct extension of cancer of floor of mouth.

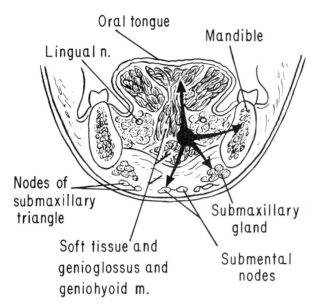

Oral tongue

Mandible

Lingual n.

Nodes of submaxillary triangle

Submaxillary gland

Soft tissue and genioglossus and geniohyoid m.

Submental nodes

Fig. 8-8. Routes of direct spread of cancer of floor of mouth.

floor of the mouth and frequently spread to involve the oral tongue, lower alveolus, and deep-lying muscles (Figures 8-7, 8-8). Submaxillary, subdigastric, and upper cervical nodes may become involved by metastases bilaterally (Figure 8-4), frequently being clinically detectable at the time of diagnosis.

Treatment

Epidermoid carcinomas of the floor of the mouth behave differently from those originating in other portions of the oral mucosa. They usually are less differentiated, frequently extend into the oral tongue and gingiva, invade muscles and mandible, invade submental lymphatics, and metastasize to submaxillary, subdigastric, and upper cervical nodes, often bilaterally. Thus, carcinoma of the floor of the mouth usually is an unfavorable lesion for surgical management, if used as a primary definitive procedure, or for radiotherapy, if used as a local oral procedure. Some limited epidermoid carcinomas of the floor of the mouth can be managed by peroral roentgen therapy or interstitial irradiation, but more advanced lesions require external irradiation to cover the entire floor of the mouth and submental soft tissues as the initial therapeutic procedure. Depending on the response, additional treatment by either surgery or local radium application may be necessary.

Over the last ten years we[5] have used a planned combined procedure with radiation therapy to be followed by radical surgery. However, with tumors of the floor of the mouth more than with any other carcinoma in the oral cavity, it has been possible to abandon the originally planned surgery because the radiation response has been sufficient to control the lesion.

Even if the carcinoma has invaded bone, preoperative irradiation has improved the control by destruction of tumor in the soft tissues, thus providing a wider tumor-free surgical margin. Sometimes the extent of surgery has been reduced, and on occasion only the involved portion of the mandible has been resected.

Results

The results depend on the extent of the primary tumor and the spread to cervical nodes. For our treatment program,[5] the two-year determinate cure rate for 43 patients was 55.3 percent and the five-year determinate cure rate for 26 patients was 42.1 percent.

Ash and Millar[3] reported a five-year survival rate of 59 percent for patients with primary lesions less than 1.5 cm in greatest dimension and an overall five-year survival rate of 40 percent. Martin and Martin[15] controlled 29 of 62 unselected patients (46.8 percent) by the use of interstitial radiation techniques. Using interstitial radium treatment of most of the primary lesions and resection of adenopathy, local irradiation failures, and radiation-produced complications, Fletcher and Mac-Comb[10] reported a five-year survival rate (Berkson-Gage method) of 67 ($\pm$5.7 percent) for 97 patients. Of this group, those without adenopathy had a five-year survival rate of 77 percent, those with adenopathy a five-year survival rate of 50 percent. Thus, regional adenopathy was controllable, even if bilateral, and seemingly less ominous than in association with oral tongue cancer. Surgical failures rarely were controlled by irradiation, although radiation failures sometimes were controlled by resection.

Thus, with treatment of each patient decided individually because of the variation in the biological behavior of carcinoma of the floor of the mouth, salvage can exceed that only recently listed in the medical literature.

Cancer of the Buccal Mucosa

The buccal mucosa covers the oral surface of the cheek from the lateral commissure of the mouth to the ascending ramus of the mandible and from lower to upper gingiva. The parotid duct opens into the oral cavity opposite the second upper molar tooth (Figure 8-9). Cancer arising in the buccal mucosa, usually of males, is much less frequent than cancer of the oral tongue,[2, 10] although exceptions have been noted in certain cultures.[11] These well-differentiated squamous cell carcinomas grossly may be plaquelike in association with leukoplakia, exophytic, nodular, infiltrative, or ulcerative. The primary tumor may spread to gingiva, "retromolar trigone," or lateral commissure of the mouth and become confused with tumors primary at those sites. The buccinator and masseter muscles may be invaded or penetrated by tumor in lymphatics draining to the superficial facial, submaxillary, or upper cervical nodes. Tumors arising in the posterior cheek often infiltrate these "deep" muscles and fascia and are more difficult to control than are lesions originating anterior to the masseter muscle. A biologically indolent, rarely metastasizing, squamous cell carcinoma (verrucous carcinoma) has been described by Ackerman.[1]

Treatment

Small cancers arising in leukoplakia may be treated effectively by local excision followed by grafting or by local irradiation. Verrucous carcinomas can be treated by conservative resection or irradiation, although change to a more aggressive tumor has been reported after irradiation.[19] More extensive primary lesions must be treated radically by resection or irradiation, or both.

Radiation therapy and surgery seem of comparable effectiveness. Irradiation is more conservative anatomically and functionally. External irradiation, peroral x-ray, and radium implantation have been effective in controlling the primary lesion.

Metastatic adenopathy is best treated surgically, although occasional control with radiation has been accomplished.

Results

"Early" diagnosis and frequent low-grade biological aggressiveness (i.e., verrucous carcinoma) can be correlated with favorable treatment results. Lampe[13] controlled 15 of 28 patients (53.6 percent) for five years with external and peroral x-ray. Paterson[18] controlled 46 of 82 patients (57 percent) for five years with radium implantation. Fletcher and MacComb[10] controlled 68 (± 6.5) percent for five years (Berkson-Gage method) by using radiation, surgery, or a combination. The prognostic influence of adenopathy was considerable for 84 percent of 45 patients without adenopathy, and 36 percent of 23 patients with adenopathy survived.[10]

Cancer of the Soft Palate and Anterior Faucial Pillar

The soft palate is a borderline structure between the oral cavity and oropharynx. It is partially formed by an extension of the posterior faucial pillars, structures of oropharyngeal origin. Cancer of the soft palate is included with cancers of the oropharynx in most texts. However, the mucosa of the inferior surface of the soft palate is an extension of the stratified squamous epithelium of the oral cavity. Except for rare mucous or salivary gland adenocarcinomas, malignant tumors of the soft palate are squamous cell carcinomas often moderately well-differentiated.

Carcinomas of the soft palate and anterior tonsillar pillar occur in two gross forms which have different clinical significance: superficial, papillary; and deeply infiltrating, ulcerative lesions.

The superficial, papillary lesion may extend over large portions of the soft palate (and anterior pillar) without infiltration. These lesions usually are responsive to radiation therapy, and often can be controlled even if the surface extent is great. However, the dose must be far higher than that necessary to cause an initial rapid gross disappearance of the lesion. Even following a high dose delivered to a tumor with a rapid initial response, there may be clinical reactivation.

The infiltrating, ulcerative type of carcinoma, which often occurs in the anterior pillar, must be distinguished from a carcinoma originating in the tonsil. Usually this is possible, although with advanced lesions the site of origin may not be evident. Carcinomas of the anterior pillar usually are highly differentiated and tend to infiltrate the tongue at the insertion of the pillar. Lack of tumor control at this junction is the most common cause of treatment failure.[20] These tumors tend to grow locally for a considerable time before metastasizing to regional nodes. Therefore, they are suitable for radical surgery.

In the more advanced tumors, which involve the palate or the post-molar mucosa, even such radical surgery frequently is followed by "recurrence" at the margins. For such lesions, radical preoperative irradiation, in an attempt to destroy the peripheral portion of the tumor, followed by radical surgery has proved advantageous.[6] Our experience over the last ten years is that when combined radical radiation therapy and radical surgery are originally planned for carcinoma of the anterior pillar, it is unwise to change this plan despite a good initial response to radiation therapy. If radiation therapy is conducted with the anticipation of radical surgery, the surgeon does not encounter any particular difficulties or complications beyond those expected with this type of major surgery. The operation should follow the irradiation within two months. However, it has been possible to operate at a later time without untoward complication.

An assessment of treatment accomplishment is difficult, for most malignant tumors involving the soft palate also involve adjacent sites, such as anterior or posterior pillars, tonsillar bed, tongue, or posterior buccal mucosa. Thus, in a study of carcinoma of the palatine arch, Schultz et al.[21] could limit tumors to a single site in only 50 of 305 patients.

Using various radiation techniques, Fletcher and MacComb[10] treated 28 patients with epidermoid carcinoma of the soft palate with a 5-year survival (Berkson-Gage method) of 60 ($\pm$10.9) percent. The survival of 17 patients with adenopathy was 53 percent. However, extensive unilateral or bilateral adenopathy was never controlled.

Cancer of the "Retromolar Trigone"

At the posterior limit of the buccal mucosa, just behind the last lower molar tooth and maxillary tuberosity, there is a triangular area which has been separated as the "retromolar trigone"[10] (Figure 8-9). Tumors originating at this site are epidermoid carcinomas which may extend to involve the mandible, lingual nerve, or muscles (glossopalatinus, buccinator, masseter, superior constrictor, internal pterygoid), often producing trismus. Extension along the pterygoid plate may involve the base of the skull.

These lesions in the retromolar mucosa are particularly unfavorable. They rarely are controlled by radiation therapy. Because of the tumor extensions, they are also unfavorable for radical surgery. Occasionally, the peripheral soft tissue extension of the tumor may be controlled by radiation therapy, thus promoting control by radical surgery.

Cancer of the Lower Gingiva

These usually well-differentiated squamous cell carcinomas frequently arise adjacent to the canine or molar teeth in older males, and consequently may be seen initially by a dentist. Cancer of the lower gingiva is comparable in frequency to cancer of the buccal mucosa.[2, 10] Although biologically indolent verrucous carcinomas may arise in this site,[1] most lesions are infiltrating, with consequent destruction of the mandible (50 percent[17]). This bone destruction may be "saucerlike" from pressure from expanding tumor or extensive ("moth-eaten") from widespread

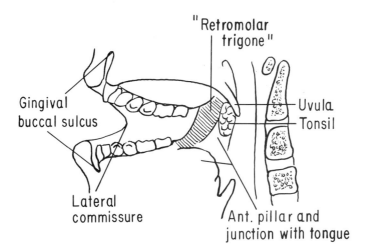

Fig. 8-9. Relationships of buccal mucosa and "retromolar trigone."

infiltration. Extensive bone destruction may follow invasion of tumor through the mental foramen. The primary tumor may extend to involve the adjacent floor of the mouth or buccal mucosa. The ipsilateral submaxillary and subdigastric nodes are frequently involved (40 percent[10]).

Treatment

In treatment planning, the high incidence of bone destruction and the frequency of cervical adenopathy must be considered. Verrucous carcinomas can be treated effectively by local resection or local irradiation. In most instances, resection would facilitate later use of dentures. In the past, evidence of bone destruction has been used as a contraindication to radiation therapy because of the possibility of mandibular necrosis. However, using orthovoltage x-ray, Lampe[13] controlled 4 of 14 lesions producing x-ray evidence of extensive bone destruction, and had clinically significant mandibular necrosis in only 1 of the 4 long-term survivors. His more recent unreported experience with ^{60}Co irradiation[12] has been even more favorable. Because local recurrence has been frequent following resection of cancers extensively destroying bone, Fletcher and MacComb[10] have advocated preoperative irradiation with an objective of sterilizing the peripheral tumor margins.

Surgery is the most effective treatment of the cervical adenopathy. Often this can be done best in continuity with resection of the primary tumor. There is no conclusive evidence that "prophylactic radical neck dissection" is profitable in this elderly population.

Results

The treatment of small lesions, those not destroying bone and most verrucous carcinomas, is effective by resection or irradiation. Comparison of past surgical and radiotherapeutic accomplishments is not valid because of patient selection. Using orthovoltage x-ray, Lampe[13] controlled 8 of 24 patients (33 percent), including a majority with extensive tumor. Using various radiotherapeutic methods, Paterson et al.[18] controlled 34 percent of 101 patients. Using radiation therapy and surgery, often in combination, Fletcher and MacComb[10] controlled 56 ($\pm$6.6 percent) (Berkson-Gage method). Their 5 YSR for 32 patients with cervical adenopathy was 46 percent.

Cancer of the Upper Gingiva and Hard Palate

Cancers of the upper gingiva and hard palate are infrequent, usually involve adjacent bone, and may be confused with malignant tumors arising in the maxillary sinus. Tumors primary on the upper gingiva usually are well-differentiated squamous cell carcinomas. Tumors arising from the mucosa of the hard palate often are mucous or salivary gland adenocarcinomas. Regional spread may be to retropharyngeal, submaxillary, and subdigastric nodes.

Treatment

Resection is preferable because of the associated bone involvement and difficulty in determining tumor extent.

REVIEW QUESTIONS

1. What are the structures of the oral cavity? Why is it important to separate these from structures of the oropharynx when considering management of the patient with cancer?

2. What histological type of cancer is most frequent in the oral cavity?

3. What improvements in application have made radiation therapy more effective in the treatment of patients with oral cancer?

4. What are the advantages of radiation therapy for patients with carcinoma of the oral tongue? When is resection preferable?

5. What is the optimal method of treatment of patients with cervical adenopathy secondary to carcinoma of the oral tongue? When should surgery be used? Are there indications for neck dissection prior to palpable identification of cervical adenopathy?

6. What factors influence control of the primary oral tongue carcinoma?

7. What is the prognostic influence of cervical adenopathy secondary to carcinoma of the oral tongue?

8. What factors hinder control of carcinoma of the floor of the mouth? How do these difficulties compare with problems of control of carcinoma of the oral tongue? What if the primary involves both sites?

9. What special problems arise when carcinomas involve the retromolar trigone? the anterior faucial pillar?

10. How often are tumors involving the soft palate limited to the soft palate? What adjacent anatomic sites usually are involved? How does this influence management and prognosis?

11. What special problems complicate management of patients with carcinoma of the gingiva?

12. What special problem may result from irradiation of the mandible? What anatomical peculiarity of the mandible may augment its vulnerability to irradiation? How should the teeth be managed in a patient with cancer of the oral cavity when radiation therapy is to be used?

BIBLIOGRAPHY

1. ACKERMAN, L. V. Verrucous carcinoma of the oral cavity. *Surgery*, 23:670–678, 1948.
2. ACKERMAN, L. V., and DEL REGATO, J. A. *Cancer: Diagnosis, Treatment and Prognosis.* Mosby, St. Louis, 4th ed., 1970.
3. ASH, C. L., and MILLAR, O. B. Radiotherapy of cancer of the tongue and floor of the mouth. *Amer J Roentgen*, 73:611–614, 1955.
4. ASH, C. L. Oral cancer: A twenty-five year study. *Amer J Roentgen*, 87:417–430, 1962.
5. BENAK, S., BUSCHKE, F., and GALANTE, M. Treatment of carcinoma of oral cavity, *Radiology*, 96:137–144, 1970.
6. BUSCHKE, F. J., and GALANTE, M. Radical preoperative roentgen therapy in primarily inoperable advanced cancers of the head and neck. *Radiology*, 73:845–848, 1959.
7. CADE, S., and LEE, E. S. Cancer of the tongue. A study based on 653 patients. *Brit J Surg*, 44:433–446, 1957.
8. DEVITO, R. Personal communication.
9. FAYOS, J. V., and LAMPE, I. Peroral irradiation of carcinoma of the oral tongue. *Radiology*, 93:387–394, 1969.
10. FLETCHER, G. H., and MAC COMB, W. S. *Radiation Therapy in the Management of Cancers of the Oral Cavity and Oropharynx.* Charles C Thomas, Springfield, Ill., 1962.
11. KHANOLKAR, V. R. Oral cancer in India. *Acta Union Int. contra Cancrum* 15:67–77, 1959.
12. LAMPE, I. Personal communication.
13. LAMPE, I. Radiation therapy of cancer of the buccal mucosa and lower gingiva. *Amer J Roentgen*, 73:628–635, 1955.
14. LEDERMAN, M. Bucco-pharyngeal cancer: A clinical study with special reference to "sulcus tumors" and classification. *Brit J Radiol*, 29:536–678, 1956.
15. MARTIN, C. L., and MARTIN, J. A. Treatment of cancer of the floor of the mouth and its cervical metastases by irradiation. *Southern Med J*, 51:1017–1025, 1958.
16. MILLBURN, L. F., and HENDRICKSON, F. R. Initial treatment of neck metastases from squamous cell cancer. *Radiology*, 89:123–126, 1967.
17. MODLIN, J., and JOHNSON, R. E. The surgical treatment of cancer of the buccal mucosa and lower gingiva. *Amer J Roentgen*, 73:620–627, 1955.
18. PATERSON, R. *The Treatment of Malignant Disease by Radiotherapy*, 2nd ed. Williams & Wilkins, Baltimore, 1963.
19. PEREZ, C., KRAUS, F., EVANS, J., and POWERS, W. Anaplastic transformation in verrucous carcinoma of the oral cavity after radiation therapy. *Radiology*, 86:108–115, 1966.
20. RIDER, W. D. Epithelial cancer of the tonsillar area. *Radiology*, 78:760–764, 1962.

21. SCHULTZ, M. D., LINTER, D. M., and SWEENEY, L. Carcinoma of the palatine arch. *Amer J Roentgen*, 89:541–548, 1963.
22. WILDERMUTH, O., and CANTRIL, S. T. Radiation necrosis of the mandible. *Radiology*, 61:771–784, 1953.

MALIGNANT TUMORS OF THE PHARYNX: RADIOBIOLOGICAL OBSERVATIONS

Analysis of the effect of irradiation on tumors originating in the pharygeal mucosa aids in understanding the interplay of biological factors influencing radiation therapy. Tumors of nearly identical histological appearance, arising in different parts of the pharynx, may grow in a dissimilar manner. Some tumors extend superficially as flat, papillary elevations of the musoca (vallecula); some diffusely invade the lymphatics in the mucosa and submucosa (tonsil); some inflltrate deeply into muscle and connective tissue (pharyngeal tongue, pyriform sinus); and some form large, nonulcerated infiltrations (pharyngeal wall). These gross variations in histologically similar tumors can be related to the structure of the mucosa and submucosa. Factors of size and abundance of lymphatics, vascularity, and connective tissue structure modify the response to irradiation (radiovulnerability) more than does the degree of histological differentiation. Radiocurability depends not only on the radiovulnerability of the tumor cells, but on tumor extent with possible invasion of neighboring tissues such as muscle or bone, and host resistance.

Appreciation of these relationships is basic to an undertanding of the biological fundamentals governing the rationale for radiation therapy. Therefore, general principles pertinent to the entire pharynx will be discussed prior to consideration of clinically specific tumors.

The pharynx extends from the base of the skull to the entrance to the cervical esophagus, and communicates with the nasal fossae, oral cavity, and larynx (Figure 8-10). Customary subdivisions are: nasopharynx (epipharynx), extending from the base of the skull to the level of the soft palate; oropharynx (mesopharynx), extending between the soft palate and the hyoid bone (epiglottis); and the hypopharynx (laryngopharynx), extending between the level of the hyoid bone and the entrance to the cervical esophagus.

Corresponding to its respiratory function, the epithelium of the nasopharynx is moderately differentiated and nonkeratinizing. In the roof and along the lateral walls, it is stratified and columnar, and adjacent to the nasal fossae it is ciliated. With age, this mucosa may become stratified squamous epithelium. On the pharyngeal surface of the soft palate, the epithelium may be more differentiated and keratinized.

The oropharynx is the junction between respiratory and digestive tracts. Its epithelium and that of the hypopharynx are similar to, although less differentiated than, the squamous epithelium of the oral cavity. The pharyngeal submucosa contains a diffuse, rich network of lymphatic vessels and lymphoid aggregates. Specific concentrations of lymphoid tissue form Waldeyer's ring (Figure 8-11). These include lymphoid follicles along the lateral walls of the nasopharynx and oropharynx, with interconnections between the palatine tonsils through the

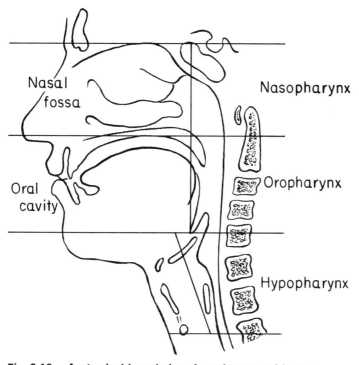

Fig. 8-10.   Anatomical boundaries of oropharynx and hypopharynx.

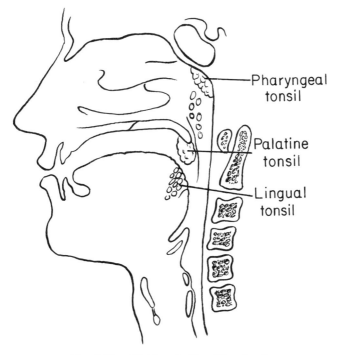

Fig. 8-11.   Waldeyer's "tonsillar ring."

pharyngeal tongue (lingual tonsil) and glossopharyngeal folds and between collections about the eustachian tubes through the pharyngeal tonsil in the roof of the
nasopharynx.

Corresponding to the diversity of normal tissues of the pharynx, there are
epidermoid carcinomas and a variant, lymphoepithelioma, and lymphosarcomas.
Because of the abundant lymphatics in the submucosa, "early" diffuse involvement
of lymphatics is characteristic of these neoplasms.

Epidermoid carcinomas predominate at all sites. Lymphoepitheliomas and
lymphosarcomas are much less frequent and arise from specific sites, such as
nasopharynx, tonsil, and pharyngeal tongue. Although lymphosarcomas initially
are localized, occasionally they are accompanied by lymphosarcoma elsewhere (i.e.,
in the stomach[1]).

It is important to recognize characteristic distributions of palpable cervical
adenopathy. In cancer of the nasopharynx, the first recognizable adenopathy is
high and posterior, below the mastoid tip. Lymphatic spread from tonsillar
neoplasms initially is palpable at the angle of the mandible. Tumors of the
hypopharynx first involve the anterior midcervical nodes.

Except for certain hypopharyngeal carcinomas, external irradiation is preferable primary treatment for tumors arising in the pharyngeal mucosa. Widespread
lymphatic involvement makes surgery inappropriate. In contrast to most oral
carcinomas, many of these tumors are sufficiently radiovulnerable to permit
destruction of the primary lesion *and* the extensive regional adenopathy.

The site of origin and the gross type of growth may be of greater prognostic
importance than the size of the tumor and its histologic differentiation. For example,
a localized carcinoma of the pyriform fossa with its tendency to infiltrate into
muscle and cartilage is controlled only occasionally, whereas a large carcinoma
of the tonsil is often curable. The pharyngeal tumors most often controlled are
those of the tonsil, aryepiglottic fold, valleculae, and nasopharynx. Tumors of
the pyriform sinus and post cricoid region, despite similarity of histological appearance, are rarely controlled.

As lymphatic spread at the time of diagnosis is assumed in most of these
tumors, regardless of whether or not it is clinically demonstrable, radical
radiation therapy must include the primary site and regional lymphatics in continuity. When the primary tumor is unilateral, as in the tonsil, treatment may be
limited to the ipsilateral side. In tumors of the nasopharynx, pharyngeal tongue,
and posterior pharyngeal wall, the treated tissue volume must include the primary
site and both sides of the neck, in continuity. Such large tissue volumes can be
irradiated more effectively with "high energy" equipment (cobalt-60, linear
accelerator, betatron), and statistically significant improvement of cure rates has
been accomplished.[2]

Reasons for failure differ for various tumor sites and types. Lymphosarcomas
usually can be controlled locally and regionally, but frequent failure results from
distant spread. Tumors of the pyriform sinus and pharyngeal tongue are less
frequently controlled at the primary site. The highly biologically aggressive tumors,
such as epidermoid carcinomas of the tonsil, pharyngeal tongue, or pyriform sinus,
if uncontrolled, rarely heal so that prognostic assessment may be made soon after
treatment. Certain lesions, such as tonsillar carcinoma and lymphosarcoma, if not
controlled, soon show evidence of tumor growth (local, regional, or distant) so
that after two years a reliable appraisal is possible. In some hypopharygeal cancers,

late appearance of distant metastases, particularly to the lung, and late local recurrence makes an appraisal doubtful even after five years.

BIBLIOGRAPHY

1. BUSCHKE, F., and CANTRIL, S. Secondary lymphosarcoma of the stomach. *Amer J Roentgen,* 49:450–454, 1943.
2. FLETCHER, G., and MAC COMB, W. *Radiation Therapy in the Management of Cancers of the Oral Cavity and Oropharynx.* Charles C Thomas, Springfield, Ill., 1962.

MALIGNANT TUMORS OF THE NASOPHARYNX

Malignant tumors of the nasopharynx are not suitable for extirpative surgery because of their anatomical inaccessibility and their biological characteristics. Tumors arising from the mucosa of the nasopharynx are controllable by radiation therapy both at the primary site and when metastatic to regional lymph nodes. Curability with currently available treatment methods thus depends on diagnosis prior to distant spread. Unfortunately, diagnostic performance has been poor despite characteristic clinical symptoms and signs, prompting Cantril and Buschke[3] to label the nasopharynx "a diagnostic blind spot." This situation has not appreciably changed since 1931 when Dr. Gordon New[8] reported that 185 operations, including 39 tonsillectomies, had been performed for relief of symptoms or signs in 194 patients prior to establishment of the correct diagnosis.

Anatomy of the Nasopharynx Correlated with Its Influence on Tumor Behavior

An understanding of anatomical relationships is essential for an understanding of the clinical findings. The nasopharynx is a chamber of 4 cm transverse, 4 cm anteroposterior, and 2–3 cm vertical dimensions (Figure 8-10). Anteriorly, it opens into the nasal fossae. Inferiorly, it is demarcated by the soft palate. The posterior wall is formed by mucosa overlying the superior constrictor muscle of the pharynx and the first and second cervical vertebrae. The posterior wall is continuous with the roof, which lies beneath portions of the occipital and basisphenoid bones and contains the pharyngeal tonsil. The lateral walls contain the eustachian tube ostia, located about 1 cm posterior to the posterior margin of the inferior turbinate and bounded posteriorly by a prominent projection (torus tubarius) and the lateral pharyngeal recess (fossa of Rosenmüller).

The epithelium over the roof and lateral walls of the nasopharynx is of respiratory type (pseudostratified columnar with goblet cells and occasionally with cilia) and is stratified squamous elsewhere. The mucosa of the roof or lateral walls may become stratified squamous with aging.

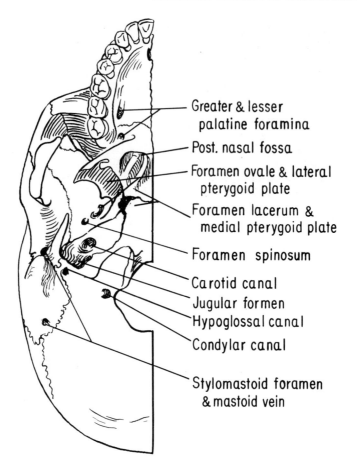

Fig. 8-12. Base of skull. Related to spread of cancer of nasopharynx
1. Foramen rotundum (not shown, anterior to foramen ovale)—contains maxillary nerve.
2. Foramen ovale—contains mandibular nerve.
3. Foramen spinosum—contains middle meningeal vessels.
4. Foramen lacerum—no contents.
5. Carotid canal—contains internal carotid artery.
6. Jugular foramen—contains internal jugular vein and cranial nerves IX, X, XI.
7. Hypoglossal canal—contains cranial nerve XII.

The posterior and lateral walls of the nasopharynx contain a strong fascia, which attaches to the base of the skull (Figures 8-12, 8-12A), and influences the spread of tumor and, consequently, the clinical presentation. Tumor may invade this fascial barrier to involve adjacent structures, i.e., levator palati muscle or parapharyngeal space, situated between the lateral pharyngeal wall and the inner surface of the ascending ramus of the mandible (Figure 8-13). The prestyloid compartment of the parapharyngeal space contains the internal maxillary artery, the inferior dental, lingual, and auriculotemporal nerves, and is immediately adjacent to the fossa of Rosenmüller and the tonsil. From this space tumor can spread to the base of the skull (foramen ovale, foramen spinosum, and great wing

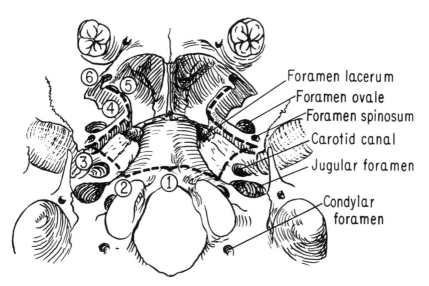

Fig. 8-12A. Attachment of pharyngeal fascia to base of skull.
1. Pharyngeal tubercle of basal occiput
2. Petro-occipital synchondrosis
3. Angular spine of sphenoid
4. Sphenopetrosal synchondrosis
5. Medial lamella of pterygoid process
6. Hamulus
(Dr. E. A. Boyden's interpretation from Rauber-Kopsch Lehrbuch, Der Anatomie IX. Auflage.)

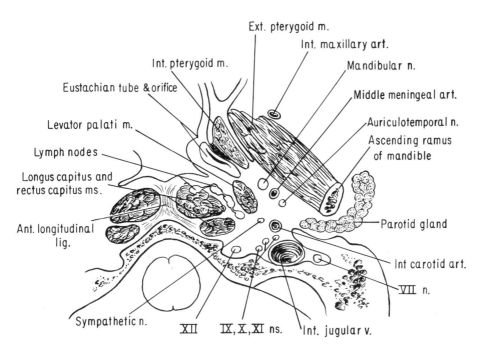

Fig. 8-13. Horizontal section through parapharyngeal space.

of sphenoid), to the parotid gland, or even inferiorly to the submaxillary gland. Sensory or motor alteration of the mandibular branch of the trigeminal nerve, trismus from invasion of the pterygoid muscles, or depression of the soft palate may follow extension of tumor into the prestyloid compartment.

The retrostyloid compartment contains the internal carotid artery, internal jugular vein, cranial nerves IX, X, XI, XII, the cervical sympathetic nerve, and lymph nodes. Thus, neoplasm can cause paresis of any of these nerves by direct invasion or compression from enlarged, tumor-bearing nodes.

The retropharyngeal compartment contains nodes, but clinical symptoms rarely result from tumor involvement.

The fossa of Rosenmüller is a common site for cancers of the nasopharynx. Tumor arising in this fossa may spread medially into the lumen of the nasopharynx (airway obstruction, bleeding, discharge), inferiorly to the oropharynx and soft palate, anteriorly to occlude the eustachian tube (serous otitis, loss of hearing), into the fascial space about the levator palati (unilateral deafness and immobility of the soft palate), or below the eustachian tube into the parapharyngeal space (see previous discussion).

Tumor may extend from the superior margin of the fossa of Rosenmüller along the bone-encased internal carotid artery canal or through the foramen lacerum to enter the cranial cavity adjacent to the cavernous sinus, and may involve cranial nerves III, IV, VI, and V (ophthalmic and maxillary branches), or destroy the greater wing of the sphenoid bone.

The abundant lymphatics of the nasopharynx, inclusive of large masses in the roof and lateral walls, drain to the retropharyngeal and deep cervical nodes (internal jugular chain, spinal acessory nerve chain, and transverse cervical artery chain; see Figures 8-14, 8-15).[7] Cervical adenopathy often is bilateral, even with a unilateral primary tumor. This combination of bilateral cervical and retropharyngeal adenopathy makes radical neck dissection futile.

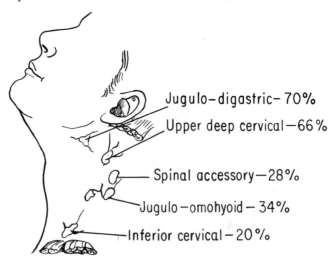

Jugulo-digastric- 70%
Upper deep cervical—66%
Spinal accessory—28%
Jugulo-omohyoid — 34%
Inferior cervical—20%

Fig. 8-14. Cervical lymph node metastases from cancer of the nasopharynx. (After Lederman, M. B., Cancer of the Nasopharynx: Its Natural History and Treatment. Courtesy of Charles C Thomas, Publ., Springfield, Ill.)

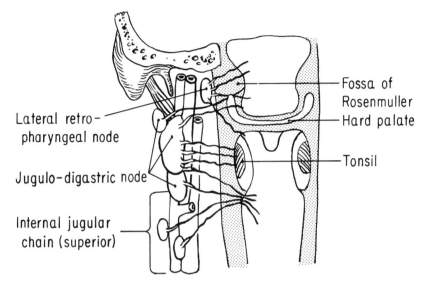

Fig. 8-15. **Nasopharyngeal lymphatics in coronal section.** (schematic from Rouviere).

Clinical Correlation

Malignant tumors primary in the nasopharynx constitute 1 to 2 percent of all cancer, and more often afflict males (5:2).[6,9,14] Although the average patient age is about 50 years, those under 40 years frequently are involved (17 percent under 40 years in Vaeth's[14] series). Orientals (except Japanese) suffer a high incidence of nasopharyngeal cancer, and a disproportionately high number have lympho-epithelioma.

The initial and only complaint in about one-third of patients is cervical adenopathy, although about one-half have noted this finding with or without other complaints, and three-fourths have detectable cervical adenopathy at the time of initial examination.[6,9,14]

Clinical findings arising from the primary tumor depend on specific site, tumor bulk, and local tumor extension. Lederman[7] found the most frequent sites of tumor to be the lateral wall and roof (Table 8-1).

The primary tumor mass may obstruct the nasal fossa (unilateral obstruction, epistaxis, discharge) or the eustachian tube (serous otitis, earache, loss of hearing).

Table 8-1. Anatomical Distribution of Tumors of the Nasopharynx*

Lateral wall	—	37.6%
Roof	—	32.6%
Posterior wall	—	15.1%
Floor	—	4.6%
Unclassified	—	10.0%

*From Lederman.[7]

Table 8-2.   Frequency of Presenting Complaint
in Cancer of the Nasopharynx

Cervical adenopathy	18.3[7] –47.5%[14]
Nasal	36.6[14]–38.5%[7]
Aural	17.0[7] –28.0%[14]
Pain (plus headache)	9.7[14]–11.5%[7]
Cranial nerve	3.2[7] – 6.0%[14]
Sore throat	4.9%[14]

Extension into the orbit may cause proptosis, diplopia, or fixation of the eye. Extension into the parapharyngeal space or cranial cavity may cause pain and specific neurological deficits (see later discussion). Thus, the patient may seek help from the neurologist, the ophthalmologist, the otolaryngologist, or the general surgeon because of a very specific clinical presentation. The frequency of various complaints is listed in Table 8-2.

Although cervical adenopathy was the first complaint of many patients (18.3[7]– 47.5 percent[14]), most patients had adenopathy at initial examination (70[7]–72 percent[14] with 30 percent bilateral), and nearly all (90 percent[4]) eventually developed it. This adenopathy usually is characteristic in location (upper deep cervical beneath the upper sternocleidomastoid muscle, apex of posterior triangle, jugulodigastric). Therefore, any patient presenting with adenopathy of this description should be considered to have cancer of the nasopharynx until proved otherwise. Inasmuch as the primary nasopharyngeal lesion may be small even with massive adenopathy and thus may not be identified, the coexistence of characteristic tumor type (biopsy of adenopathy) and specifically distributed cervical adenopathy makes treatment as cancer of the nasopharynx more rational than neck dissection.

Neurological complications may be frequent, characteristic, and serious. In a recent study,[13] 16 percent presented with neurological findings (diplopia, facial paresthesia, visual loss), and 30 percent ultimately had neurological complications. The cranial nerves can be damaged by direct extension of tumor or by pressure from adenopathy in an enclosed space. Thus, cranial nerves V and VI are at particular risk following extension through the base of the skull via the canal for the internal carotid artery, the foramen lacerum, and the foramen ovale, and those cranial nerves emerging from the skull through the posterior fossa (IX, X, XI, XII) are vulnerable to extracranial spread of tumor to the retroparotid space or retropharyngeal lymph nodes. Cranial nerves II, III, and IV may be involved by tumor in the anterior cavernous sinus or superior orbital fissure. The olfactory nerve (I) may be involved in the nasal cavity or above the cribiform plate. The facial nerve may be involved after it leaves the stylomastoid foramen. Horner's syndrome may follow pressure on the sympathetic chain (carotid or prevertebral). Many syndromes related to specific nerve involvement have been described and are thoroughly discussed in other texts.[1,7]

Pain, either characteristic or ill-defined, often is a prolonged diagnostic problem for both patient and physician. This may result from nerve irritation, bone destruction, or infection, and may be distributed along any branch of the trigeminal nerve, the skull vertex, or the occiput, or may be earache incident to obstructive serous otitis.

X-ray examination may document a soft tissue mass (which should be directly visible) or bone destruction. This latter finding may be noted in about 10 percent of those examined,[14] may involve the foramen lacerum, pterygoid process, body and great wing of the sphenoid, or carotid canal,[5,7] and is prognostically ominous. It is important not to "overinterpret" the radiographs. Indistinctness of the tip of the petrous pyramid has been reported erroneously as evidence of tumor invasion of bone. Therefore, reports of curability despite bone involvement must be accepted with reservation. Certainly unequivocal radiographic evidence of massive bone destruction is indicative of incurability. Bone invasion is most frequent with well-differentiated epidermoid carcinomas, and may occur incident to small primary lesions.

Pathologic Findings

The primary tumor may be very small, it may be exophytic and bulky even without mucosal ulceration, it may be lobulated, or it may be flat and ulcerated.

There is no widespread acceptance of a classification of malignant tumors arising from the respiratory and stratified squamous epithelium and lymphoid structures of the nasopharynx. These tumor types include: epidermoid carcinoma; lymphosarcoma; reticulum cell sarcoma; lymphoepithelioma; transitional cell carcinoma; plasmacytoma. Thus, there is a wide variation in tumor types reported from different institutions or from the same institution over a period of time. A few reported series are listed in Table 8-3.

In addition to the high incidence of spread to regional lymph nodes, there may be widespread lymphatic metastases (often with the lymphomas) or hematogenous metastases (i.e., to bone with lymphoepithelioma).

Treatment

The anatomy of the primary tumor site and the likelihood of retropharyngeal and bilateral cervical adenopathy eliminates surgery as a treatment method. Fortunately, these tumors are radioresponsive to tolerable doses and, thus, these patients are potentially radiocurable even with large cervical adenopathy.

Table 8-3. Histopathology (Incidence) of Malignant Tumors of the Nasopharynx

	University of California (Vaeth[14])	Mayo Clinic (Thomas and Waltz[13])	M. D. Anderson (Fletcher and Million[4])
Epidermoid carcinoma	17.1%	33.3%	47.3%
Transitional cell carcinoma	40.3%	—	—
Lymphoepithelioma	30.5%	46.3%	37.5%
Lymphosarcoma	4.9%	4.6%	8.9%
Adenocarcinoma	2.4%	—	0.9%
Plasmacytoma	—	—	0.9%
Melanosarcoma	1.2%	—	—
Miscellaneous sarcoma	3.6%	—	—

Technique

The unpredictability of dosage necessary for eradication of tumor in these potentially curable patients leads to use of radiation doses just within tolerance of the adjacent structures. The likelihood that retropharyngeal and bilateral cervical lymphatics are tumor-bearing necessitates vigorous irradiation of both sides of the neck above the clavicles concurrent with treatment of the entire nasopharynx, inclusive of the bony roof and posterior wall, plus any local extensions of tumor, i.e., nasal fossa, orbit, cavernous sinus, parapharyngeal space.

Optimal irradiation of this large tissue volume to high dose can be accomplished only with an external radiation source, which should be of supervoltage energy. Dose supplementation at the primary site through isotope applicators occasionally is of value.

Complications of Treatment

Inclusion of vital structures (i.e., base of brain, cervical spinal cord) as well as bone, which may be destroyed by tumor, in the vigorously irradiated volume results in a substantial incidence of morbidity. This morbidity, acceptable with curative objective, must be accounted for when palliation is being considered.

Complications during or shortly following treatment with proper technique include dry mouth from suppression of the parotid and submaxillary glands, sore throat from pharyngeal reaction, and skin reaction in the external auditory canals and serous otitis media.

The serious complications occur later. Thus, the salivary change plus direct irradiation of teeth result in frequent, characteristic alveolar-junction caries. Therefore, many radiotherapists recommend pretreatment extraction of all unhealthy teeth plus those teeth in the direct radiation beam.[4] Bone necrosis usually is self-limiting if the tumor is controlled. However, this complication in the auditory canal may constitute a lifelong problem.

The major morbidity and occasional mortality are related to changes in the brain stem and cervical spinal cord. We have recognized transitory clinical findings attributed to cervical cord damage in about 5 percent of the patients treated with 800 kv and 2 Mev x-ray for 30 years. Fletcher and Million[4] report four "authenticated cases" of radiation myelitis with three deaths in 112 patients treated between 1948 and 1960. Scanlon et al.[10] report a single fatality attributed to radiation myelitis, six months post-treatment, in a series of 142 patients. This unwelcome sequela can be minimized by limitation of the segment of spinal cord irradiated and by prolongation of the overall treatment time when using daily increments.[15]

Results

There is a well-documented prognostic relationship with tumor type, tumor extent, and adequacy of treatment. Females often fare better than males, although Scanlon et al.[10] found no correlation between prognosis and sex or primary site, or between type and duration of presenting clinical findings.

Overall five-year tumor-free survivals of about 30 percent have been reported for several years (Vaeth,[14] 28.2 percent; Smedal and Watson,[12] 33.3 percent; Scanlon et al.,[10] 30 percent). Recent data from treatment centers with modern

Table 8-4. Correlation of Survival at Five Years and Histopathological Tumor Type

Tumor Type	Vaeth[14]	Author Fletcher and Million[4]	Scanlon et al.[10]
Epidermoid carcinoma	3/14 (21.4%)	–	–
Transitional cell carcinoma	10/33 (30.3%)	–	–
Total epidermoid	13/47 (27.7%)	12/36 (33%)	35/119 (29%)
Lymphoepithelioma	6/25 (24.0%)	14/35 (40%)	–
Lymphosarcoma	3/4 (75.0%)	4/8 (50%)	2/5 (40%)
Adenocarcinoma	0/2 (–)	1/1 (–)	2/5 (40%)

equipment and aggressive treatment policies indicate further improvement (Fletcher and Million,[4] 38 percent absolute 5-year survival).

The correlation of prognosis with a histopathological type of tumor is difficult because of the variations in classification previously discussed. In several series, patients with lymphoepithelioma had the best survival incidence,[5,7,10] although in others[2,4,14] there was no significant difference between lymphoepithelioma and epidermoid carcinoma. When the epidermoid carcinoma is well-differentiated, a higher dose may be required for local tumor control.[4,11]

Although each series includes only a small number, patients with lymphosarcoma often have the most favorable survival incidence.[4,7,14]

Table 8-4 lists the correlation of survival and tumor type in several series. Correlation between series must be done with reservation.

The high incidence of regional adenopathy makes prognostic correlation applicable to most patients with cancer of the nasopharynx. It is significant that patients with bilateral cervical adenopathy frequently are curable by radiotherapy, for this is in marked contrast to a lower incidence of cure in patients with oral and hypopharyngeal cancers with cervical adenopathy. Lederman[7] reported no difference in survival at five years for patients with or without cervical adenopathy, whereas Vaeth,[14] Fletcher and Million,[4] and Scanlon et al.[10] found that the survival rate was worse with bilateral adenopathy than when nodes were detected unilaterally (Table 8-5).

Invasion of the base of the skull or cranial nerve paresis secondary to tumor greatly reduce the chance for survival. Distant metastases, i.e., below the clavicle, make the patient incurable.

Table 8-5. Correlation of Survival at Five Years to Cervical Adenopathy

Spread	Vaeth[14]	Author Fletcher and Million[4]	Scanlon et al.[10]
No adenopathy	12/23 (52.2%)	2/7 (29%)	– (67%)
Unilateral adenopathy	9/34 (26.4%)	12/26 (46%)	11/46 (24%)
Bilateral adenopathy	2/25 (8.0%)	12/37 (32%)	5/35 (14%)

Radiation dose has an influence on both local tumor control and survival. Recent trends to higher dosage have resulted from improved equipment and altered philosophy of treatment. Fletcher and Million[4] had no local failure of tumor control in the nasopharynx since using doses of 6,500 rads with megavoltage equipment. Scanlon et al.[10] had a five-year survival incidence of 23 percent with less than 5,000 R and 35 percent with more than 5,000 R.

The incidence of reappearance of tumor in the nasopharynx has been reported as 20–35 percent of patients irradiated.[4, 14] This reactivation of tumor may be noted more than five years post-treatment,[4, 5, 14] and usually can be related to low dosage (100 percent "local recurrence" with less than 4,000 R[16]). However, we have seen "recurrence" (or new tumor?) as late as 13 years following high radiation dosage. Some of these patients can be re-treated successfully, although the risk of radiation squelae is increased. Re-treatment with external irradiation, in our experience, has been unsatisfactory. However, local "recurrences" have been treated effectively with radium in an intracavity applicator.

REVIEW QUESTIONS

1. Correlate the following clinical presentations with regional spread of cancer arising in the nasopharynx:
   a. Unilateral nasal obstruction and epistaxis
   b. Inability to rotate one eye laterally
   c. Unilateral ophthalmoplegia and blindness
   d. Unilateral hearing loss and serous otitis
   e. Trismus
   f. Unilateral paralysis and depression of the soft palate
   g. Unilateral paresis of cranial nerves IX, X, XI, XII
   h. Horner's syndrome.

2. Explain why such specific clinical presentations might be confusing for the physician.

3. How often is cervical adenopathy discovered by the patient? by the physician on initial examination? How often is cervical adenopathy bilateral? Is the patient with cervical adenopathy curable?

4. What are the two most likely primary tumor sites in a 35-year-old male with unilateral deep upper cervical adenopathy? What if biopsy of these enlarged nodes is interpreted as poorly differentiated epidermoid carcinoma? lymphosarcoma? lymphoepithelioma? What would you do if no primary tumor was identified on physical examination?

5. What is the most frequent histological type of cancer arising in the nasopharynx? What other tumor types may be found there? Does this spectrum of tumor types arise from any other structure?

6. What are the most frequent sites of metastases from cancer arising in the naso-pharynx? How does this influence radiation therapy?

7. Which histological tumor types arising in the nasopharynx are controllable by radiation therapy? How frequent is local tumor control? Is this dose related? Does the incidence of local control vary with histological tumor type?

8. What is the prognosis for patients with cancer of the nasopharynx? How is prognosis affected by cervical adenopathy? by invasion of the base of the skull? by distant metastases?

BIBLIOGRAPHY

1. ACKERMAN, L. V. and DEL REGATO, J. A. *Cancer: Diagnosis, Treatment and Prognosis*, 4th ed. Mosby, St. Louis, 1970.
2. BACLESSE, F. Les cancers du rhinopharynx. Etude radiographique. Résultats éloignés par la radiothérapie. *Ann Otolaryng* (Paris), 73:509–520, 1956.
3. CANTRIL, S. T., and BUSCHKE, F. J. Malignant tumors of the nasopharynx. A diagnostic blind spot. *West J Surg Obstet Gynec*, 54:494–496, 1946.
4. FLETCHER, G. H. *and* MILLION, R. R. Malignant tumors of the nasopharynx. *Amer J Roentgen*, 93:44–55, 1965.
5. GODTFREDSON, E. Ophthalmologic and neurologic symptoms of malignant nasopharyngeal tumors: Clinical study comprising 454 cases with special reference to histopathology and possibility of earlier recognition. *Acta Otolaryng* (Stockholm), 59:19–323, 1944.
6. KRAMER, S. The treatment of malignant tumors of the nasopharynx. *Proc Roy Soc Med*, 43:867–874, 1950.
7. LEDERMAN, M. *Cancer of the Nasopharynx: Its Natural History and Treatment.* Charles C Thomas, Springfield, Ill., 1961.
8. NEW, G. B. Highly malignant tumors of the nasopharynx and pharynx. *Trans Amer Acad Ophthal Otolaryng*, 36:39–44, 1931.
9. PARKER, R. G. Malignant tumors of the upper airway: Selective use of radiation therapy. *Radiol Clin* (Basel), 33:47–59, 1964.
10. SCANLON, P. W., RHODES, R. E., JR., WOOLNER, L. B., DEVINE, K. D., and MC BEAN, J. B. Cancer of the nasopharynx. One hundred forty-two patients treated in the 11-year period 1950–1960 *Amer J Roentgen*, 99:313–325, 1967.
11. SCHMIDT, M. C. Cancer of the nasopharynx. *Radiology*, 78:751–759, 1962.
12. SMEDAL, M. I., and WATSON, J. R. Treatment of cancer of the nasopharynx with two million volt radiation. *S Clin N Amer*, 39:669–675, 1959.
13. THOMAS, J. E., and WALTZ, A. G. Neurological manifestations of nasopharyngeal malignant tumors. *JAMA*, 192:103–106, 1965.
14. VAETH, J. M. Nasopharyngeal malignant tumors: 82 consecutive patients treated in a period of twenty-two years. *Radiology*, 74:364–372, 1960.
15. VAETH, J. M. Radiation-induced myelitis. In: *Progress in Radiation Therapy*, 3rd ed., F. Buschke, Ed, Grune & Stratton, New York, 1965.
16. WANG, C. C., and SCHULTZ, M. D. Management of locally recurrent carcinoma of the nasopharynx. *Radiology*, 86:900–903, 1966.

CANCER OF THE OROPHARYNX

The oropharynx (mesopharynx) is a chamber common to the digestive and respiratory passages. It extends from the soft palate to the level of the hyoid bone (tip of epiglottis) and is demarcated from the oral cavity by the circumvallate papillae of the tongue, the anterior faucial pillars and soft palate (Figure 8-16). In order of frequency, cancer involves the pharyngeal tongue and valleculae, tonsil, and lateral and posterior pharyngeal walls, including the posterior pillars.[1]

A spectrum of tumor types arises from the oropharyngeal mucosa. The most frequent type is epidermoid carcinoma of less histological differentiation than is common in the oral cavity. These tumors may be deeply infiltrative and ulcerative, or may spread superficially along the mucosa without infiltration of underlying tissue. A variety of epidermoid carcinoma with lymphoid collections in both primary and metastatic sites (lymphoepithelioma, Regaud-Schmincke tumor) may originate from the pharyngeal tongue or tonsil. Lymphosarcomas, which may arise from the abundant lymphoid tissue, especially that in Waldeyer's ring, are most frequent in the tonsil. These tumors are bulky without ulceration, often producing anatomical distortion or even partial obstruction without destruction of adjacent normal structures.

A high incidence of extensive, bulky, cervical adenopathy is characteristic. This adenopathy is often bilateral, especially from tumors primary in the pharyngeal tongue or valleculae.

General Principles of Management

At the time of diagnosis, most primary lesions are large, often crossing the midline, and associated with extensive cervical adenopathy, frequently bilateral. Lymphoepitheliomas and lymphosarcomas frequently metastasize widely "early" in the clinical course. These biological facts contraindicate treatment by surgery.

These tumors are radiovulnerable both at the primary site and in regional nodes. In comparison to cancers of the oral cavity, failure more frequently is due

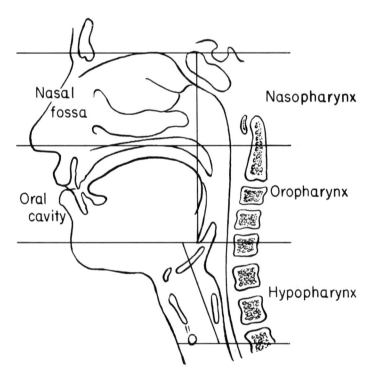

Fig. 8-16.   Anatomical boundaries of the oropharynx.

to distant metastases in the presence of control of the primary site and regional adenopathy. Adequate radiation therapy must include the primary site and regional nodes in continuity. Therefore, external irradiation is necessary. For tumors of the pharyngeal tongue and valleculae, both cervical regions, at least to the clavicle, must be treated. Such radical radiation therapy is accompanied by substantial sequelae. When large segments of the cervical spinal cord are heavily irradiated, radiation myelitis is a rare sequela. Minimization of irradiation of the cervical spinal cord must be a factor in the selection of the technique of treatment.

Cancer of the Pharyngeal (Base, Posterior One-Third) Tongue

The pharyngeal (base, posterior one-third) tongue, posterior to the lingual V (circumvallate papillae), has a different developmental origin and anatomy than the oral (anterior two-thirds, mobile) tongue. The difference in tumor types and biological behavior with consequent differences in clinical course, treatment, and prognosis make separation from cancer of the oral tongue necessary.

Clinical studies of cancer of the pharyngeal tongue have been further confused by arbitrary inclusion of tumors primary in the vallecula or glossopharyngeal sulcus, although separation often is impossible.

The pharyngeal tongue is a muscular structure with an overlying squamous epithelium less differentiated than that of the oral tongue. A large number of sub-, mucosal lymphoid collections make the surface irregular and give origin to tumor types not found in the oral tongue. The pharyngeal tongue is a surprisingly mobile structure (as visualized on cineradiographic study), and limitation of motion by tumor infiltration is the basis of interference with speech and swallowing. The lymphatics of the pharyngeal tongue are independent of the oral tongue, with drainage through the lateropharyngeal wall below the faucial tonsil to subdigastric nodes. This drainage, particularly from tumors located near the midline, may be to the contralateral cervical nodes.

Cancer primary in the pharyngeal tongue usually occurs in males beyond "middle age" and constitutes about one-fourth of all cases of cancer of the tongue. Eighty percent of these tumors are poorly differentiated squamous cell carcinomas, and about 15 percent are well-differentiated epidermoid carcinomas.[5] Lymphoepitheliomas, lymphosarcomas, and adenocarcinomas of the tongue occur infrequently. Epidermoid carcinomas of the base of the tongue may deeply infiltrate the muscles of the tongue so that their true extent is difficult to estimate by clinical examination. The infrequent lymphoepitheliomas and lymphosarcomas are often bulky.[1] In Marcial's series,[5] only 7.5 percent of the primary lesions were less than 3 cm, and only one-third were grossly limited to the pharyngeal tongue, while one-fifth extended to the oral tongue and one-half to the surrounding structures, such as epiglottis, tonsil, and anterior pillar (Figure 8-17).

The primary lesion may be large and yet cause insignificant symptoms until there is ulceration. It may then cause sore throat, dysphagia, pain, or voice change.[2] Because of this silent development, bilateral involvement of deep cervical nodes is commonly found on first examination or represents the presenting symptom of the disease. Cancer of the pharyngeal tongue is second to cancer of the nasopharynx as an undetected source of cervical adenopathy.[4] The primary tumor may be overlooked, even during careful examination for an undetected primary, because on

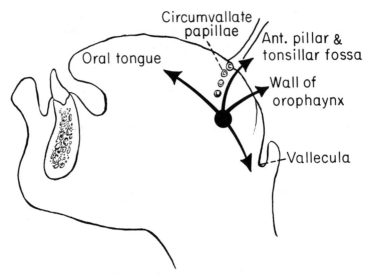

Fig. 8-17.   Routes of direct spread of cancer of pharyngeal tongue.

mirror examination the lesion may be misinterpreted as lymphoid hyperplasia of the lingual tonsil. In these instances the palpable induration may be more impressive than the mirror findings.

Marcial reported cervical adenopathy at the time of initial examination in 80 percent of patients, with bilateral adenopathy in 50 percent.[5] In primary lesions extending to the oral tongue or surrounding structures, the incidence of cervical adenopathy exceeded 90 percent.[5]

Treatment

The primary treatment of cancer of the pharyngeal tongue is external irradiation for reasons previously discussed. Poorly differentiated epidermoid carcinomas, lymphoepitheliomas, and lymphosarcomas, are potentially controllable by radiation therapy, both at the primary site and in the cervical nodes. Radiation treatment must include en bloc the pharyngeal tongue, local extensions, and both sides of the neck to the clavicle.

Results

Even with such aggressive treatment, the majority of primary sites and cervical adenopathies are not controlled, although useful palliation often results. Well-differentiated epidermoid carcinomas are rarely controlled by external irradiation and usually cannot be treated with interstitial methods.

Results reported in the literature have been confusing because of variations of included patients (i.e., extensions to oral tongue, glossopharyngeal sulcus) and treatment methods. Although more aggressive irradiation is now possible with "supervoltage" apparatus, continued application to extensive local primary and regional metastatic disease limits an improved performance.

The overall gross five-year survival rates have been between 10 and 20 percent. However, with more aggressive treatment now possible, Fletcher and MacComb[4] report a five-year survival (Berkson-Gage method) of 32 (±5.8 percent), including a 21 percent survival of 62 patients with cervical adenopathy from epidermoid carcinoma.

Local and regional control of lymphosarcomas is more likely, but death from generalized spread of tumor is frequent (4 of 12 patients survived five years[1]).

Although it is important to separate malignant tumors of the pharyngeal tongue from those of the oral tongue, cancers occasionally "straddle" the intervening junction. These tumors usually are moderately well-differentiated and have a bad prognosis because of infrequent local control and high frequency of lymphatic spread.

Carcinoma of the Vallecula

Carcinomas arising in the valleculae may be more radiocurable than those originating from the mucosa of the neighboring pharyngeal tongue, thus making the differentiation clinically important. These cancers usually spread superficially to the adjacent epiglottis, lateral pharyngeal wall, and tongue rather than infiltrate deeply. Although the cervical nodes frequently are involved, these poorly differentiated carcinomas are radiovulnerable at both primary and metastatic sites.

Carcinoma of the Pharyngeal Wall

Carcinomas of the lateral pharyngeal wall most frequently originate in the lateral portion of the pharyngoepiglottic fold. They may be deeply ulcerated and spread along the pharyngeal wall to involve the epiglottis and pyriform fossa. These tumors usually are poorly differentiated carcinomas associated with extensive, deep mid-cervical adenopathy that may still be controlled by radiation therapy.

Carcinomas of the posterior pharyngeal wall characteristically protrude, and frequently are ulcerated. These may be more radiovulnerable and radiocurable than retropharyngeal carcinomas in the hypopharynx, which occasionally extend into the esophagus.

Reported therapeutic results are scarce. Fletcher and MacComb[4] report a five-year survival rate (Berkson-Gage method) of 32 (±8 percent) of 48 patients. Post-treatment persistence at the primary site is frequent.

Cancer of the Tonsil

Much confusion has resulted from the failure to separate malignant tumors arising in the tonsil and tonsillar bed from those originating in the anterior faucial pillar, for these latter tumors are well-differentiated epidermoid carcinomas which have the characteristics of oral rather than oropharyngeal cancer.

A unilaterally enlarged tonsil in an adult must be considered a malignant tumor until proved otherwise. Biopsy of the usually ulcerated lesion, contrary to prevalent misconception, does not "spread" the disease, and involves much less risk than the delay of observation with or without use of antibiotics. In nonulcerated lymphosarcoma, which can be suspected and usually diagnosed clinically, radiation therapy should follow biopsy.

The majority of malignant tumors of the tonsil and tonsillar bed are poorly differentiated epidermoid carcinomas which usually are firm, exophytic, and ulcerated and may spread superficially to involve the anterior or posterior pillars, soft palate, lateral pharyngeal tongue, and lateral pharyngeal wall (Figures 8-18, 8-19). If there is extensive destruction of the pillar and palate, the origin probably is in those sites rather than in the tonsil. Another source of confusion is the nasopharyngeal tumor which extends inferiorly into the tonsillar fossa and masquerades as a primary tonsillar neoplasm.

Tumor extension to the pharyngeal tongue or lateral pharyngeal wall has serious prognostic implication.[7]

Upper cervical (subdigastric) adenopathy is nearly always present at the time of diagnosis and often is the first clinical finding. Metastatic tumor may progressively involve the submaxillary, deep cervical, and supraclavicular nodes, but may still be controllable by irradiation. Distant metastases, especially to liver and lung, occur in 5 to 10 percent of patients.[6]

Treatment

Radiation therapy requires delivery of moderately high doses to a large tissue volume which includes the primary site and the ipsilateral lymphatic drainage area down to the clavicle in continuity. Thus, treatment can only be delivered with external irradiation, preferably from a supervoltage source. Radium implantation can be used to augment the dosage at special sites, such as residua in the adjacent tongue or pharyngeal wall.

Results

Fletcher and MacComb[4] reported a five-year survival rate (Bergson-Gage method) of 34 ($\pm$6.8 percent) for 66 patients with epidermoid carcinoma of the tonsil. Of 51 patients with adenopathy, 26 percent survived as compared with 62 percent of 15 patients without adenopathy.[4]

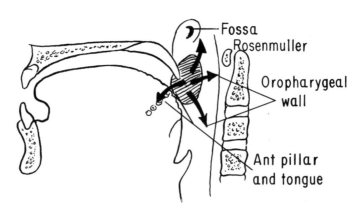

Fossa Rosenmuller

Oropharygeal wall

Ant pillar and tongue

Fig. 8-18.   Routes of direct spread from cancer of tonsil.

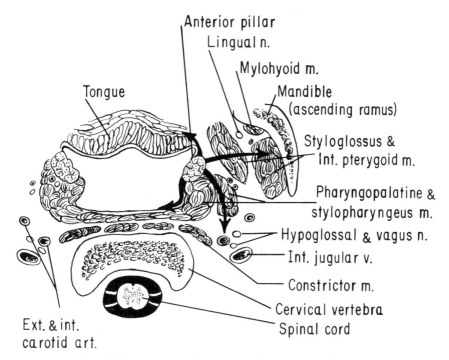

Fig. 8-19.   Routes of direct spread from cancer of tonsil.

Lymphoepitheliomas can be separated as an infrequent type of epidermoid carcinoma having specific histologic characteristics and biological behavior. These tumors create treatment problems similar to those of epidermoid carcinoma, although they have a greater tendency to metastasize widely, particularly to bone.

Lymphosarcoma of the tonsil is much less frequent than epidermoid carcinoma. The highest incidence is between 50 and 60 years of age. The gross appearance of the more common form is sufficiently characteristic for clinical diagnosis. This smooth, spherical enlargement of one tonsil may stretch the anterior pillar. It is more rubbery in consistency than carcinoma. Prior to ulceration, it is painless. This gross appearance may be as characteristic as the histological findings, which sometimes are equivocal and misleading. A less frequent form of lymphosarcoma is ulcerated and spreads along the lateral pharyngeal wall.

Massive cervical adenopathy, often bilateral, is present in most patients at the time of diagnosis. However, because of the rapid growth of lymphosarcomas, rather large primary lesions may be detected prior to the development of palpable regional metastases.

For patients with lymphosarcoma arising in the tonsil, radiation therapy with an external source must include a large volume, including both cervical regions and the primary site, as well as Waldeyer's ring. The effective dosage is close to that required for epidermoid carcinomas. Ennuyer and Bataini[3] reported a collected five-year survival rate of 37 percent (52 of 150 patients) using medium volt x-ray therapy. Most deaths are due to widespread lymphoma, usually without recurrence in the irradiated volume.

REVIEW QUESTIONS

1. What are the anatomical limits of the oropharynx? What structures are included?

2. How do the usual histological types of oropharyngeal cancer differ from cancers arising in the oral cavity? How do these differences affect patient management?

3. What are the differences between cervical adenopathy associated with oropharyngeal cancer and oral cavity cancer? How do these differences influence patient management?

4. Why must carcinomas of the pharyngeal tongue be separated from those of the oral tongue in considering treatment and prognosis?

5. What specific problems compromise treatment and prognosis of patients with carcinoma of the pharyngeal tongue? Why is surgery rarely applicable? Can radiation therapy control the regional adenopathy? How often? Does this vary with tumor type?

6. What confusion results from grouping cancers arising in "the tonsillar region?" What is the embryological origin of the tonsil and tonsillar fossa? What tumor types arise from the tonsil? the anterior tonsillar pillar? What are the differences in associated cervical adenopathy? How do these differences influence patient management?

BIBLIOGRAPHY

1. ACKERMAN, L. V., and DEL REGATO, J. A. *Cancer: Diagnosis, Treatment and Prognosis*, 4th ed. Mosby, St. Louis, 1970.
2. DALLEY, V. M. The place of radiotherapy in the treatment of tumors of the base of the tongue. *Amer J Roentgen*, 93:20–28, 1965.
3. ENNUYER, A., and BATAINI, J. P. Les tumeurs de l'amygdale et de la région velopalatine. Maison et Cie, Paris, 1956.
4. FLETCHER, G. H., and MAC COMB, W. S. *Radiation Therapy in the Management of Cancers of the Oral Cavity and Oropharynx*. Charles C Thomas, Springfield, Ill., 1962.
5. MARCIAL, V. Carcinoma of the base of the tongue. *Amer J Roentgen*, 81:420–429, 1959.
6. MOSS, W. T. *Therapeutic Radiology*, 3rd ed. Mosby, St. Louis, 1969.
7. RIDER, W. D. Epithelial cancer of the tonsillar area. *Radiology*, 78:760–764, 1962.

CANCER OF THE HYPOPHARYNX (LARYNGOPHARYNX)

The hypopharynx is that segment of the digestive tract posterior and lateral to the larynx between the free portion of the epiglottis (hyoid bone) and the mouth of the esophagus (lower border of cricoid cartilage) (Figure 8-20). Malignant tumors, usually poorly differentiated epidermoid carcinomas, arise from the piriform fossae, post-cricoid mucosa, aryepiglottic folds, and posterior hypopharyngeal walls. Baclesse[1] has classified cancer of the hypopharynx into those more favorable lesions arising in the upper (membranous) segment, including the aryepiglottic fold and upper lateral and posterior pharyngeal walls, and those prognostically ominous lesions arising in the inferior (osteocartilaginous) segment, including the piriform sinus, post-arytenoid, and post-cricoid regions, and mouth of the esophagus. In the former group the primary lesion is frequently fungating and bulky. Moss[2] correlates the incidence of adenopathy and the primary site as: free portion of epiglottis and aryepiglottic fold, 68 percent; lateral and posterior pharyngeal walls, 50 percent; piriform sinus, 71 percent and epiesophagus, 44 percent.

There are curious geographic and sex correlations in patients with malignant tumors of the hypopharynx. In France, Italy, and the Mediterranean countries the most frequently involved site is the piriform sinus in men. In the Scandinavian countries post-cricoid carcinoma in women (usually with Plummer–Vinson syndrome) is most frequent. In the Anglo-Saxon countries the incidence is between these extremes.[3]

Carcinomas arising in the *piriform sinus* are the most common of the hypopharyngeal cancers. The primary tumor often is initially "silent," but eventually invades the larynx and/or the thyroid cartilage and often eventually involves the carotid artery (Figure 8-21). Three-fourths of these patients develop midcervical adenopathy, usually unilaterally, and this often is the presenting clinical finding. Permanent control of either primary site or regional adenopathy with radiation or surgery is unlikely. Therefore, there is prognostic importance in separation of these tumors from those frequently curable tumors arising on the aryepiglottic folds.

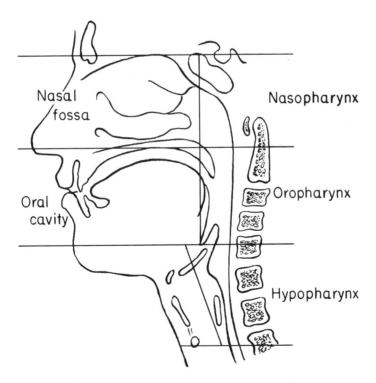

Fig. 8-20.   Anatomical boundaries of the hypopharynx.

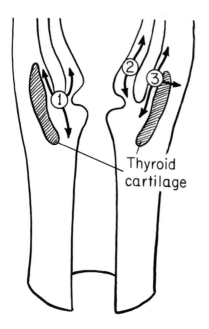

Thyroid
cartilage

Fig. 8-21.   Routes of direct spread from carcinomas of the pyriform sinus.
1.   Base of sinus with extension to subglottic
     region or lateral or medial wall.
2.   Medial wall with involvement of larynx.
3.   Lateral wall with spread to cartilage and
     adjacent soft tissues in the neck.

Carcinomas of the *aryepiglottic fold* are often included with cancers of the larynx. These exophytic primary lesions and their frequent ipsilateral midcervical adenopathy are controllable by radiation therapy or surgery.

Malignant tumors of the *post-cricoid region* usually are moderately to well-differentiated epidermoid carcinomas. They may invade cartilage-containing structures (i.e., larynx or trachea), carotid artery, or jugular vein, and may extend into the cervical esophagus. Cervical adenopathy is frequent. Control by radiation therapy or radical surgery is infrequent. Hypopharyngeal carcinomas of the posterior and lateral walls are similar to the corresponding lesions in the oropharynx, but have a poorer prognosis.

Epidermoid carcinomas of the hypopharynx are infrequently controlled by either radiation therapy or surgery alone. Radiation control of the primary lesion is compromised by destruction of neighboring cartilage-containing structures, poor repair, infection, and edema. Adequate resection usually requires removal of the larynx and pharyngeal wall accompanied by a neck dissection. Such extensive surgery frequently is not applicable. However, since in selected patients tumor control by radical surgery (pharyngolaryngectomy) may be possible after radiation failure, it is important to conduct radiation therapy so that it does not preclude radical surgery. It is important that surgeon and radiotherapist repeatedly re-evaluate these patients during the course of irradiation.

REVIEW QUESTIONS

1.   What are the limits of the hypopharynx? What structures are included?

2.   What is the usual histological tumor type?

3. How does the regional adenopathy vary with primary tumor site?

4. Which cancers of the hypopharynx have the best prognosis with current treatment methods?

BIBLIOGRAPHY

1. BACLESSE, F. Roentgentherapy in cancer of the hypopharynx. *JAMA*, 140:525–529, 1949.
2. MOSS, W. T. *Therapeutic Radiology*, 3rd ed. Mosby, St. Louis, 1969.
3. LEDERMAN, M. Post-cricoid carcinoma. *J Laryng*, 72:397–405, 1958.

CARCINOMA OF THE LARYNX

In 1922, at the International Congress of Otolaryngology in Paris, the French radiotherapist, Henri Coutard, reported 6 patients free of laryngeal cancer following x-ray therapy.[19] These patients, with extensive laryngeal cancer, had been considered inoperable by an outstanding laryngological surgeon. Three of these patients were still free of tumor 16 years after treatment. For the first time it was demonstrated that x-ray therapy had a definite role in the primary, curative treatment of patients with cancer. Therefore, 1922 can be considered the year of birth of modern radiation therapy and the beginning of its slow recognition as a clinical specialty.

Since then, large numbers of patients with laryngeal cancer have been treated in radiotherapy centers throughout the world. Based on this experience, indications have developed for the interrelated use of surgery and radiation therapy in the management of patients with this disease. Wherever equal surgical and radiotherapeutic competence is available, these indications for use are recognized and accepted.

The rationale for treatment of patents with laryngeal carcinoma is based on the biology of the tumor and the anatomical peculiarities of the structures involved.

Anatomy and Tumor Classification

The use of radiation therapy has made obsolete the differentiation between carcinomas of the extrinsic and intrinsic larynx, for the original purpose of this distinction was to separate those cancers limited to the larynx—and thus curable by total laryngectomy—from those extending beyond the larynx. Confusion has resulted from the inclusion of tumors arising from the adjacent pharyngeal mucosa, but involving the larynx. These tumors should be included with carcinomas of the hypopharynx. The following discussion includes only tumors originating from the mucosa of the larynx.

For effective study of the biology of cancer of the larynx, its clinical presentations, and its treatment, supraglottic, glottic, and subglottic divisions must be differentiated (Figures 8-22, 8-23, 8-24). Each division has a different mucosa, submucosa, and lymphatic drainage, and tumors involving each site behave differently.

The *glottis*, or true vocal cord, is covered by well-differentiated squamous epithelium and is devoid of lymphatics.

The *supraglottis,* consisting of laryngeal ventricle, false cord, arytenoid, aryepiglottic fold, laryngeal surface and free border of the epiglottis, is covered by cylindrical epithelium in the young. With aging, much of this cylindrical epithelium is replaced by squamous epithelium. Thus, in the adult, the epiglottis, the aryepiglottic fold and, less consistently, the false cord, as well as the true cord, are covered by squamous epithelium. The mucosa and submucosa are rich in lymphatics.

The *subglottis* arbitrarily extends from the undersurface of the true vocal cord to the lower margin of the cricoid cartilage. The epithelium is a transition from the squamous epithelium of the true cord to the ciliated epithelium of the trachea.

Corresponding to these mucosal and submucosal variations, malignant tumors arising from the true vocal cord nearly always are well-differentiated epidermoid carcinomas which do not spread to regional lymph nodes until they have extended beyond the cord. Malignant tumors arising from the supraglottic and subglottic

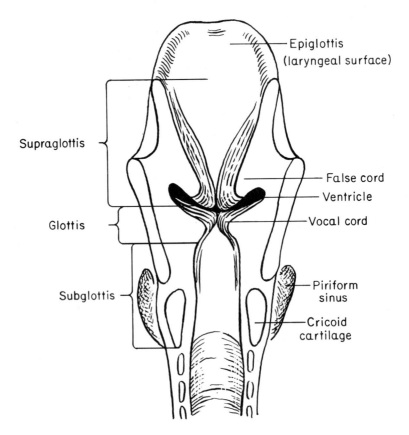

Fig. 8-22.   Anatomical divisions of the larynx.   (posterior view).

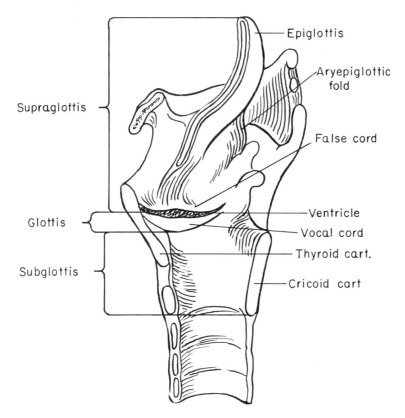

Fig. 8-23. Anatomical divisions of the larynx. (sagittal view).

portions are usually less differentiated, and tend to spread extensively through the regional lymphatics.

The lymphatic drainage of the normal larynx nearly always is into the ipsilateral cervical nodes.[18] The incidence of regional cervical node metastases varies with (1) the primary tumor site (Figure 8-25); (2) the extent of the primary tumor, being of higher incidence with larger tumors, particularly with extralaryngeal

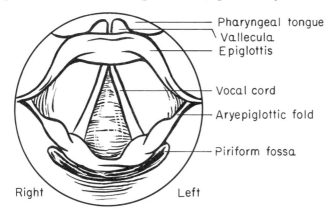

Fig. 8-24. Indirect (mirror) view of the larynx.

extension; (3) the histological differentiation, being of higher incidence with less differentiated tumors; and (4) previous treatment failure which may reflect a biologically more aggressive tumor. The orderly pattern of spread may be disturbed by previous treatment or by metastases themselves.

Tumors of Specific Sites and Their Treatment

Carcinoma of the true *vocal cord* is the most frequent laryngeal cancer.[8, 12] Inasmuch as the true vocal cord does not have a lymphatic drainage, these highly differentiated squamous cell carcinomas do not metastasize to regional nodes until they have extended beyond the cord. This biological curiosity allows careful observation of the response to irradiation without risk of progression of tumor beyond control by surgery. It also permits irradiation of small tissue volumes to high dose with little risk of sequelae.

These carcinomas may extend anteriorly across the commissure, posteriorly to involve the arytenoid, laterally and superiorly to involve muscles and ventricle, and inferiorly to the subglottic region. Extension into adjacent muscle or arytenoid results in limitation of vocal cord mobility. Thus, vocal cord immobility, although it may at times be caused by edema, is a serious prognostic finding.

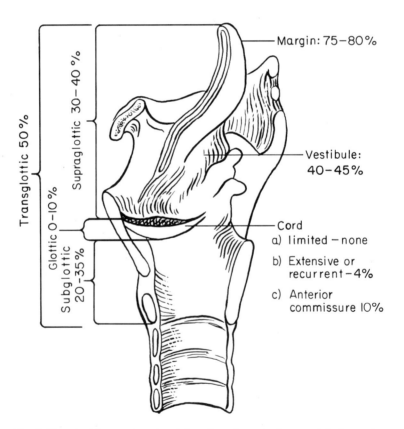

Fig. 8-25.   Incidence of regional lymph node metastases related to primary tumor site.   (After Baclesse,[20] Kuhn et al.,[11] McGavran.[15])

The predominant and often exclusive symptom of vocal cord cancer is persistent hoarseness. Pain, either spontaneous or with manipulation of the thyroid cartilage, is indicative of infection with or without invasion of cartilage by tumor.

The following staging of carcinoma of the glottis (modified after that of Nielsen and Strandberg[17]) has proved useful because the different stages correspond directly to the magnitude of the necessary surgical procedure and therefore to the functional result following surgery as compared with radiation therapy.

The staging proposed by the American Joint Committee on Cancer Staging and End Results Reporting (1962)[1] includes all laryngeal cancers. Inasmuch as the problems of glottic, supraglottic and subglottic cancers are different, separate staging for glottic carcinomas is helpful to the clinician.

Clinical Staging of Carcinoma of the Vocal Cord

Stage I (Figure 8-26):

> The carcinoma involves the anterior two-thirds of one vocal cord (or less), does not extend into the anterior commissure and does not extend to the arytenoid. The cord mobility is normal. There is no palpable cervical adenopathy.
>
> *(This tumor can be controlled equally well by radiation therapy or cordectomy, but the quality of voice is better following radiation therapy.)*

Stage II (Figures 8-27, 8-28):

> The carcinoma involves one or both vocal cords and the anterior commissure. The cord mobility is normal or only slightly reduced. There is no palpable cervical adenopathy.
>
> *(Radiation therapy is almost as effective as for Stage I carcinomas, while the necessary surgery is laryngectomy.)*

Stage III (Figures 8-29 to 8-31):

> The carcinoma extends to the arytenoid, the vestibule or the subglottic region. The vocal cord is fixed. There is no palpable cervical adenopathy.
>
> *(The prognosis is reasonably good with total laryngectomy. Radiation therapy is likely to fail, but in selected situations may be tried with laryngectomy reserved for treatment failure.)*

Stage IV (Figure 8-32):

> The carcinoma is extensive within the larynx and/or extends beyond the anatomic limits of the larynx. The vocal cord is fixed. Cervical adenopathy is palpable and presumed to be tumor-related.
>
> *(These patients are not curable by radiation therapy. Surgery if applicable, may have to be pharyngolaryngectomy. Planned preoperative irradiation may be worth a trial.)*

When epidermoid carcinomas are limited to the anterior two-thirds of a normally movable vocal cord (no involvement of anterior commissure or arytenoid), either radiation therapy or limited resection (cordectomy) can control the tumor

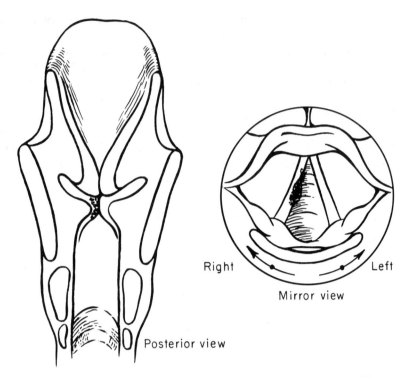

Right   Left

Mirror view

Posterior view

Fig. 8-26. Stage I Glottic Carcinoma.   Tumor limited to anterior ⅔ of a freely movable vocal cord.

Table 8-6.   Vocal Cord Cancer, Stage I
(Operable by Partial Resection)
(Treated by Radiation)

| Source | 5-year Survival Rate | |
	Absolute	Determinate
Schultz (1963)	78/88 (89%)	78/88 ? (89%)
Robbins (1963)	60/73 (82%)	60/65 (92%)
Sheline (1958)	24/30 (80%)	24/26 (92%)
Nielsen (1944)	15/16 (94%)	15/15
Schall (1945)	12/13 (92%)	12/13 ? (92%)
Lederman (1951)	10/12 (83%)	10/12 ? (83%)
Lenz (1947)	6/7 (85%)	6/7 (85%)
Garland (1952)	6/6	6/6
Cantril, Buschke (1952)	5/6 (83%)	5/5
Leborgne (1948)	4/4	4/4
Evans (1952)	3/3	3/3
Parker (1965)	3/3	3/3
Total	226/261 (86%)	226/247 (91%)

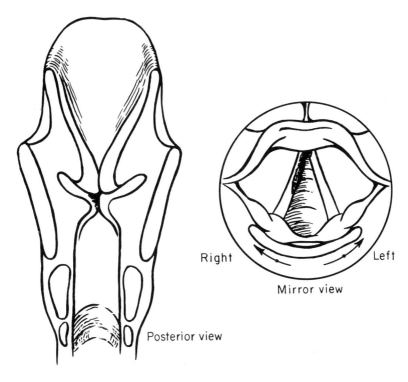

Fig. 8-27. Stage II Glottic Carcinoma. Tumor limited to anterior ⅔ of one vocal cord and the anterior commissure. Vocal cord motion normal or slightly impaired.

Right

Left

Mirror view

Posterior view

in at least 90 percent of patients (Table 8-6). However, the voice is better following radiation therapy, being normal in 80 percent[7] and useful in the rest.

The overall cure rate for these limited tumors can be improved by resection of lesions uncontrolled by primary irradiation. In the past, resection in heavily irradiated tissue has usually meant laryngectomy. However, partial resections (cordectomy) have been accomplished without difficulty in the irradiated larynx,[3,7,10] and with the use of modern "tissue-sparing techniques"[3] partial resections will be performed with increasing frequency. This treatment policy of primary radiation therapy followed by resection of failures has resulted in overall tumor control in more than 95 percent of patients with carcinoma of the true cord, Stage I, with maximal preservation of laryngeal function (Table 8-7).

Table 8-7. Vocal Cord Cancer, Stage I and II
(Surgical Treatment of Radiation Failures)
(Cord limited lesions)

Source	Failures R. T.	Surgical Attempts	Control 5 yrs.	Overall 5-year Survival Rate
Schultz (1963)	10/88 (11%)	8	7	85/88 (96.5%)
Nielsen (1937)	5/66 (7%)	?	2	63/66 (95.4%)

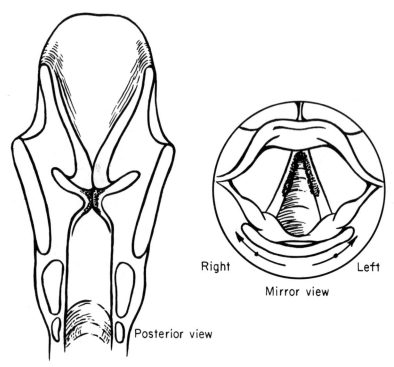

Right Left

Mirror view

Posterior view

Fig. 8-28. Stage II Glottic Carcinoma. Tumor limited to anterior ⅔ of both vocal cords and the anterior commissure. Vocal cord motion normal or slightly impaired.

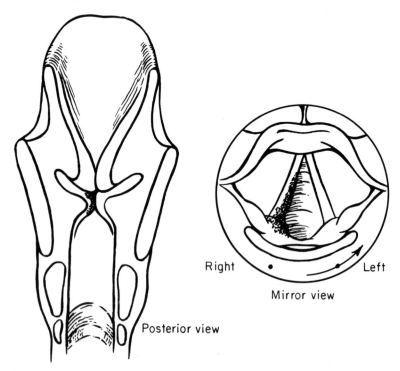

Right Left

Mirror view

Posterior view

Fig. 8-29. Stage III Glottic Carcinoma. Tumor extends to the arytenoid. Vocal cord fixed.

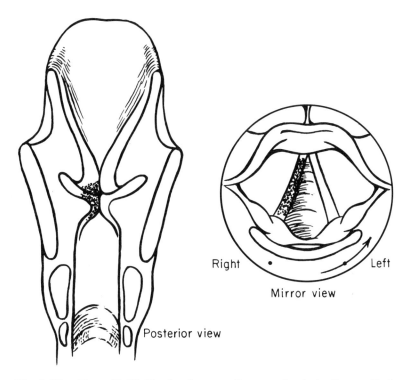

Fig. 8-30. Stage III Glottic Carcinoma. Tumor extends to the vestibule. Vocal cord fixed.

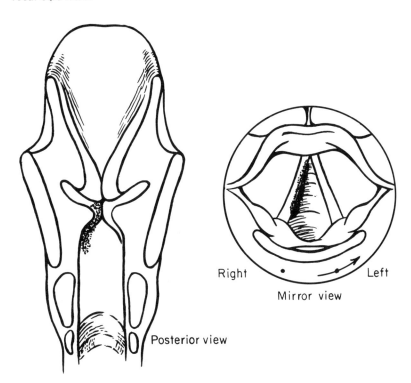

Fig. 8-31. Stage III Glottic Carcinoma. Tumor extends to subglottic region. Vocal cord fixed.

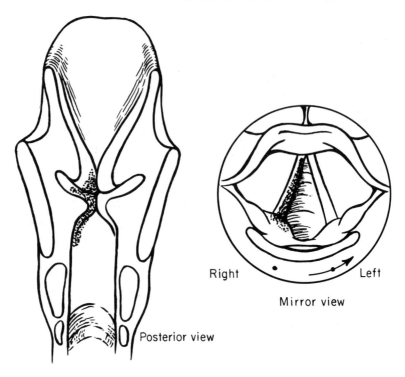

Fig. 8-32. Stage IV Glottic Carcinoma. The tumor is extensive within the larynx (involves arytenoid, vestibule, and subglottic regions) and/or extends beyond the anatomic limits of the larynx. The vocal cord is fixed. The adenopathy is palpable and presumed to be tumor-related.

Carcinomas limited to the posterior third of the true vocal cord, although infrequent, deserve mention. These lesions often are not amenable to cordectomy. In our experience, if cord mobility is unimpaired, radiation therapy is as effective as it is for cancer involving the anterior vocal cord.[6,24] Vaeth[24] reported three-year control of 7 of 8 lesions restricted to the posterior one-third of a movable cord, whereas the single failure was controlled by laryngectomy. When arytenoid mobility is decreased, the effectiveness of radiation therapy is reduced. Lenz[14] controlled 2 of 3 with partial fixation and 4 of 21 with complete fixation.

When the carcinoma involves one movable cord and the anterior commissure (Stage II), the effectiveness of primary irradiation is not compromised[6,21,22,24] (Table 8-8). Inasmuch as resection need be more extensive, usually total laryngectomy, the functional preservation possible with radiation therapy should be exploited. Likewise, the effectiveness of radiation therapy remains high when carcinoma involves both movable vocal cords with or without involvement of the intervening anterior commissure (Stage II)[6,24] (Table 8-9).

When the motion of the cancer-bearing vocal cord is impaired (Stages II and III), the effectiveness of radiation therapy is reduced (Table 8-10). Primary laryngectomy provides a higher incidence of tumor control. However, 40 to 50 percent of these tumors can be controlled by irradiation.[4] If laryngectomy is reserved for those larynxes not reverting to grossly normal appearance by three months after

Table 8-8. Vocal Cord Cancer, Stage II
(Involvement of One Cord & Anterior Commissure)

Source	5-year Survival Rate	3-year Survival Rate
Lenz (1941)	2/3 (absolute)	
Wang & Schultz (1963)	22/27 (determinate) 81%	
Nielsen (1951)	26/31 (absolute) 84%	
Vaeth (1965)	—	10/11* (absolute) 90%
Parker (1965)		
Cord movable	2/2	4/4
Cord motion impaired	—	1/2
Cord fixed	—	0/0

*Failure controlled surgically.

Table 8-9. Vocal Cord Cancer, Stage II
(Both Cords & Anterior Commissure)

Source	5-year Survival Rate
Lenz (1947)	2/3
Robbins (1954)	16/21 (absolute) 76%
Vaeth (1965)	6/9* (absolute) 67%
Parker (1965)	1/1

*One failure controlled surgically.

irradiation, the overall incidence of control will compare with primary laryngectomy, but at least 4 of 10 larynxes will be preserved (Table 8-11).

Thus, radiation therapy is of particular value for all patients with Stage II and for some with Stage III glottic carcinomas because a policy of primary irradiation, with reservation of surgery (laryngectomy) for radiation therapy failures, results in tumor control comparable to that of primary laryngectomy without added treatment-produced complications and with preservation of many larynxes.

If the true vocal cord is fixed by extensive tumor, especially if there is extension to adjacent structures or adenopathy, radiation therapy is ineffective, and primary resection is indicated. Even though an infrequent cancer of this description may slowly resolve and be controlled by irradiation, the potential risk of the escape of tumor from possible surgical control makes deferment of laryngectomy for a trial of radiation therapy highly questionable.

Table 8-10. Vocal Cord Cancer, Stage III
(Impaired Motion)
(Primary Radiation Therapy)

Source	5-year Survival Rate	
	Absolute	Determinate
Robbins (1960)	20/47 (43%)	20/40 (50%)
Wang & Schultz (1963)	33/78 (42%)	33/67 (49%)

Table 8-11.   Vocal Cord Cancer
(Operable by Laryngectomy)
(Primary Radiation Therapy)

Source	No. Patients	% Total Patients	Radiation Therapy	5-year Survival Rate (Absolute) Laryngectomy	Total
Cutler (1944)	48	30%	25/48 (52%)	—	52%
Harris (1954)	50	43%	28/50 (56%)	—	56%
Lederman (1951)	200	68%	64/200 (32%)	23 (12%)	44%
Nielsen (1951)	78	32%	33/78 (42%)	13 (17%)	59%
Sheline (1958)	43	34%	30/43 (67%)	1 (2%)	69%
Cantril, Buschke (1952)	36	62%	14/36 (38%)	5 (13%)	51%
Total	455		194/455 (42%)	42 (9%)	51%

Malignant tumors of the *supraglottis (vestibulum)*, usually epidermoid carcinomas of slight to moderate histological differentiation, often involve several structures, i.e., epiglottis, aryepiglottic fold, ventricular band, and ventricle, by the time of diagnosis and have a high incidence of regional adenopathy.

Carcinomas arising from the free border and laryngeal surface of the *epiglottis* are often exophytic, partially filling the airway and making visualization of the endolarynx difficult. Anterior extension through the epiglottic cartilage into the pre-epiglottic space is frequent and ocasionally may be palpable and visible between the upper margin of the thyroid cartilage and the hyoid. Anatomical distortion from such anterior tumor extension may be visualized by lateral radiographs exposed with "soft tissue technique" (Figure 8-33). At the time of recognition, most carcinomas of the epiglottis (incidence 30[15]–80 percent[11]) are accompanied by sizable regional (upper anterior cervical) adenopathy.

The common clinical indications of this type of epiglottic carcinoma are hoarseness and dyspnea, either of which may appear suddenly. In contrast to the constant hoarseness caused by carcinoma of the vocal cord, hoarseness associated with epiglottic carcinomas may vary with tumor extent and edema. Pain is infrequent even with extensive tumor.

These bulky, exophytic tumors of the epiglottis (or aryepiglottic fold) are suitable for irradiation,[5,21] and the regional adenopathy, often bilateral, can be controlled in a majority of patients. The results are compiled in Table 8-12.

Carcinoma of the epiglottis may present in another form, as an infiltrating, ulcerative lesion. The dominant symptom is pain aggravated by swallowing. Even if controlled by radiation therapy, cartilage necrosis is probable and slough of at least a portion of the epiglottis is likely. Loss of the free portion of the epiglottis is of no functional consequence. However, if the base of the epiglottis and adjacent tissue are involved, serious problems with impairment of laryngeal mobility and nonhealing necrosis may be aggravated by irradiation.

Data of results of radiation therapy of carcinomas of the *aryepiglottic fold* or arytenoid are scarce. Robbins[20] reported control of 2 of 5 limited lesions and 3 of 10 advanced lesions associated with extension into the hypopharynx and

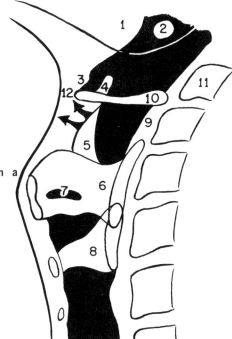

Fig. 8-33. Laryngeal anatomy as seen on a lateral projection x-ray.
1. Pharyngeal tongue
2. Mandible
3. Vallecula
4. Tip of epiglottis
5. Aryepiglottic fold
6. Thyroid cartilage
7. Ventricle
8. Cricoid cartilage
9. Prevertebral soft tissue
10. Hyoid
11. Cervical vertebra
12. Pre-epiglottic space

regional adenopathy. Lederman[13] controlled 5 of 19 lesions of the aryepiglottic fold. Lenz[14] controlled 3 of 11 lesions involving the epiglottis and aryepiglottic fold.

Carcinomas arising in the *false cord* usually do not alter the voice (hoarseness, quality change) until they extend to involve the arytenoid. Edema is frequent, resulting in anatomical distortion, intermittent dyspnea from encroachment on the airway, and frequent failure to identify tumor by biopsy. In these circumstances

Table 8-12. Cancer of Epiglottis
(Radiation Therapy)

Source	Site	5-year Survival Rate
	Posterior Surface	
Robbins (1960)		10/14
Parker (1965)		1/1
	Tip	
Robbins (1960)		2/2
Parker (1965)		1/1
	Extensive	
Robbins (1960)		3/54
	Unclassified	
Nielsen (1951)		5/10

it may be necessary to obtain multiple biopsies to establish the diagnosis. Sizable regional adenopathy is frequent.

Carcinomas arising in the lateral *ventricle* are quiescent until tumor extension results in encroachment on the airway, alteration of the adjacent false cord, or tumefaction in the neck. Regional adenopathy is frequent.

Cancers of the ventricle and false cord are epidermoid carcinomas of moderate histological differentiation, usually are locally extensive at the time of diagnosis, occasionally invade adjacent cartilage, and frequently are associated with regional adenopathy. Tumors involving the ventricle and false cord may be considered together, for neoplasm frequently involves both at the time of diagnosis, and separate data are not available. Robbins controlled 6 of 7 lesions without palpable adenopathy and 2 of 3 advanced local lesions with regional adenopathy.[20]

There is a diversity of opinion among experienced radiotherapists concerning the effectiveness of irradiation of carcinoma involving the *subglottic* mucosa. Many believe that radiation therapy rarely is effective for these tumors. Schulz[22] states that such therapeutic faintheartedness is "another one of the myths which have crept into our therapeutic scripture." Such differences in opinion may result from a variation in concept. There may be a difference in biological behavior between epidermoid carcinomas originating on the vocal cord and extending to minimally involve the adjacent subglottic mucosa and those tumors primary in the subglottic mucosa extending superiorly to involve the cord. The latter extend submucosally, invade cartilage and ulcerate, and rarely are suitable objects of radiation therapy. McGavran et al.[15] believe that most subglottic cancers originate on the vocal cords and thus are the less ominous lesions which can be controlled by irradiation. A range of reported results is listed in Table 8-13.

Technique of Radiation Therapy

In few malignant tumors treated with radiation is meticulous technique so important. This has been documented for a long time and yet is ignored by many. Carcinomas of the vocal cord were cured by irradiation before there was any physical measurement of dose. Dr. Coutard and his disciples depended on the biological response assessable by direct visualization. The control of cord-limited cancers has not noticeably improved with quantitative and qualitative specification of radiation

Table 8-13.   Cancer Involving Subglottic Region (Radiation Therapy)

Source	5-year Survival Rate (absolute)
Lenz (1947)	1/3 (33%)
Schultz (1957)	7/13 (53%)
Lederman (1951)	3/10 (30%)
Robbins (1963)	7/20 (35%)
Nielsen (1951)	1/10 (10%)
Total	19/56 (34%)

dosage and development of modern photon generators, although tissue tolerance has improved.

Often it is not appreciated that the techniques of treatment for lesions limited to the cord and for those originating in the supraglottic or subglottic regions are different. Since carcinomas that have not extended beyond the true cord do not metastasize to nodes, very small tissue volumes can be treated to high doses. This requires daily control by an experienced radiotherapist. In contrast, lesions originating in supra- or subglottic mucosa or extending into this mucosa need treatment fields sufficiently large to include the ipsilateral cervical nodes.

Although it is possible to adequately treat these patients with orthovoltage x-ray (Coutard used even more archaic equipment), better quality radiation and adequate protraction of daily treatment (i.e., 800 rads per week in five equal increments) permit treatment without significant morbidity. Previously, massive mucosal reactions, which were considered necessary for tumor response, caused greater morbidity than cordectomy. It now has been documented that such reactions can be avoided without jeopardizing tumor control.[3, 25]

The potential benefit of "tissue-sparing" apparatus can be realized only through adherence to long-established treatment principles. Many surgeons have documented that resections can follow competently administered radiation therapy. This includes cordectomy,[5, 7, 10] laryngectomy,[5, 26] and laryngopharyngeal resections with node dissections.[9] The sucess of such ventures depends upon the competence of both radiation therapist and surgeon, the extent of the tumor, the presence of residual tumor, and the post-irradiation interval. However, such sucess is not entirely recent, for Nielsen[16] reported post-orthovoltage irradiaton laryngectomies without an increase in the incidence of fistulas in 1951.

Although concepts are subject to change, several absolute contraindications to radical radiation therapy persist: (1) lack of professional competence; (2) involvement of thyroid or cricoid cartilage by tumor, necrosis, or infection; (3) extensive subglottic carcinoma with ulceration and cartilage invasion; (4) arytenoid fixation by tumor; (5) previous unsucessful radical radiation therapy.

Complications and Sequelae of Radiation Therapy

During the early years of radiation therapy of patients with laryngeal carcinoma, when medium voltage x-ray was the best available and when our knowledge of the time-dose relationship and tissue tolerance was still insufficient, complications were frequent. The most dreaded complications were laryngeal edema and necrosis of cartilage. Today with correct indications for treatment and with adequate technique, such complications can be avoided.

Radiation-produced changes are related to (1) the skill of the therapist, (2) the extent of the tumor, (2) concurrent or pre-existing laryngeal disease, and (4) previous treatment.

No sophistication of physical dosimetry or development of treatment apparatus can supersede frequent, careful examination of the patient by the radiotherapist so that treatment can be adjusted to the individual response.

Sequelae of radiation therapy can be correlated with dose-time-volume relationships. Disproportionately high dosage, short overall treatment time, large daily increments, and large irradiated tissue volumes will be followed by unnecessary complications. Fletcher and Klein[7] recorded a 7 percent incidence of edema or necrosis with irradiation of large tissue volumes (35 to 40 sq cm fields) to 5,000+ rads in four weeks—6,000+ rads in 5½ weeks. Over half of these sequelae subsided with conservative management, but 2 percent eventually required tracheostomy and laryngectomy. For many years we have treated limited carcinomas of the vocal cord with a protraction and quality of radiation that avoided a visible mucositis.[3, 25] If comparable to other clinical situations, patients so treated should have few, if any, late sequelae. As Lederman has emphasized, patients who do not have trouble during treatment usually will not have late complications.[13]

REVIEW QUESTIONS

1. What are the three anatomical divisions of the larynx? What structures are included in each division? What are some anatomical differences that have significance in the biological behavior and consequently the management of cancer involving these structures?

2. What are the common symptoms and signs of carcinoma of the epiglottis? How do these differ from the symptoms and signs of vocal cord cancer? What is the incidence of regional adenopathy in patients with cancer of the epiglottis? Is this adenopathy likely to be bilateral? Are these cancers radiocurable?

3. How do cancers of the false cord or ventricle present clinically? Why are these tumors usually locally extensive when discovered?

4. What is the usual clinical presentation of patients with cancer limited to the vocal cord? Is regional adenopathy frequent? Why? Why is loss of normal mobility of the vocal cord an important prognostic indicator?

5. What is your understanding of subglottic carcinoma? How are these tumors diagnosed?

6. What is the major advantage of radiation therapy in the management of patients with laryngeal cancer? What are the disadvantages?

7. What is the expected incidence of control of carcinoma limited to the vocal cord? How is this performance altered by restriction of cord mobility? by extension across the anterior commissure?

8. List four absolute contraindications to radical radiotherapy of laryngeal cancer. What are some contraindications to surgery?

9. Why should carcinomas limited to a normally mobile vocal cord be irradiated in a small tissue volume?

10. What are some complications of radiotherapy of laryngeal cancer? What factors alter this incidence of treatment-produced complications?

BIBLIOGRAPHY

1. American Joint Committee on Cancer Staging and End Results Reporting, 1962.
2. BACLESSE, F. Carcinoma of the larynx. *Brit J Radiol*, Suppl. 3, 1949.
3. BUSCHKE, F., and VAETH, J. M. Radiation therapy of carcinoma of the vocal cord without mucosal reaction. *Amer J Roentgen*, 89:29–34, 1963.
4. CANTRIL, S. T. Radiation therapy in cancer of the larynx: A review. *Amer J Roentgen*, 81:456–474, 1959.
5. CANTRIL, S. T. Radiation therapy in cancer of the larynx. *Amer J Roentgen*, 83:17–20, 1960.
6. FLETCHER, G. H. Personal communication, 1965.
7. FLETCHER, G. H., and KLEIN, R. Dose-time-volume relationships in squamous cell carcinoma of the larynx. *Radiology*, 82:1032–1042, 1964.
8. FOXEN, E. H. M. Endolaryngeal carcinoma: A survey of 206 cases. *J. Laryng*, 71:787–799, 1957.
9. GOLDMAN, J. L., and SILVERSTONE, S. M. Combined radiation and surgical therapy for cancer of the larynx and laryngopharynx. *Trans Amer Acad Ophthal Otolaryng*, 65:496–507, 1961.
10. HARRIS, W., SILVERSTONE, S. N., and KRAMER, R. Roentgen therapy for cancer of larynx and laryngopharynx: Twenty years' experience. *Amer J Roentgen*, 71:813–825, 1954.
11. KUHN, A. J., DEVINE, K. D., and MACDONALD, J. R. Cervical metastases from squamous cell carcinoma of the larynx. *Laryngoscope*, 67:169–190, 1957.
12. LEDERMAN, M. The classification and staging of cancer of the larynx. *Brit J Radiol*, 25:462–471, 1952.
13. LEDERMAN, M. Place of radiotherapy in treatment of cancer of the larynx. *Brit Med J*, 1:1639–1646, 1961.
14. LENZ, M. Roentgen therapy in cancer of larynx. *JAMA*, 139:117–121, 1947.
15. MCGAVRAN, M. H., BAUER, W. C., and OGURA, J. H. The incidence of cervical lymph node metastases from epidermoid carcinoma of the larynx and their relationship to certain characteristics of the primary tumor. *Cancer*, 14:55–66, 1961.
16. NIELSEN, J. Functional results and permanence of cure following roentgentherapy of intralaryngeal carcinomas. *J Fac Radiol*, 3:29–34, 1951.
17. NIELSEN, J., and STRANDBERG, O. Roentgen treatment in cancer of the larynx. *Acta Radiol*, 23:189–208, 1942.
18. PRESSMAN, J. J., SIMON, M. B., and MORRELL, C. M. Anatomic studies related to dissemination of cancer of the larynx. *Cancer*, 14:1131–1138, 1961.
19. REGAUD, C., COUTARD, H., and HAUTANT, A. Contribution au traitement des cancers endolaryngés par les rayons-X. X Congrés International d'Otologie, Paris, 19–22, Juillet, 1922.
20. ROBBINS, R. Indications for radiation therapy in laryngeal cancer. *Amer J Roentgen*, 83:21–24, 1960.
21. ROBBINS, R. Personal communication, 1965.
22. SCHULTZ, M. D. Personal communication, 1965.
23. SHELINE, G. E., and STONE, R. S. Carcinoma of the larynx. *Ann Otol*, 67:1066–1073, 1958.
24. VAETH, J. M. Personal communication, 1965.
25. VAETH, J. M., and BUSCHKE, F. Radiation therapy of carcinoma of the vocal cord without mucosal reaction. *Amer J Roentgen*, 97:931–932, 1966.
26. WANG, C. C., and SCHULZ, M. D. Cancer of the larynx. Its management by radiation therapy. *Radiology*, 80:963–972, 1963.

CANCER OF THE NASAL FOSSA AND PARANASAL SINUSES

Malignant tumors arising in the mucosa of the nasal fossa and paranasal sinuses constitute less than 1 percent of all cancer in the human. Familiarity with the pathology, clinical course, and treatment however is essential for any physician assuming responsibility for these patients, because the patient's fate usually depends on initial management.

Although a broad histological spectrum of tumor types is common to both nasal fossa and paranasal sinuses, and both sites may be involved in any patient, distinct differences in anatomy, biological behavior of tumor, and clinical presentation require separate discussions of tumors primary in each site.

Nasal Fossa

It is essential to determine whether tumors occupying the nasal fossa originate in the mucosa or extend from the adjacent paranasal sinuses, nasopharynx, oral cavity, or skin.

Clinical Presentation

Malignant tumors primary in the nasal fossa usually occur in older males (average 60 years; males 2:1).[13]

Patients with these tumors present with unilateral nasal obstruction, abnormal nasal discharge, bleeding, and, when the tumor is extensive, pain.

Tumor Types.　　Most malignant tumors originating in the nasal mucosa are *epidermoid carcinomas* of varying degrees of differentiation. Two major types of tumor can be distinguished grossly: (1) Bulky, exophytic, polypoid lesions which may grow rapidly and cause unilateral nasal obstruction as the presenting symptom. These tumors may be very radioresponsive both at the primary site and when metastatic to regional nodes. (2) Ulcerating, deeply infiltrating carcinomas which may involve any part of the mucosa or mucocutaneous junction.

Well-differentiated epidermoid carcinomas must be distinguished from squamous cell papillomas, for the latter should be treated surgically.

Lymphosarcomas may rapidly obstruct the nasal fossa. Mucosal ulceration is not frequent. Regional and distant lymph nodes often become involved.

Malignant melanomas may be bulky with consequent obstruction, discharge, and bleeding.

Esthesioneuroepitheliomas (olfactory neuroblastomas) are rare tumors arising from the olfactory mucosa. They may obstruct the nasal fossa, invade local structures, and metastasize via lymphatics or blood vessels.[2]

Other malignant tumors, infrequently seen, are *plasmacytoma, sarcoma,* and *adenocarcinoma* of mucous or salivary gland origin.

Spread of Tumor (Figure 8-34).　　Primary malignant tumors of the nasal fossa spread by direct extension to the maxillary and ethmoid sinuses and nasopharynx; to retropharyngeal, submaxillary, cervical, and, occasionally, to distant nodes; and infrequently via the blood stream.

Treatment

Radiation therapy is the anatomically conservative treatment method. Thus, when comparably effective, it has advantage over surgery. Well-differentiated epidermoid carcinomas can be treated effectively by local irradiation or resection. With extensive or less differentiated epidermoid carcinomas, the advantages of radiation therapy should be exploited. Regional (retropharyngeal, cervical) metastases to lymph nodes from poorly differentiated tumors can be controlled by irradiation.

Surgery is preferable for the treatment of adenocarcinomas of mucous or salivary gland origin and melanoma, although, if these lesions are not resectable, local irradiation to high dosage often proves beneficial.

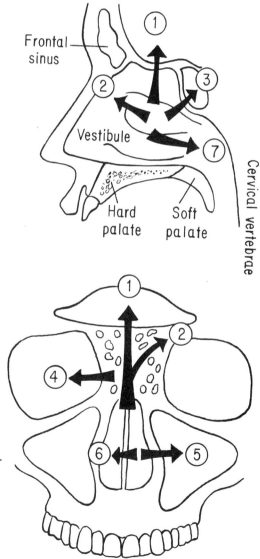

Fig. 8-34. Routes of Spread of Malignant Tumors of Nasal Fossa.
1. Anterior cranial fossa
2. Ethmoid sinuses
3. Sphenoid sinus
4. Orbit
5. Maxillary sinus
6. Other nasal fossa
7. Nasopharynx

Treatment Results and Prognosis

The importance of separating tumors primary in the nasal fossa from tumors arising in adjacent sites, but involving the nasal fossa, is documented in our series,[13] in which only 2 of 14 patients died of uncontrolled epidermoid carcinoma primary in the nasal fossa, a survival incidence far better than for patients with cancers primary in the paranasal sinuses or nasopharynx.

Adenocarcinomas of mucous or salivary gland origin may recur locally, often after a long interval. Malignant melanomas rarely are permanently controlled, but may respond sufficiently for palliation.

Plasmacytomas may be controlled locally. Ennuyer et al.[8] reported control of 6 of 14 patients at 5 years, and Lindberg[11] reported radiation-produced control of 3 patients over 5 years. However, appearance of tumor at other sites is frequent even after long intervals (a 13-year interval in a patient in our series).

Olfactory esthesioneuroblastomas apparently require aggressive treatment for local control.[2, 11] There are no data from a series of adequately radiation treated patients followed for long periods.

Paranasal Sinuses

Nearly all malignant tumors primary in the paranasal sinuses arise from the mucosa of the maxillary sinus. A few tumors arise in the ethmoid sinuses, and these structures often are involved by extensions of tumor primary in the maxillary sinus. Primary tumors of the sphenoid and frontal sinuses are very rare.

Patients may be of a wide age range (30 to 84 years, with an average of 55 years)[5] and usually are males (3:2).[5]

Clinical Presentation

A knowledge of the complex anatomy of the paranasal sinuses is basic to an understanding of the symptoms and signs produced by tumor. Clinical recognition usually follows extension of tumor from these bone-encased, pneumatic cavities (Figure 8-35). Thus, at the time of diagnosis, most patients have "locally advanced" cancer with bone destruction, infection, and involvement of adjacent vital structures. Inasmuch as many of these patients die with locally uncontrolled tumor without distant spread, the effectiveness of available treatment, surgery and radiation therapy, turns on diagnosis before the tumor is so extensive. This will require a high level of suspicion of every persistent or unilateral or unusual change in the sinuses, with consequent frequent direct exploration. X-ray examination rarely is diagnostic until there is bone destruction, and such an appraisal almost uniformly underestimates tumor extent.

Carcinoma primary in the maxillary sinus may obstruct the ostium, with consequent symptoms and signs of sinusitis.

Clinical findings related to tumor extension may be characteristic and predictable, based on the anatomy. The following discussion is based on that of Bunting.[4]

The maxilla is cone-shaped with the apex formed by the zygomatic process, and the base by the nasal wall. The maxillary sinus has three walls: anterolateral, post-

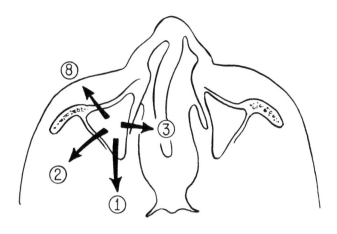

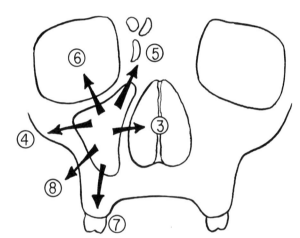

Fig. 8-35. Routes of Spread of Carcinoma of Maxillary Sinus.
1. Pterygopalatine fossa
2. Infratemporal fossa
3. Nasal fossa
4. Zygoma
5. Ethmoid sinuses
6. Orbit
7. Alveolus and palate
8. Cheek

erolateral, and medial. The maxilla has frontal, zygomatic, palatal, and alveolar processes.

The anterolateral wall forms the anterior alveolar process and transmits the infraorbital nerve. Tumor extension in this region may produce swelling and anesthesia of the cheek.

The posterolateral wall forms the anterior margin of the infratemporal fossa (superior dental vessels and nerves) and the pterygopalatine fossa (sphenopalatine ganglion and maxillary nerve). Tumor extension here may produce trismus and even temporal swelling. Further extension in the pterygopalatine fossa may involve the base of the skull.

The roof of the antrum is the floor of the orbit. Destruction of this thin bony partition may result in proptosis, fixation of the globe, diplopia, or corneal ulceration.

Superior-medial extension involves the ethmoid sinuses, lying between the orbit and the nasal cavity.

Extension of tumor medially into the nasal fossa may produce unilateral obstruction, discharge, and bleeding. Superiorly, involvement of the nasolacrimal duct may cause epiphora.

The palatal process of the maxilla forms part of the floor of the nasal fossa and the hard palate. The maxilla also forms the alveolar process so that the roots of several teeth (canine to third molars) may communicate with the sinus. Consequently, tumors may produce toothache, loosening of the teeth, and distortions of the hard palate and gingivobuccal sulcus.

Pathologic Findings

A broad spectrum of histological tumor types include epidermoid carcinoma (40–50 percent), transitional cell carcinoma, lymphoepithelioma; adenocarcinoma, lymphosarcoma and rarely plasmocytoma.

Metastases usually involve regional (cervical, retropharyngeal, preauricular) nodes, but may spread to distant nodes or distant sites through the bloodstream. The incidence of recognized distant spread has increased in our series[5] as control of the primary tumor has increased.

Classification by Site and Extent

Ohngren[12] attempted to estimate the behavior and prognosis of malignant tumors of the maxillary sinus based on their site and extent. The least ominous were anterior-inferior-medial tumors, the worst, superior-posterior-medial tumors. Those tumors of anterior-inferior-lateral or superior-posterior-lateral sites were considered of intermediate aggressiveness. Ohngren's "malignancy plane," extending from the inner canthus to the angle of the mandible, separated anterior-inferior tumors, considered of moderate malignancy, from posterior-superior tumors, considered more malignant.

Baclesse[1] used x-ray studies to divide maxillary sinus cancers into those of the infrastructure, those of the suprastructure, those of the endosinus, and those of the maxillary-ethmoid region. He divided ethmoid tumors into an anterior group extending into the frontal-nasal angle, a central group extending into the nasal fossa, and a posterior group extending into the sphenoid.

Although when tumors can be accurately classified they may conform to Ohngren's predictions,[12] application of such classifications has had serious limitations because of the frequency of extensive tumor[5,7] and inadequate definition by standard methods of evaluation.

Treatment

Carcinomas arising in the maxillary sinus characteristically become extensive locally prior to the detection of regional or distant metastases.[16] Therefore, currently available local treatment methods, surgery and radiation therapy, may be curative if local tumor control is accomplished.

The use of radiation therapy should be selective, relating to tumor type, extent, and general condition of the patient.

Surgery is the mainstay of treatment for the most frequent tumor type, moderate to well-differentiated epidermoid carcinoma, as well as for adenocarcinoma. Preoperative irradiation probably improves the incidence of local tumor control[6, 10] and may favorably alter some tumors so they may become removable by maxillectomy.

Many of these patients will not be candidates for maxillectomy because of tumor extent (across the midline, into the pterygopalatine fossa) or because of their poor general health. Tumor in a few of these patients may be controlled by radiation therapy, but usually palliation is a welcome accomplishment.

Poorly differentiated carcinomas, lymphomas and lymphoepitheliomas and plasmocytomas can be controlled by radiation therapy both at the primary site and in regional nodes. This high level of local control (12 of 15 in our series)[5] in patients often dying of disseminated tumor makes the morbidity of radical resection unnecessary.

Treatment Technique.   Modern, high energy equipment (^{60}Co, ^{137}Cs, linear accelerator) is essential because a high radiation dose usually is required for tumor control; bone surrounds and usually is involved by the primary tumor; collimation of the radiation beam is necessary to reduce dosage to adjacent vital structures, i.e., eyes, brain stem.[14]

When the roof of the maxillary sinus is involved, the orbit must be treated with consequent high risk of eye problems. This risk has prompted many to advocate orbital exenteration. However, with protection of the cornea, many patients retain use of the irradiated eye for the duration of their lives.[15] This corneal protection must be done with care, for superior extensions of the sinus and tumor also may be "protected."[4]

Prior to irradiation of the maxillary sinus, it is essential that adequate, dependent drainage be established surgically. This requires a sizable opening through the hard palate, for Caldwell-Luc and nasal fossa fenestrations rarely continue to function. Since instituting this time-honored basic surgical principle about 1948, our patients' tolerance to radical radiation therapy has been much better. This opening also allows adequate visual assessment of response to treatment, and may continue to serve for many years of follow-up examination.

Except for those patients to be treated by maxillectomy with or without neck dissection, irradiation of the regional lymphatics should be considered in the treatment planning, for metastases from radiosensitive primary tumors can be controlled.[5, 7]

As in the management of patients with other cancers, a critical part of the treatment technique is the cooperation between surgeon and radiotherapist, starting with the initial pretreatment evaluation and persisting throughout treatment and the follow-up period.

Radiation-produced Complications.   Complications of radical radiotherapy are frequent and occasionally are serious because of necessary high dose, bone involvement, and presence of adjacent structures, i.e., eyes, teeth. These include bone necrosis (8 of 47),[5] particularly about the palatal stoma, and eye problems inclusive of conjunctival and corneal irritation and occasional lens change in long-term survivors. In retrospect, in only 2 of 22 of our patients[15] did preirradiation enucleation seem advisable.

Results

Prognosis should be correlated with primary tumor site, tumor extent, condition of the patient, and adequacy of treatment. Patients with limited tumors and tumors confined to the anterior-inferior sinus (Ohngren) apparently fare best with adequate treatment.[5,9] Results of both radiotherapy and surgery have improved with better treatment techniques. However, there are minimal data to document the accomplishments of either. Deeley and Morrison[7] report a three-year survival of 44 percent of 30 patients with carcinoma of the maxillary sinus treated with supervoltage x-ray since 1953. We[5] had 10 survivors from 33 patients with epithelial tumors of the antrum treated with supervoltage x-ray between 1937 and 1957. Seventeen of these 33 primary tumors were controlled. As local tumor control has improved, more patients have died of metastases three to five years following treatment.[5]

Radiotherapy and surgery now can be combined without significantly increased morbidity, and survivals of 40[6] to 45 percent[10] have been reported.

Regional adenopathy, incident to radiation-responsive primary tumors, can be controlled by vigorous irradiation, as reported by Deeley and Morrison,[7] who succeeded in 3 of 7 patients.

A major contribution of radiation therapy is relief of tumor-produced problems, i.e., pain, bleeding, proptosis, in more than 50 percent of patients who eventually die with uncontrolled cancer.

REVIEW QUESTIONS

1. What are the reasons for separating cancer of the nasal fossa from cancer of the paranasal sinuses? Is this always possible? Why?

2. What histological types of tumor arise from the mucosa of the nasal fossa? from the paranasal sinuses? from the nasopharynx?

3. What is the basic advantage of radiation therapy in the treatment of patients with carcinoma of the nasal fossa?

4. Which paranasal sinus is most frequently affected by cancer?

5. Can you relate the likely clinical presentation to specific extensions of tumor from the maxillary sinus? What clinical presentation is likely to lead the patient to the ophthalmologist? to the dentist? to the otolaryngologist? to the neurologist?

6. When tumors arise in the anterior-inferior part of the maxillary sinus, is the prognosis better or worse than for tumors arising postero-superiorly? How often can such an estimate of primary site be made at the time of diagnosis?

7. For which tumor type in the maxillary sinus is surgery the most useful? What is the operation of choice? How often is this possible? What are the limitations?

8. In what situations is radiation therapy useful for patients with cancer of the maxillary sinus?

9. Why are the complications of radiation therapy more frequent than for treatment of most major cancers? How can these complications be minimized?

10. What is a representative tumor-free survival incidence for patients with carcinoma of the maxillary sinus with use of current treatment? How can this be improved?

11. On standard roentgenographs of the paranasal sinuses, cancer frequently is not suggested as a diagnosis until there is evidence of bone destruction. What other x-ray findings should arouse suspicion of cancer? Considering the anatomical configuration of the paranasal sinuses, what x-ray examinations might be most sensitive in documenting destruction of bone?

BIBLIOGRAPHY

1. BACLESSE, F. Les épithéliomes du sinus maxillaire supérieur (à l'excursion de ceux de l'ethmoide et des fosses nasales). Importance de la classification topographique. Résultats éloignés obtenus par roentgenthérapie seule. *Bull Cancer* (Paris), 36:277–284, 1949.
2. BECKER, M. H., and JACOX, H. W. Olfactory esthesioneuroepithelioma. Experiences in the management of a rare intranasal malignant neoplasm. *Radiology*, 82:77–83, 1964.
3. BOONE, M. L. M., HARLE, T. S., HIGHOLT, H. W., and FLETCHER, G. H. Malignant disease of the paranasal sinuses and nasal cavity. Importance of precise localization of extent of disease. *Amer J Roentgen*, 102:627–636, 1968.
4. BUNTING, J. S. Anatomical influence in megavoltage radiotherapy of carcinoma of maxillary antrum. *Brit J Radiol*, 38:255–260, 1965.
5. CANTRIL, S. T., PARKER, R. G., and LUND, P. K. Malignant tumors of the maxillary sinus. Correlative study of clinical, anatomical and pathologic aspects of supervoltage roentgentherapy *Acta Radiol* [*Ther*], 58:105–128, 1962.
6. DALLEY, V. M. Malignant disease of the antrum. *Brit J Radiol*, 32:278–285, 1959.
7. DEELEY, T. J., and MORRISON, R Treatment of malignant disease of nasal sinuses by supervoltage radiotherapy. *J Laryng*, 77:43–49, 1963.
8. ENNUYER, A., BATAINI, P., HELARY, J., and CHAVANNE, G. Les plasmacytomes de voies aérodigestives supérieures. A propos de 248 cas dont 19 traités à la Fondation Curie. *Ann Radiol* (Paris), 6:741–768, 1963.
9. JESSE, R. H. Preoperative versus postoperative radiation in treatment of squamous carcinoma of paranasal sinuses. *Amer J Surg*, 110:552–556, 1965.
10. LARSSON, L., and MARTENSSON, G. Carcinoma of the paranasal sinuses and the nasal cavities. *Acta Radiol* [Ther.], 42:149–172, 1954.
11. LINDBERG, R. Unusual tumors of the head and neck. *Radiology*, 86:1090–1095, 1966.
12. OHNGREN, L. G. Malignant tumours of the maxillo-ethmoidal region. *Acta Otolaryng* (Stockholm), Suppl. 19, 1933.
13. PARKER, R. G. Carcinoma of the nasal fossa. *Amer J Roentgen*, 80:766–774, 1958.
14. PARKER, R. G., WOOTTON, P., and BURNETT, L. Dosage to important sites in radiation therapy of tumors about the head and neck. *Amer J Roentgen*, 90:240–245, 1963.
15. PARKER, R. G., BURNETT, L. L., WOOTTON, P., and MCINTYRE, D. J. Radiation cataract in clinical therapeutic radiology. *Radiology*, 82:794–798, 1964.
16. WINDEYER, B. W., and WILSON, C. P. Tumors of nose and nasal sinuses. In: *British Practice in Radiotherapy*. E. R. Carling and B. W. Windeyer, Eds, Butterworth, London, 1955.

CANCER OF THE THYROID

The availability of radioactive iodine stimulated a renewed interest in cancer of the thyroid gland. Quickly recognized therapeutic limitations of ^{131}I unfortunately have obscured a potentially significant contribution of external beam irradiation to the care of these patients.

Assessment of the treatment of patents with thyroid cancer is difficult because of the infrequency of tumor, the broad spectrum of tumor types, the extremely variable natural history of these cancers, and the multitude of therapeutic applications.

Cancer of the thyroid is more frequent in females and in those over 40 years. There are special problems in the young host, in whom the course usually is long and indolent; and in the elderly host, in whom the course usually is short and violent.

The actual incidence of thyroid cancer is uncertain (approximately 1 percent of all cancer[16]), for there are very real problems of diagnosis related to the frequently long, innocuous biological course and the resemblance of well-differentiated follicular carcinomas to normal thyroid and small cell carcinomas to lymphoma. In a recent autopsy study,[22] in 90 of 193 patients, thyroid cancer had been unsuspected prior to death. The risk of cancer is greatest for patients with a nontoxic, "single" nodule (10–20[4]), and is progressively less for patients with nontoxic nodular goiter, toxic nodular goiter, and toxic diffuse goiter. The reported incidence in nodular goiter has varied widely (2[26,29]–25 percent[8]).

The etiological relationship of irradiation of the anterior neck of infants to the development of thyroid carcinoma has been of interest and concern. Although direct proof of cause and effect is lacking, strong circumstantial evidence includes a higher incidence of irradiation in the histories of patients with thyroid cancer[32] and a higher incidence of thyroid cancer in those patients irradiated.[3,15] Cancers arise in previously irradiated thyroids after a mean interval of about 10 years, shorter for those under 6 years and longer for those over 11 years.[18] The interval between irradiation and diagnosis and the incidence of thyroid cancer are dose-related.[18,25] This risk of radiation-induced thyroid carcinoma should be eliminated in current practice, for there is no indication for irradiation of benign conditions in the neck and upper chest of children.

Anatomical Relationship

The clinical presentation, treatment planning, and often the course have close relationship to the regional anatomy. The thyroid gland is in intimate relationship to the overlying skin and soft tissue, trachea, esophagus, recurrent laryngeal nerve, carotid artery, and jugular vein (Figure 8-36). Regional lymphatic spread may be unilateral or bilateral involving midline nodes, nodes adjacent to the jugular vein, or nodes in the anterior superior mediastinum (Figure 8-37).

Clinical Presentation

The most common finding is a nodule or mass in the thyroid (85 percent[6]). Many patients have noted a recent change in a goiter present for many years. A

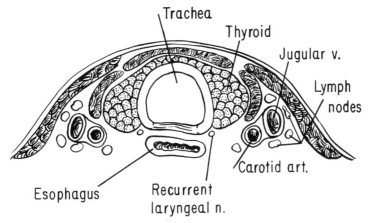

Fig. 8-36. Anatomical relationships of the thyroid gland. Transverse section of the neck at the level of the third tracheal ring to show relationship of thyroid gland to important adjacent structures.

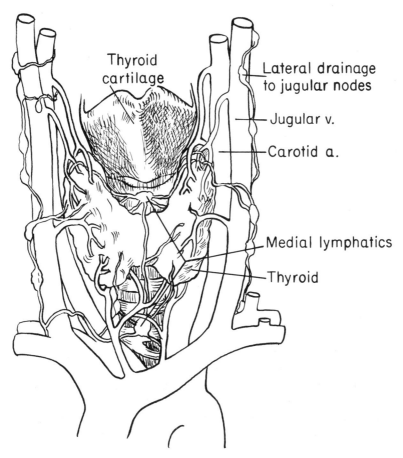

Fig. 8-37. Lymphatic drainage of thyroid gland.

feeling of local pressure, hoarseness, local pain, bleeding, and partial airway obstruction usually indicates local invasion by undifferentiated thyroid cancer. Symptoms and signs, even initially, may be related to metastases, i.e., pain from bone involvement, dyspnea, or cough from pulmonary involvement. The diagnosis frequently is established only when the thyroid cancer is extensive.[30] Small, localized thyroid carcinomas often are unsuspected during life.[22]

The differential diagnosis includes benign thyroid nodule, thyroiditis, and metastasis.

Pathology and Classification

The plethora of schemes for classifiying cancer of the thyroid incriminates each for its shortcomings. Classifications based on structure vary from the simple, such as that proposed by Windeyer,[30] to the detailed, as proposed by Warren and Meissner.[28] The highly variable biological behavior was the basis of the classification of Frantz.[11]

The system used here will suffer the shortcomings of simplicity.

I. Differentiated carcinomas

   A. Papillary adenocarcinoma
   B. Follicular adenocarcinoma
   C. Mixed type of adenocarcinoma

II. Undifferentiated carcinoma

   A. Giant cell carcinoma
   B. Small cell carcinoma (diffuse and compact)
   C. Cuboidal cell carcinoma
   D. Mixed type of carcinoma

III. Miscellaneous malignant tumors

   A. Hürthle cell carcinoma
   B. Epidermoid carcinoma
   C. Lymphoma
   D. Fibrosarcoma
   E. Metastatic tumor

Approximately 75 percent of all thyroid carcinomas are differentiated[28] and have long life histories.[11]

Papillary adenocarcinoma, the most frequent type of thyroid cancer, often arises in young hosts, including children; progresses slowly; may be multicentric, frequently metastasizes to regional lymph nodes; infrequently spreads through the blood vessels and rarely takes up ^{131}I in useful quantity.

Follicular (alveolar) adenocarcinoma is less frequent, varies from the well-differentiated form resembling normal thyroid except for vascular invasion to a poorly differentiated form; usually progresses slowly, but on occasion may kill rapidly; usually spreads through the blood stream and in differentiated form takes up [131]I.

Undifferentiated carcinomas are pleomorphic with cells described as small (diffuse or compact), cuboidal, spindle-shaped, spheroidal, or giant in form. This type of cancer is most frequent in the older patient and often is rapidly growing with local infiltration of adjacent tissues and structures and widespread hematogenous and lymphatic metastases leading to early death (25 percent dead within one month and 50 percent dead within four months of their first visit[13]).

Primary epidermoid carcinoma of the thyroid is rare (less than 1 percent of thyroid cancer[28]), and little is known of its biologic behavior.

The Hürthle cell is considered an altered thyroid epithelial cell.[28] Foci of these cells may be found in any type of thyroid cancer. Little is known of the behavior of malignant tumors primarily composed of Hürthle cells.

Fibrosarcomas arising from thyroid stroma are rare, but might behave as they do elsewhere.

Lymphosarcomas arising in the thyroid are rare and would require differentiation from diffuse small cell carcinomas, which might be more locally aggressive and less responsive to irradiation.

Metastases to the thyroid are rare, being found in less than 2 percent of 1,000 autopsies on patients with cancer.[1] Metastases usually arise from breast and lung cancers.

A former concept of "lateral aberrant thyroid" tumors has been discredited. There is evidence that these tumors are metastases from undetected primary carcinomas in the thyroid gland.[5,14,27]

Staging

Treatment planning and prognosis depend on extent as well as type of tumor. The components of clinical (and surgical) staging are:

1. Primary site: Whether the tumor is limited to the thyroid or has invaded beyond the capsule locally
2. Regional lymphatics: Whether the nodes are palpable, fixed, unilateral or bilateral
3. Distant spread:

Treatment

Therapy should be specific for each patient based on the type and extent of tumor and the age and general condition of the patient.

Surgery

Papillary and follicular carcinomas without local extension beyond the thyroid and any regional adenopathy should be primarily removed surgically. However, there is no unanimity of opinion for type or extent of operation. Clark, Ibanez, and White,[7] on the basis of whole organ studies, found cancer in multiple sites within the thyroid in 64 of 80 patients treated for the first time, and thus documented a rationale for complete removal of the thyroid. Frazell and Foote[12] found that 113 of 115 patients with "clincially positive or doubtful" cervical adenopathy had tumor in nodes, whereas 41 of 67 patients without palpable adenopathy had tumor in nodes, thus encouraging routine radical neck dissection. Most of these tumor-bearing nodes were in the mid, lower, and upper jugular chain, but submaxillary, accessory chain, juxtathyroid, and anterior mediastinal nodes also were involved. However, Crile, Suhrer, and Hazard[9] reported that conservative surgery consisting of "complete" local removal of the primary tumor plus removal of grossly involved regional nodes produced excellent results for patients with papillary and follicular adenocarcinomas.

The value of surgery alone for thyroid cancers invading adjacent structures or of surgery of any form for undifferentiated thyroid carcinomas is doubtful.[2,20]

Radiation Therapy

Treatment may be by an external beam, preferably of supervoltage quality, or, when applicable, by use of radioactive iodine (^{131}I). Although the latter has been emphasized in the medical literature, it has benefited only about half of that small proportion (10–15 percent) of patients with carcinomas that retain sufficient isotope to warrant a therapeutic trial.[6] Uptake of therapeutic consequence usually is limited to well-differentiated follicular adenocarcinomas, either in primary or metastatic sites. Well-differentiated papillary and undifferentiated carcinomas rarely take up appreciable amounts of ^{131}I.[17] The uptake of ^{131}I in metastases from thyroid carcinomas may be increased by a prolonged preparation including initial ablation of the normal functioning thyroid gland by surgical removal, or large doses of ^{131}I, followed in about two months by TSH or thiouracil prior to the administration of the therapeutic dose of ^{131}I. A dose of 1μ Ci per gram of tumor has been estimated to deliver the equivalent of 40,000–100,000 rads to the tissue within a few millimeters of the beta ray emitting isotope, while 1 mCi of ^{131}I delivers 1 rad to the blood and the equivalent of 0.5 rad total body dose.[19] Treatment-related complications, which increase with increasing doses of ^{131}I and vary with the site of tumor, include myxedema, bone marrow depression, bladder irritation, reactions in the salivary glands, radiation pneumonitis (with pulmonary metastases), and, on rare occasions, leukemia.[6,19]

All types of thyroid carcinomas may be sufficiently responsive to make external irradiation of the necessary tissue volume, inclusive of the thyroid and adjacent structures and nodes, feasible and worthwhile. Doses of 6,500 rads in six to seven weeks with supervoltage radiation are easily tolerated.

Therefore, the anterior neck, and sometimes the anterior superior mediastinum, should be irradiated postoperatively whenever resection has been incomplete, regardless of tumor type. External irradiation is the primary treatment of choice for patients with undifferentiated carcinomas of the thyroid, especially when local extension is producing problems. Also local irradiation can be an effective palliative agent for relief of problems caused by metastases, particularly to bone.

Medical Treatment

In 1937 T. P. Dunhill[10] wrote that he had found that orally administered desiccated thyroid was effective in controlling well-differentiated thyroid carcinomas, presumedly because of pituitary suppression. This material, in adequate dosage, i.e., 0.20 grams per day, has proved very valuable in long-term suppression of thyroid carcinoma and should be used routinely after definitive treatment.

Results

Cancers localized to the thyroid or even metastatic to regional lymph nodes should be cured by adequate surgery. Thus, using total thyroidectomy plus radical or modified neck dissections in about half the patients, Clark, Ibanez, and White[7] reported that 81 of 94 (86.2 percent) primarily treated patients survived five years, and 25 of 30 (83.3 percent) survived ten years. Crile, Suhrer, and Hazard[9] reported 34 of 39 patients (87.2 percent) living without evidence of carcinoma more than five years after conservative operations (excision of the primary tumor and grossly involved lymph nodes) for papillary adenocarcinoma.

Smedal, Salzman, and Meissner[24] studied 59 patients with differentiated thyroid carcinoma irradiated because of residual tumor after conservative resection. Eight were pure follicular adenocarcinomas, one was a pure papillary carcinoma, and 50 were mixed follicular and papillary carcinomas. Thirty-seven of the 59 patients were alive and well more than five years after treatment, although 9 had died with uncontrolled tumor, and 11 had died of intercurrent disease. Four of the 9 tumor-related deaths were among the 8 patients with "pure" follicular carcinomas. All four had pulmonary metastases. Control improved with use of supervoltage quality radiation and higher doses.

Frazell and Foote[12] reported that 10 of 23 patients with inoperable thyroid papillary adenocarcinoma survived more than five years after radiation therapy. Windeyer[30] found marked regression or disappearance of tumor mass in 10 of 24 patients with papillary adenocarcinoma and noted that doses in excess of 4,000 R were necessary. Sheline, Galante, and Lindsay[21] found that locally persistent papillary adenocarcinoma can remain nondetectable for as long as 25 years after external irradiation.

Windeyer[30] found follicular adenocarcinomas to be less responsive to external irradiation than papillary adenocarcinomas, with appreciable regression in only 4 of 20 patients. Likewise, Sheline et al.[21] found a less consistently favorable response in follicular carcinoma, but 5 of 8 patients survived 5 to 28 years after local irradiation.

In only a small proportion of patients with undifferentiated carcinoma (3 of 57[30]) is total surgical ablation possible. Smedal and Meissner[23] treated 44 patients with undifferentiated thyroid carcinomas with 2 mv x-ray to doses of 4,800 to 6,000 R, and had local control in 28. Both the incidence of local control and the average survival were better for patients with compact small cell, cuboidal cell, or mixed tumors than for diffuse small cell or giant cell tumors. Patients in the favorable groups have lived as long as 10 years, but no patient with giant cell carcinoma has lived longer than 18 months. Windeyer[30] noted definite responses to irradiation in 51 of 93 patients. Sheline et al.[21] had no tumor-free survivors; all 5 patients with giant cell carcinoma died within two months of diagnosis and treatment.

Following various methods of treatment, Winship[31] reported that 17 percent of 334 children with thyroid carcinoma have died with uncontrolled cancer.

However, he cautions that, due to the frequent slow growth of thyroid carcinoma, 20-year follow-up studies are necessary.

REVIEW QUESTIONS

1. Why is it difficult to evaluate the treatment of patients with thyroid cancer?

2. What are the problems of identifying thyroid carcinoma?

3. Which palpable abnormality of the thyroid has the highest correlation with malignant tumor?

4. Should there be any risk of medical radiation-induced thyroid cancer in children? Why?

5. What is the most frequent histologic type of thyroid cancer? What is its usual biological course?

6. Which histological type of thyroid cancer accumulates ^{131}I in therapeutically significant amounts? What fraction of patients with thyroid cancer has been benefited by therapeutic use of ^{131}I?

7. What is a "lateral aberrant thyroid" tumor?

8. When is surgery preferable for patients with thyroid cancer? What are the limitations of the method?

9. What type of operation is appropriate for patients with carcinoma limited to the thyroid?

10. Which radiotherapeutic modality, ^{131}I or external beam, is most frequently beneficial for patients with thyroid cancer? Have you seen a patient so treated?

11. When is external irradiation advisable in the treatment of patients with thyroid carcinoma? How should this use vary with tumor extent? tumor type? age of patient?

12. What is the rationale for using daily dessicated thyroid for patients with thyroid carcinoma?

BIBLIOGRAPHY

1. ABRAMS, H. L., SPIRO, R., and GOLDSTEIN, N. Metastases in carcinoma. Analysis of 1,000 autopsied cases. *Cancer*, 3:74–85, 1950.
2. ACKERMAN, L., and DEL REGATO, J. A. *Cancer: Diagnosis, Treatment and Prognosis*, 4th ed. Mosby, St. Louis, 1970.
3. ARCHER, V. E., and SIMPSON, C. L. Semi-quantitative relationships of radiation and neoplasia in man. *Health Phys*, 9:45–56, 1963.
4. BEIERWALTES, W. H. Treatment of hyperthyroidism and thyroid cancer with ^{131}I. *Northwest Med*, 63:871–877, 1964.

5. BLACK, B. M. Papillary adenocarcinoma of the thyroid gland, so-called lateral aberrant thyroid tumors. *West J Surg*, 56:134–144, 1948.

6. BRISTER, G. H., ALBRIGHT, E. C., JAESCHKE, W. H., and VERMUND, H. Factors influencing survival in 100 patients with thyroid malignancy. *Wisconsin Med J*, 63:111–122, 1964.

7. CLARK, R. L., IBANEZ, M. L., and WHITE, E. C. What constitutes an adequate operation for carcinoma of the thyroid? *Arch Surg (Chicago)*, 92:23–26, 1966.

8. COLE, W. H., MAJARAKIS, J. D., and SLAUGHTER, D. P. Incidence of carcinoma of the thyroid in nodular goiter. *J Clin Endocr*, 9:1007–1011, 1949.

9. CRILE, G., JR., SUHRER, J. G., JR., and HAZARD, J. B. Results of conservative operations for malignant tumors of the thyroid. *J Clin Endocr*, 15:1422–1431, 1955.

10. DUNHILL, T. P. The surgery of the thyroid gland. *Trans Med Soc London*, 60:234–282, 1937.

11. FRANTZ, V. K. Pathology of the thyroid. In: *The Thyroid*. S. C. Werner. Hoeber-Harper, New York, 1955.

12. FRAZELL, E. L., and FOOTE, F. W., JR. Papillary cancer of the thyroid: Review of 25 years of experience. *Cancer*, 11:895–922, 1958.

13. GRAHAM, J. M., and MCWHIRTER, R. Carcinoma of the thyroid. *Proc Roy Soc Med*, 40:669–680, 1947.

14. KING, W. L. M., and PEMBERTON, J. DE J. So-called lateral aberrant thyroid tumors. *Surg Gynec, Obstet*, 74:991–10001, 1942.

15. LATOURETTE, H. B., and HODGES, F. J. Incidence of neoplasia after irradiation of the thymic region. *Amer J Roentgen*, 82:667–677, 1959.

16. LINDEN, G. Cancer of thyroid gland. *Proc Nat Cancer Conf*, 4:671–674, 1960.

17. MARINELLI, L. D., FOOTE, F. W., JR., HILL, R. F., and HOCKER, A. F. Retention of radioactive iodine in thyroid carcinomas: Histopatholgic and radioautographic studies. *Amer J Roentgen*, 58:17–32, 1947.

18. RAVENTOS, A., and WINSHIP, T. The latent interval for thyroid cancer following irradiation. *Radiology*, 83:501–508, 1964.

19. ROSE, R. G., and KELSEY, M. P. Radioactive iodine in diagnosis and treatment of thyroid cancer. *Cancer*, 16:896–913, 1963.

20. SHELINE, G. E. The present status of radiation therapy in carcinoma of the thyroid. In: *Progress in Radiation Therapy*, Vol. I. F. Buschke, Ed, Grune & Stratton, New York, 1958.

21. SHELINE, G. E., GALANTE, M., and LINDSAY, S. Radiation therapy in the control of persistent thyroid cancer. *Amer J Roentgen*, 97:923–930, 1966.

22. SILLIPHANT, W. M., KLINCK, G. H., and LEVITIN, M. S. Thyroid carcinoma and death: Clinicopathologic study of 193 autopsies. *Cancer*, 17:513–525, 1964.

23. SMEDAL, M. I., and MEISSNER, W. A. The results of x-ray treatment in undifferentiated carcinoma of the thyroid. *Radiology*, 76:927–935, 1961.

24. SMEDAL, M. I., SALZMAN, F. A, and MEISSNER, W. A. The value of 2 MV roentgenray therapy in differentiated thyroid carcinoma. *Amer J Roentgen*, 99:352–364, 1967.

25. TOYOOKA, E. T., PIFER, J. W., CRUMP, S. L., DUTTON, A. M., and HEMPELMANN, L. H. Neoplasms in children treated with x-rays for thymic enlargement. II. Tumor incidence as a function of radiation factors. *J Nat Cancer Inst*, 31:1357–1377, 1963.

26. VANDER, J. B., GASTON, E. A., and DAWBER, T. R. Significance of solitary nontoxic thyroid nodules; preliminary report. *New Eng J Med*, 251:970–973, 1954.

27. WARREN, S., and FELDMAN, J. D. The nature of lateral "aberrant" thyroid tumors. *Surg Gynec Obstet*, 88:31–44, 1949.

28. WARREN, S., and MEISSNER, W. A. Tumors of the thyroid gland. Section IV, Fascicle 14, *Atlas of Tumor Pathology*. A.F.I.P., Washington, D.C., 1953.

29. WATT, C. H., and FOUSHEE, J. C. The incidence of carcinoma in nodular thyroids in southwest Georgia. *J Med Ass Georgia*, 40:414–417, 1951.

30. WINDEYER, B. W. Cancer of the thyroid and radiotherapy. Mackenzie Davidson Memorial Lecture. *Brit J Radiol*, 27:537–552, 1954.

31. WINSHIP, T. Carcinoma of the thyroid in childhood. *Pediatrics*, 18:459–466, 1956.

32. WINSHIP, T., and ROSVOLL, R. V. Childhood thyroid carcinoma. *Cancer*, 14:734–743, 1961.

9

TUMORS
OF THE CENTRAL
NERVOUS SYSTEM

Selective therapeutic use of ionizing radiation can benefit many patients with malignant tumors involving the central nervous system. At times treatment may be curative. Even temporary relief of clinical problems may improve the quality of limited survival. Assessment of the past performance of radiation therapy is uncertain, for only a limited number of tumors of a broad biological spectrum have been vigorously treated and followed. The application of radiation has been hindered by difficulties in tumor identification and classification, inadequate anatomical definition of tumor extent, and uncertainty of the radiation tolerance of the central nervous system.

Primary tumors of the brain and spinal cord have unique characteristics which require revision of the usual concepts of malignancy. Histologically, "benign" neoplasms may be "malignant" because of their involvement of a critical structure or growth within a closed cavity with resultant profound physiological change, i.e., obstruction of cerebrospinal fluid and regional pressure changes with secondary gliosis, necrosis, and atrophy. Primary intracranial malignant tumors usually arise from supporting structures of the central nervous system, not from the nerve cells. Thus, more than half of primary intracranial tumors are gliomas. Intracranial tumors may be single or multifocal, but nearly always remain localized to the brain. If metastases occur, they are implanted along the routes of the cerebrospinal fluid, not through lymphatics or blood vessels. Tumor implants in the surgical incision are, for practical purposes, unknown.

Intracranial tumors comprise about 2 percent of all primary malignant tumors in humans.[8] They are disproportionately more frequent in children and adults between 40 and 60 years of age.

Primary intracranial tumors are of broad biological spectrum and involve many sites which have different functions. Each tumor may vary in its composition in different parts and at different times during its evolution. Thus, classification is difficult. In this discussion, a classification suggested by Bailey[1] will be used:

A. Tumors of the encephalon (glioma, neuroma)
B. Tumors of the covering cells (meningioma)
C. Tumors of the hypophysis (pituitary adenoma, craniopharyngioma)
D. Dysgerminomas (pinealoma, chordoma)

190

GENERAL PRINCIPLES OF RADIATION THERAPY OF TUMORS
OF THE CENTRAL NERVOUS SYSTEM

All tumors of the central nervous system are radioresponsive to some degree, ranging from the sensitive medulloblastoma and pinealoma to the minimally sensitive, well-differentiated astrocytoma and well-differentiated meningioma. However, necessary conservation of adjacent normal central nervous system tissue restricts the clinical usefulness of radiation therapy. Misconceptions unnecessarily further limiting the usefulness of radiation therapy persist because of a lack of understanding of tumor biology and radiation tolerance of the central nervous system. Many of the changes in normal central nervous system tissue, i.e., edema and necrosis, often attributed to radiotherapy or surgery, may be produced by tumor growth.[8] Bouchard[8] emphasizes that there are no pathognomonic structural changes produced by irradiation of the central nervous system. Little is known about physiological changes produced by radiation as used clinically, but there is sufficient knowledge of the radiation tolerance of the central nervous system[29, 42, 50] for guidance in clinical radiation therapy. This range of tolerance varies from the less tolerant, radiosensitive brain stem (suggested dose limitation—4,500 rads in five weeks[37]) through the more tolerant sites, i.e., cerebral motor cortex (suggested dose limitations—6,000 rads in six weeks[37]) to the least important and more tolerant sites, i.e., frontal cerebrum (suggested dose limitation—6,000 to 7,000 rads in six to seven weeks[37]). These tolerances are reduced with irradiation of large tissue volumes and reduction of overall treatment times and number of treatment increments.

The management of patients with tumors of the central nervous system is determined by tumor type, location and extent, and, in part, by necessary diagnostic procedures, especially surgery for identification of tumor and decompression of the brain.

Radiation therapy may be used as a complement to incomplete resection (glioblastoma multiforme, some pituitary tumors) or as the primary definitive treatment following biopsy (medulloblastoma), or when the diagnosis must rest on clinical evidence (pinealoma, brain-stem glioma, pituitary adenoma). In contrast to many therapeutic regimens in which preoperative irradiation is preferable, radiation therapy of tumors of the central nervous system usually follows surgery because of the necessity of exploration to establish the diagnosis, define the site and extent, and provide necessary decompression.

Anatomical site and extent of tumor often determine resectability and thus indirectly influence the use of radiation therapy. Surgery is preferable when resection of tumor and adjacent normal tissue will not threaten the patient's life or produce an unjustifiable disability. Thus, resection is indicated for many tumors involving the cerebellum, nondominant temporal or frontal lobes, or even dominant prefrontal or anterior temporal lobe cortex, but it usually is contraindicated for tumors involving the sensory or motor cortex, speech or visual centers, hypothalamus, brain stem, and spinal cord. Radiation therapy is indicated for highly responsive tumors regardless of site, because of the advantage of conserving normal central nervous system tissue; for responsive tumors known to frequently metastasize along the central nervous system axis (medulloblastoma, ependymoma); for sensitive tumors which cannot be resected because of location (brain stem); and for sensitive tumors incompletely resected because of extent and site (glioblastoma multiforme).

Radiation therapy can be started within days following the craniotomy, whenever the patient can cooperate and the wound is healing satisfactorily. Treatment usually lasts several weeks and can be continued on an outpatient basis. Properly administered radiation therapy should not produce clinically significant edema of the central nervous system, neurological deficits, or "radiation sickness." Paradoxically, clinical improvement most likely due to the surgical decompression often appears early during radiation therapy and may be incorrectly attributed to the irradiation.

RADIATION THERAPY OF SPECIFIC TUMORS

Most primary intracranial tumors are *gliomas,* 75 percent being of astrocytic origin.[8] *Glioblastoma multiforme,* the most frequent and most biologically aggressive glioma, usually involves the cerebrum of males 30 to 50 years of age. Many clinicians believe that if a patient with glioblastoma multiforme survives for many years after treatment, the diagnosis was incorrect. In 176 patients treated primarily by liberal, but incomplete, resection followed by vigorous irradiation, Bouchard[8] reported a five-year survival rate of 7 percent. However, he emphasized improvement in the "quality of survival" with a return to "normal life" for most of the duration of survival in 75 percent of patients. If radiation therapy is to be used, it must include a large tissue volume, because of the poorly demarcated, infiltrating tumor. This large tissue volume must be irradiated to substantial dosage, i.e., 4,500 to 6,000+ rads in five to eight weeks.

There is little conclusive evidence that radiation therapy favorably influences the course of well-differentiated *astrocytomas.* Long tumor-free survivals can be related to adequate resection. In infratentorial astrocytomas, common in children, the five-year survival rate may be 75 to 80 percent[33] of those treated surgically.

Oligodendrogliomas constitute about 5 percent of all tumors of the central nervous system and about 10 percent of all gliomas.[26]

The most frequent site of origin is the white matter of the frontal lobes.[26] These tumors may be large and cystic (20 percent[26]) at the time of diagnosis, and the majority may contain calcium (intercellular and vascular) detectable by x-ray. Evaluation of the contribution of radiation therapy, nearly always used after incomplete resection, is difficult because of the infrequency of the tumor, its usually protracted natural history, and lack of comparable groups treated by different regimens. Sheline et al.[44] report an apparent improvement in survival at five years for their patients vigorously irradiated (5,000 rads in 45 to 50 days) after incomplete resection.

Ependymomas are predominantly tumors of children and young adults. Primary tumors may arise from ependymal cells lining the ventricles of the brain, the central canal of the spinal cord, the ventriculus terminalis of the conus medullaris of the spinal cord, or in scattered foci in the filum terminale and cerebral hemispheres.[26] Supratentorial primary tumors have no anatomical site predilection, are less frequent, and have a worse prognosis than infratentorial primary tumors, which usually arise from the floor or roof of the fourth ventricle.[26] Primary tumors may become "large" prior to clinical detection, usually based on symptoms and signs of internal obstruction of cerebrospinal fluid. Almost 60 percent of spinal cord gliomas, particularly those in the lumbosacral region, are ependymomas.[26]

Surgical removal is rarely complete, and such attempts often result in unacceptable operative morbidity and mortality. Many ependymomas respond well to irradiation, and vigorous treatment following partial resection seems instrumental in improved long-term survival rates with minimal treatment-produced neurological sequelae. Phillips, Sheline, and Boldrey[41] submitted evidence that survival rates were dose-related. Thus, 13 of 15 patients receiving more than 4,500 rads in 5 to 6 weeks survived more than 5 years without clinical evidence of tumor. Although their good survival rates persisted at 10 to 20 years post-treatment, recurrences 10 years post-treatment have been reported by Kricheff et al.[28] Those tumors involving ventricular surfaces may "seed" along the cerebrospinal axis. Although the clinical incidence of such "seeding" increases with the thoroughness of the diagnostic search,[43] the possible sequelae secondary to irradiation of the entire central nervous system axis have deterred routine "prophylactic" treatment.

Medulloblastomas are highly malignant tumors comprising about 25 percent of all intracranial tumors in children.[20] In childhood (peak incidence five to ten years[18]), these tumors usually arise in the midline of the cerebellum, whereas in the young adult they may arise from a cerebellar hemisphere or possibly even be supratentorial.[7] Medulloblastoma has the greatest tendency of any intracranial tumor to form implantation metastases intracranially or intraspinally.[12] Differentiation from other malignant intracranial tumors in children, such as ependymoblastomas, oligodendrogliomas,[12] and alveolar sarcomas,[48] may be difficult.

Since medulloblastoma was first defined by Bailey and Cushing in 1925,[2] there was unabated pessimism regarding its prognosis until it was recognized[39] that this tumor, because of its biological behavior, represents a radiotherapeutic problem entirely and that surgery should be limited to biopsy for diagnosis and decompression if necessary. "The evidence suggests that medulloblastoma of the cerebellum may be a curable disease and that cure is possible only with irradiation."[30]

Because of the tendency of implantation of tumor cells transported in the cerebrospinal fluid, it is now generally acepted that treatment, in an attempt to accomplish permanent control, must include both the brain and spinal cord. There is still some difference of opinion whether, in the absence of clinical signs or symptoms indicating cord involvement, the cord should be given the same dose as that given the known primary lesion in the posterior fossa. The rationale accepted by those who suggest a smaller dose to the cord is that disseminated tumor cells that have not been well-established as metastatic foci may be destroyed with smaller doses. This question is important because—apart from the risk of cord damage by high doses of irradiation—one of the difficulties of radical therapy is the effect on the hematopoietic tissue. However, with sufficient protraction of treatment, marrow depression rarely necessitates discontinuation of treatment or significantly alters the anticipated therapeutic course.

Such aggressive treatment must be justified by histological proof of tumor. Whether such proof is best obtained by a limited biopsy procedure[40] or by partial resection with decompression remains unanswered.

Brain damage, possibly caused by late radiation injury, has become clinically manifest in at least 3 of Lampe and McIntyre's first 7 survivors,[30] appearing as late as 7½ years after treatment. From later experiences with more protracted irradiation, it is likely that these sequelae can be minimized. Lampe[30] has suggested that some of the late manifestations of brain damage might be related to the initial hydrocephalus rather than to the irradiation.

Table 9-1. Results of Radiation Therapy in Medulloblastoma

Institution	No. Pts.	Living "Without Tumor" at 3 Yrs.	Living "Without Tumor" at 5 Yrs.	Normal at 5 Yrs.	Technique	
					Dose	Tissue Volume
U. of Michigan[48]						
1938–1950	30	—	6 (20%)	3 (10%)	2,500 R/7–10 days[30]	entire CNS
1950–1958	8	—	5 (62%)	2 (25%)	5,000–6,000 R/55–65 days	entire CNS
1938–1958	38	—	11 (28%)	5 (13%)		
Montreal Neurological Hospital						
1939–1953[9]	41	29.2%	19.5%		4,500–5,000 R/45–50 days[9]	entire CNS
1939–1958[8]	50	36.0%	27%			
Manchester Holt Radium Institute[38]						
1932–1953	31	55%	41%	41% (?)	3,000 R/3 wks.[39] 3,500 R/5 wks.	entire CNS

Considering that until recently medulloblastoma was considered "hopeless," the results of treatment—with adequate dose and inclusion of the entire central nervous system—are encouraging (Table 9-1). Although figures in the individual series are too small to be statistically meaningful, it is certain that a number of children can be saved and will live useful lives. These results contradict such recent statements as: "There is no adequate treatment for medulloblastoma."[18]

Gliomas of the optic nerve and chiasm are uncommon astrocytic tumors (1 percent of brain tumors[25]), usually diagnosed in children. Although the natural history of this neoplasm may be unpredictable, it slowly enlarges, with eventual involvement of the intraorbital and intracranial portions of the optic nerve. Complete surgical removal of the tumor rarely is feasible and results in unilateral blindness.

There is little reported experience with vigorous use of irradiation, but tumor control and even restoration of vision has been attributed to treatment.[49] However, we have noted lack of clinically measurable tumor progression and even intermittent visual improvement for as long as eight years prior to tumor reactivation in untreated patients.

Tumors of the midbrain and brain stem are a specific problem because of location. Tumors of the midbrain involve structures between the posterior third ventricle and the pontine protuberance, and consequently may affect important motor and sensory nerve fibers routed through the pons to the medulla.[8] These tumors are nearly always gliomas, comprising about 15 percent of primary intracranial gliomas.[8] Tumors of the midbrain rarely can be biopsied, so radiation therapy is licensed by clinical diagnosis. Local irradiation often should be preceded by a surgical shunt, which in itself may be a major palliative gesture. Reliable radiotherapeutic experience is sparse. In a group of 37 patients irradiated, Bouchard[8] noted frequent, early clinical improvement, with ultimate survival of 17 patients for more than five years and 7 of 17 patients for more than ten years. Although those patients dying of uncontrolled neoplasm usually had documented gliomas, any diagnostic errors inclusive of benign masses, would likely be in the surviving group.

Brain-stem gliomas are rapidly fatal, if untreated. Histological documentation rarely is available prior to treatment, but an expanding brain-stem lesion with appropriate clinical findings usually is a glioma. Again, useful radiotherapeutic experience is sparse, and diagnostic errors tend to favorably influence the prognosis by inclusion of benign lesions among the survivors. Bouchard[8] reported 8 of 34 patients (30 intensively irradiated) living and well from 5 to 21 years after treatment. Substantial radiation dosage, i.e., 5,000 to 6,000 rads, probably necessary for gliomas, can be safely delivered to the primary site and local tumor extensions, if adequately protracted, i.e., 50 to 60 days.[8]

Following Béclère's first report of the x-ray treatment of *pituitary adenomas* in 1909,[5] radiation therapy became established as the preferable primary treatment method for most of these tumors. This reputation was based on a good performance record, which included a high rate of clinically measured tumor control and avoidance of treatment-produced mortality or significant morbidity. Most of the early recorded experience was accumulated with use of orthovoltage x-ray equipment with its inherent limitations of modest depth doses, selective bone absorption, and production of severe skin reactions with permanent epilation. The resultant inadequate tumor doses and treatment-produced sequelae can now be avoided, but their memory continues to give birth to lasting misconceptions.

The evaluation of treatment results has been hindered by inadequate irradiation (particularly by use of repeated courses with small dosage), occasional diagnostic error, a variability and chronicity of progression of the adenomas, and difficulty of objective measurement of accomplishment. Thus prejudices regarding treatment methods persist, as noted in the 1942 statement of Dyke and Davidoff:[22] "There is some tendency on the part of radiotherapists and neurological surgeons to show preference for their own type of therapy."

Pituitary adenomas are among the few abnormalities in which the therapeutic radiologist has not insisted on pretreatment biopsy proof. This has been reasonable because of a high level of diagnostic performance, at least for chromophobic and eosinophilic adenomas, based on clinical and laboratory findings, and formerly because of a substantial mordibity and occasional mortality incident to surgical exposure of the pituitary. However, improvements in neurological surgery have, for practical purposes, eliminated these risks.

The clinical diagnosis of pituitary adenoma is based on three groups of findings: ophthalmologic signs; roentgenologic changes in the sella; and symptoms and signs of endocrinopathy.

The characteristic ophthalmological changes, most frequent in chromophobic adenomas, are bilateral, temporal quadrant visual field defects. However, visual field changes may be unilateral or more extensive in one eye, or may be bizarre and not diagnostic.

The characteristic sellar enlargement seen roentgenologically may occasionally be associated with other tumors or even with increased intracranial pressure. Conversely, the sella may be of normal appearance despite a pituitary adenoma, as noted by Sosman,[47] in 20 percent of acromegalic patients and in 7 percent of patients with chromoprobic adenomas.

The clinical detection of degenerative cystic change, with or without hemorrhage, recorded in 10 to 40 percent[23,36] of pituitary adenomas is not of high order, resulting in a diagnostic uncertainty of importance, for such changes are the predominant biological cause of failure of radiation therapy.

Another cause of failure of radiation therapy has been the difficulty in clinically identifying craniopharyngiomas masqerading as pituitary adenomas. In the past, when craniopharyngiomas were ineffectively treated, this distinction was of little practical importance. However, the development of effective radiotherapeutic techniques for craniopharyngiomas has made it necessary to identify (often by surgery) pituitary lesions prior to treatment.

Three radiation treatment modalities have been used. The largest experience has been with radiation from an external source (x-ray, gamma ray). "Supervoltage" sources (^{60}Co, accelerator, betatron) have eliminated the inherent limitations of orthovoltage equipment. Necessary doses of 4,500–5,000 rads can be delivered to the pituitary fossa in a single five- to six-week course without difficulty.

Irradiation with heavy particles (alpha particles, protons) has been pioneered by Lawrence and associates.[32] Doses of 10,000 to 12,000 rads delivered in 6 to 11 days have resulted in complete destruction of the contents of the pituitary fossa. Similar results have followed implantation of the pituitary with various radioactive isotopes (radon, yttrium-90). Useful as such pituitary ablation can be in the treatment of patients with widespread, hormone-dependent cancer (breast, prostate), destruction of remnants of normal pituitary associated with benign adenomas is not desirable. The risk of damage to the chiasm, optic nerves, and adjacent structures associated with these procedures makes them contraindicated when conventional procedures (supervoltage radiation therapy), which are safe and effective, are available.

Therapeutic accomplishment must be objectively measured by preservation of vision, hopefully with reversal of recent visual loss, and arrest or favorable modification of glandular dysfunction. Documented data from well-treated patients are not plentiful.

Whereas eosinophilic adenomas may be more radiation-responsive than chromophobic adenomas,[10] currently available techniques allow comparably successful treatment of both.[10,15]

Sheline et al. reported clinical control of 73 percent (8 of 11) of patients with chromophobic adenomas[45] and of 78 percent (14 of 18) of patients with eosinophilic adenomas[46] with use of adequate doses of radiation.

Experience with radiation treatment of basophilic pituitary adenomas has been sparse [21,24,34,47] because of the rarity of the neoplasm and the diagnostic difficulties in separation from nontumorous endocrine disturbances. It would seem that basophilic pituitary adenomas are responsive to doses used in the treatment of other pituitary adenomas. In fact, Cushing's syndrome has been effectively treated with smaller doses to the pituitary.[47] Although only a few will respond to irradiation, a trial may be justified prior to adrenal surgery unless an adrenal tumor has been demonstrated.

Visual field defects from pressure on the optic nerves and chiasm from extra-sellar tumor extension can be reversed with irradiation. Correa and Lampe[15] reported a return to normal visual fields in 20 percent (11 of 55) and improvement in 40 percent (22 of 55) of patients receiving pituitary irradiation. Colby et al.[14] documented that 82.4 percent (28 of 34) of patients with visual impairment of less than one-third improved or their vision remained stationary, and 52.4 percent (11 of 21) of patients with visual field defects greater than two-thirds improved with pituitary irradiation. However, such favorable responses may not be detectable for several weeks after treatment, and improvement may slowly continue for many months. Therefore, immediate surgical decompression is essential if visual field deterioration has been rapidly progressing, or if a major visual defect exists at time of diagnosis and further visual loss would be dangerous. In long-existing visual defects with optic nerve degeneration, treatment of any type cannot produce reversal of the basic nerve damage.

Favorable alteration of endocrinopathy is more difficult to measure. Sheline[46] reported improvement in 77 percent (13 of 17) of those acromegalics receiving doses of over 3,500 rads to the pituitary in a single four- to six-week course, as measured by reversal of skeletal changes, visceral hypertrophy, evidence of hyper-metabolism, decreased carbohydrate tolerance, and elevated blood-serum phosphorus. Correa and Lampe[15] reported regression in 2 and arrest of changes in 17 of 29 acromegalics treated by pituitary irradiation. More sophisticated testing, such as measurement of plasma growth hormone levels,[4] may allow better evaluation in the future.

Results are dose-related. Thus, Correa and Lampe[15] reported "satisfactory" results in 79.3 percent (23 of 29) of patients receiving doses greater than 4,000 rads in a single four- to six-week course, although the performance fell off to 44.4 percent (12 of 27) if the dose was less than 2,500 rads. Sheline[45] found recurrences in patients with chromophobic adenomas in 3 of 5 treated with radiation only and in 6 of 19 irradiated postoperatively with doses considerably less than 4,000 rads, but there were no recurrences in 6 receiving only radiation and in only 1 of 27 irradiated postoperatively with doses exceeding 4,000 rads. Likewise, in the treatment of patients with acromegaly, endocrine hyperactivity and signs of pressure on structures adjacent to the sella were controlled in 26 to 29 percent of patients receiving less than 3,500 rads and in 77 to 78 percent of patients receiving over 3,500 rads.[46]

Biological causes of failure of radiation therapy of pituitary adenomas include intratumor cysts (10 to 40 percent[23, 36]) and hemorrhage; very large tumors (which may invade surrounding vital structures and are more likely to be cystic); rapid tumor growth; and other tumors, i.e., craniopharygioma, masquerading as pituitary adenomas.

The major technical cause of failure is inadequate dosage. This may result from lack of conviction by the therapist, limitations of equipment, or inaccuracy of delivery of radiation to a small target. In the past, the error of an inadequate physical dose frequently was compounded by reducing its biological equivalent through administration in multiple, interrupted courses. This discarded custom of treatment in multiple courses also has been incriminated in the production of unnecessary radiation sequelae.[45, 46]

In an assessment of treatment-produced sequelae, it must be remembered that pituitary adenomas are benign tumors albeit they may produce disastrous effects. Absence of serious sequelae is the hallmark of correctly administered radiation therapy. In Sheline's [45, 46] extensive experience, in no patient could death be attributed to irradiation, and there was no major complication in any patient treated in single, uninterrupted course.

Based on this evidence, the following indications and contraindications for the treatment of chromophobic and eosinophilic pituitary adenomas seem reasonable:

1. Radiation therapy, with a tumor dose of 4,500–5,000 rads delivered in a five- to six-week uninterrupted course, is the primary procedure of choice when the clinical diagnosis seems correct, when visual defects are minimal or more extensive but stationary, and when the endocrinopathy is minimal and not rapidly progressive.

The conclusions of Sheline (therapeutic radiologist) and Boldrey (neurosurgeon)[45] based on an extensive experience were: "With proper patient selection and early operative decompression for the radiation failures, the error in clinical diagnosis presents less risk than the mortality and morbidity of operative intervention. Furthermore, if vision is not severely threatened, there is time to await response to irradiation."

2. Primary surgery is indicated when there is diagnostic uncertainty, when there is rapid visual loss, when there is sizable extrasellar extension of tumor, when there is substantial or rapidly progressive endocrinopathy, and when pituitary irradiation has failed. Vigorous irradiation of the pituitary fossa should follow resection of the gland, when purposely incomplete.

Optimal care for these patients requires the close cooperation of endocrinologist, neurosurgeon, ophthalmologist, and therapeutic radiologist from the time of evaluation for treatment through the long critical period of close post-treatment observation.

Craniopharyngiomas (suprasellar cyst, hypophyseal duct tumor, Rathke's pouch tumor) are primary intracranial growths (comprising 2 to 4 percent of intracranial tumors[8]) arising in the hypophyseal region, usually above the sella. Children with dystrophia adiposogenitalis (Fröhlich's syndrome) frequently are affected. These histolocally benign growths, containing squamous epithelial-lined cysts, are "malignant" by position. Adequate resection nearly always results in unacceptable complications. Although for many years neurosurgeons and therapeutic radiologists considered radiation therapy of little value, Kramer et al.[27] have accumulated evidence that surgery limited to decompression of the cyst followed by vigorous local irradiation (5,000 rads in 5 weeks to 7,000 rads in 7½ weeks) results in long-term clinical control in most patients. With modern techniques such doses can be introduced into a well-defined volume without excessive dose to any single portion of normal brain.

Chordomas are tumors, histologically resembling embryonic notochord, arising from notochordal rests along the vertebral column.[26] The two frequent sites are: basisphenoid, where extension of tumor may involve pons, sellar contents, hypothalamus, or nasopharynx; and sacrococcygeal. Complete resection usually is impossible. Vigorous irradiation, on occasion, may have produced growth restraint in these relentless, but slow-growing tumors.

Pinealomas are infrequent tumors (0.5 to 2.0 percent of intracranial neoplasms[8]), usually arising in children or young adults. Because of prohibitive operative mortality, diagnosis must be established clinically (with a differential consideration of gliomas and cysts of the third ventricle, craniopharyngiomas, and pituitary tumors, extensions from cerebellar tumors[19]).

Symptoms and signs resulting from obstruction of the aqueduct of Sylvius can be relieved by a shunt. These tumors have gained a reputation of being radiosensitive, although the evidence is inconclusive. Useful radiotherapeutic experience is lacking because the diagnosis remains unsubstantiated in most survivors. Most radiotherapeutic failures prove to be tumors other than pinealoma. Spinal cord metastases from primary intracranial pinealomas are sufficiently infrequent (2 of 36 patients[19]) that irradiation of the central nervous system axis seems unnecessary.

Hemangioblastomas and hemangioendotheliomas are true neoplasms usually arising in the cerebellum and growing as a mural nodule in a cyst.[26] Complete surgical removal often is possible. However, recurrent lesions tend to become increasingly vascular, often associated with polycythemia,[17] and more aggressive biologically. Because of the potential malignant character of these tumors, Bouchard[8] recommends postoperative irradiation.

Metastases to the brain affect up to 10,000 patients in the United States annually.[11] The common primary tumor sites are: bronchus (31 to 34 percent); breast (13 to 39 percent); gastrointestinal tract (16 percent); kidney (8 percent); skin (7 percent); and thyroid (4 percent).[11, 13] Metastases account for 4.1 percent[39] to 26.3 percent[16] of brain tumors and are found in about 5 percent of patients with cancer at autopsy.[51] Such metastases are multiple in 70 percent of patients afflicted[51] and are likely to coexist with metastases to other sites. As metastases to the brain usually are multiple, treatment, if indicated, should include the entire brain. Occasionally isolated foci causing incapacitating disability can be selectively treated.

In their series of 218 patients, Chu and Hilaris[13] estimated that 77.8 percent of those completing radiation therapy to the entire cranium benefited by relief of related symptoms and signs, with an average remission of 4.7 months and average survival of 6.6 months. Favorable responses were more frequent with doses exceeding 3,000 rads (250 kvp, HVL of 2.0 mm Cu, method of calculation not stated) delivered in three weeks, and were highly satisfactory with primary cancer of the breast (86 percent) and lung (83.3 percent). Second and even third treatment courses proved successful.

Tumors of the spinal cord and its membranes are similar in type, but different in incidence, when compared with intracranial tumors, probably reflecting differences in the quantity of medullary tissue and cord coverings. About 25 percent of these tumors are extradural, 25 percent are intramedullary, and 50 percent are extramedullary but intradural.[3] In a study of 979 intraspinal neoplasms,[26] the most common tumors were: neurilemoma, 29.9 percent; meningioma, 25.9 percent; and intramedullary glioma, 22.5 percent. The affected sites were: thoracic, 48.5 percent; lumbar, 25.5 percent; cervical, 19 percent; sacral, 6 percent; and multiple, 1 percent.

The usefulness of radiation treatment of spinal cord tumors is poorly defined, for few therapeutic radiologists have had an opportunity to treat even a modest number of affected patients. The indications for radiation therapy depend on tumor type, site and extent, and the resulting clinical problem. Useful clinical guides of the radiation tolerance of the spinal cord are available,[6, 42, 50] although such tolerances may be reduced by local tumor-produced changes.

Intramedullary tumors of the spinal cord usually are ependymomas or astrocytomas, rarely oligodendrogliomas or other types.[26] About 50 percent of spinal cord gliomas arise in the conus medullaris or filum terminale.[26] Initial treatment nearly always is surgical for biopsy, attempted resection, or decompression. Ependymomas may be usefully radioresponsive and possibly radiocurable. Astrocytomas, oligodendrogliomas, and other gliomas nearly always are "low-grade" malignancies, and patients may enjoy long survival periods, regardless of treatment, although vigorous local irradiation may delay or avert tumor-produced problems.[8]

Extramedullary-intradural tumors usually are "benign" (i.e., meningioma, neurinoma, dermoid tumor, lipoma), and radiation therapy has no value. An exception would be the treatment of metastases of medulloblastoma or ependymoma.

Extradural tumors usually are malignant. These may be lymphomas, often extending from adjacent sites, or carcinomatous metastases, most frequently arising from cancer of the breast or lung. The definitive, although palliative, treatment usually is local irradiation. However, if at the time of diagnosis there is progressive or even unmeasured neurological deficit, surgical decompression should precede irradiation, for the reduction of tumor produced by irradiation may be too slow to avoid cord damage from pressure or vascular insufficiency. A possible exception is the use of chemotherapy followed by irradiation for patients with lymphomas. This program, which may avoid laminectomy, requires very careful, frequent neurologic observation of the patient so that surgical decompression can be instituted if there is no rapid, favorable response.

REVIEW QUESTIONS

1. List several unique characteristics of tumors of the brain and spinal cord. What is the clinical importance of each? What is your definition of a "malignant" tumor of the brain?

2. At what ages are intracranial tumors most frequent? Compare the incidence, primary site, and common tumor types in children and adults.

3. What limits the total dose of radiation to the brain? What is the least radiation-tolerant structure in the normal brain? How may this vary when tumor is present?

4. Histological verification of tumor should be a requisite of radiation therapy. In what circumstances may this be impractical in patients with intracranial tumors? If diagnostic errors result from lack of histological verification, how may this affect the results of treatment?

5. What general types of CNS tumors are favorable objects of radiation therapy?

6. When radiation therapy and surgery are combined in the treatment of humans with malignant intracranial tumors, why is the irradiation usually postoperative?

7. Does technically correct irradiation of the intracranial contents produce "radiation sickness" in the human?

8. What is the most likely explanation when a patient with a brain tumor becomes worse clinically within 24 hours after the first treatment? When he suddenly becomes worse clinically after two weeks of treatment?

9. What is the most frequent intracranial tumor? Does it arise from nerve cell or supporting tissue? List several examples of this general tumor type.

10. What is the objective of radiation therapy for patients with glioblastoma multiforme? How can this be measured?

11. What gliomatous tumors are radio curable?

12. What are the advantages of supervoltage radiation therapy of pituitary adenomas? What are the disadvantages? What is the clinical tumor control rate? What are the causes of failure?

13. How is pituitary adenoma diagnosed clinically? What is the accuracy of such diagnosis? What are the likely sources of error?

14. When should surgery have preference over radiation therapy in management of patients with pituitary adenomas? Why?

15. Until recently, craniopharyngiomas were considered "radioresistant." Now there is evidence that these tumors can be controlled by irradiation. Why has this attitude changed? Have you seen such patients? How were they treated?

16. What malignant tumors most frequently metastasize to the brain? Are these patients

ever curable? Except for attempts to relieve a suddenly appearing neurological defect, why is treatment of a single metastasis in the brain usually ill-advised?

17. What are the similarities and differences of tumor types affecting brain and spinal cord?

18. What part of the spinal cord is most frequently involved?

19. How would you manage a patient with sudden clinical appearance of spinal cord deficit secondary to tumor? What if these changes occurred in a patient with lymphosarcoma?

20. Why is it difficult to accurately assess the potentials of radiotherapy of patients with CNS tumors based on past performance?

BIBLIOGRAPHY

1. BAILEY, P. *Intracranial Tumors*, 2nd ed. Charles C Thomas, Springfield, Ill., 1948.
2. BAILEY, P., and CUSHING, H. Medulloblastoma cerebelli: A common type of midcerebellar glioma of childhood. *Arch Neurol* (Chicago), 14:192–223, 1925.
3. BASSETT, R. C., KAHN, E. A., SCHNEIDER, R. C., and CROSBY, E. C. *Correlative Neurosurgery*. Charles C Thomas, Springfield, Ill., 1955.
4. BECK, P., SCHWALCH, D. S., PARKER, M. L., KIPNIS, D. M., and DAUGHADAY, W. H. Correlative studies of growth hormone and insulin plasma concentrations with metabolic abnormalities in acromegaly. *J Lab Clin Med*, 66:366–379, 1965.
5. BECLERE, M. Le traitement médical des tumeurs hypophysaires du gigantisme et de l'acromégalie par la radiothérapie. *Bull Soc Med Hop Paris*, 27:274–293, 1909.
6. BODEN, G. Radiation myelitis of the cervical cord. *Brit J Radiol*, 21:464–469, 1948.
7. BODIAN, M., and LAWSON, D. The intracranial neoplastic diseases of childhood. *Brit J Surg*, 40:368–392, 1953.
8. BOUCHARD, J. *Radiation Therapy of Tumors and Diseases of the Nervous System*. Lea & Febiger, Philadelphia, 1966.
9. BOUCHARD, J., and PIERCE, C. B. Radiation therapy in the management of neoplasms of the central nervous system, with a special note in regard to children: Twenty years' experience, 1939–1958. *Amer J Roentgen*, 84:610–628, 1960.
10. BUSCHKE, F. Radiotherapy of pituitary adenomas. *West J Surg Obstet Gynec*, 58:271–278, 1950.
11. CHAO, J. H., PHILLIPS, R., and NICKSON, J. J. Roentgen-ray therapy of cerebral metastases. *Cancer*, 7:682–689, 1954.
12. CHRISTENSEN, E., and ALS, E. Medulloblastoma. *Acta Psychiat Scand*, Suppl. 108:87–100, 1956.
13. CHU, F. C. H., and HILARIS, B. B. Value of radiation therapy in the management of intracranial metastases. *Cancer*, 14:577–581, 1961.
14. COLBY, M. Y., JR., GAGE, R. P, SVIEN, H. J., and KEARNS, T. P. Evaluation of results of radiation treatment of pituitary chromophobe adenomas producing visual impairment. *Radiology*, 3:195–200, 1964.
15. CORREA, J. M., and LAMPE, I. The radiation treatment of pituitary adenomas. *J Neurosurg*, 19:626–631, 1962.
16. COURVILLE, C. B. *Pathology of the Central Nervous System: A Study Based upon a Survey of Lesions Found in a Series of Forty Thousand Autopsies*, 3rd ed. Pacific Press, Mountain View, Calif., 1950.
17. CRAMER, F., and KINSEY, W. The cerebellar hemangioblastomas. Review of 53 cases with special reference to cerebellar cysts and the association of polycythemia. *Arch Neurol* (Chicago), 67:237–252, 1952.
18. CRUE, B. L. *Medulloblastoma*. Charles C Thomas, Springfield, Ill., 1958.

19. CUMMINS, F. M., TAVERAS, J. M., and SCHLESINGER, E. B. Treatment of gliomas of the third ventricle and pinealomas. With special reference to the value of radiotherapy. *Neurology* (Minneap), 10:1031–1036, 1960.

20. DARGEON, H. W. *Tumors of Childhood*. Hoeber-Harper, New York, 1960.

21. DOHAN, F. C., RAVENTOS, A., BOUCOT, N., and ROSE, E. Roentgen therapy in Cushing's syndrome without adrenocortical tumor. *J Clin Endocr*, 17:8–32, 1957.

22. DYKE, C. G., and DAVIDOFF, L. M. *Roentgen Treatment of Diseases of the Nervous System*. Lea & Febiger, Philadelphia, 1942.

23. HENDERSON, W. R. Pituitary adenomata: Follow-up study of surgical results in 338 cases (Dr. Harvey Cushing's series). *Brit J Surg*, 26:811–921, 1939.

24. JOHNSEN, S. F. Roentgen irradiation of the pituitary in Cushing's syndrome, with brief discussion of pathogenisis of the syndrome. *Acta Med Scand*, 144:165–188, 1952.

25. KAHN, E. A., BASSET, R. C., SCHNEIDER, R. C., and CROSBY, E. C. *Correlative Neurosurgery*, pp. 214–231. Charles C Thomas, Springfield, Ill., 1955.

26. KERNOHAN, J. W., and SAYRE, G. P. Tumors of the Central Nervous System. Section X, Fasc. 35 and 37, Atlas of Tumor Pathology, A.F.I.P.

27. KRAMER, S., SOUTHARD, M., and MANSFIELD, C. M. Radiotherapy in the management of craniopharyngiomas: Further experience and late results. *Amer J Roentgen*, 103:44–52, 1968.

28. KRICHEFF, I. I., BECKER, M., SCHNECK, S., and TAVERAS, J. M. Intracranial ependymomas: Study of survival in 65 cases treated by surgery and irradiation. *Amer J Roentgen*, 91:167–175, 1964.

29. LAMPE, I. Radiation tolerance of the central nervous system. In: *Progress in Radiation Therapy*, Vol. I. F. Buschke, Ed, Grune & Stratton, New York, 1958.

30. LAMPE, I., and MAC INTYRE, R. S. Medulloblastoma of the cerebellum. *Arch Neurol* (Chicago), 62:322–329, 1949.

31. LAMPE, I., and MAC INTYRE, R. S. Experiences in the radiation therapy of medulloblastoma of the cerebellum. *Amer J Roentgen*, 71:659–668, 1954.

32. LAWRENCE, J. H., TOBIAS, C. A., BORN, J. L., GOTTSCHALK, A., LINFOOT, J. A., and KLING, R. P. Alpha particle and proton beams in therapy. *JAMA*, 186:236–245, 1963.

33. LIEBNER, E. J., PRETTO, J. S., HOCHHAUSER, M., and KASSARABA, W. Tumors of the posterior fossa in childhood and adolescence. *Radiology*, 82:193–201, 1964.

34. LINFOOT, J. A., LAWRENCE, J. H., BORN, J. L., and TOBIAS, C. A. The alpha particle or proton beam in radiosurgery of the pituitary gland for Cushing's disease. *New Eng J Med*, 269:597–601, 1963.

35. LIVINGSTON, K. E., HORRAX, G., and SACHS, E., JR. Metastatic brain tumors. *Surg Clin N Amer*, 28:805–810, 1948.

36. MOGENSON, E. F. Chromophobe adenoma of pituitary gland; follow-up study on 60 surgical patients with special reference to endocrine disturbances. *Acta Endocr* (Kobenhavn), 24:135–152, 1957.

37. MOSS, W. T. *Therapeutic Radiology*, 3rd ed. Mosby, St. Louis, 1969.

38. PATERSON, E. Malignant tumors of childhood. *J Fac Radiol*, 9:170–174, 1958.

39. PATERSON, E., and FARR, R. F. Cerebellar medulloblastoma: Treatment by irradiation of the whole central nervous system. *Acta Radiol*, 39:323-336, 1953.

40. PEIRCE, C. B., CONE, W. V., BOUCHARD, J., and LEWIS, R. C. Medulloblastoma: Non-operative management with roentgen therapy after aspiration biopsy. *Radiol*, 52:621–632, 1949.

41. PHILLIPS, T. L., SHELINE, G. E., and BOLDREY, E. Therapeutic considerations in tumors affecting the central nervous system: Ependymomas. *Radiology*, 83:98–105, 1964.

42. PHILLIPS, T. L., and BUSCHKE, F. Radiation tolerance of the thoracic spinal cord. *Amer J Roentgen*, 105:659–664, 1969.

43. SAGERMAN, R. H., BAGSHAW, M. A., and HANBERG, J. Considerations in treatment of ependymoma. *Radiology*, 84:401–408, 1965.

44. SHELINE, G. E., BOLDREY, E. B., KARLBERG, P., and PHILLIPS, T. L. Therapeutic considerations in tumors affecting the central nervous system: Oligodendrogliomas. *Radiology*, 82:84–89, 1964.

45. SHELINE, G. E., BOLDREY, E. B., and PHILLIPS, T. L. Chromophobe adenomas of the pituitary gland. *Amer J Roentgen*, 92:160–173, 1964.

46. SHELINE, G. E., GOLDBERG, M. B., and FELDMAN, R. Pituitary irradiation for acromegaly. *Radiology*, 76:70–75, 1961.

47. SOSMAN, M. C. Cushing's disease—Pituitary basophilism (Caldwell lecture, 1947). *Amer J Roentgen*, 62:1–32, 1949.

48. SMITH, R. A., LAMPE, I., and KAHN, E. A. The prognosis of medulloblastoma in children. *J Neurosurg*, 18:91–97, 1961.

49. TAVERAS, J. M., MOUNT, L. A., and WOOD, E. H. The value of radiation therapy in the management of gliomas of the optic nerves in chiasm. *Radiology*, 66:518–528, 1956.

50. VAETH, J. Radiation-induced myelitis. In: *Progress in Radiation Therapy*, Vol. III. F. Buschke, Ed, Grune & Stratton, New York, 1965.

51. WILLIS, R. A. *The Spread of Tumours in the Human Body*, 2nd ed Butterworth, London, 1952.

10

CARCINOMA
OF THE BREAST

In the treatment of "operable" carcinoma of the breast, radiation therapy has played a secondary role. However, of the total number of patients suffering from the disease, only a minority (about 30 percent) is fortunate enough to remain free of manifestations of progressive tumor following surgery alone. Many patients with inoperable or surgically uncontrolled disease require treatment, either in an attempt to retard tumor progression or for palliation. In many such situations, judiciously administered radiation therapy is the most reliable and effective therapeutic method. Some surgeons and radiotherapists of considerable experience believe that even in "operable" situations, adjuvant radiation therapy is of value. Thus, a significant number of patients with carcinoma of the breast will be treated with radiation at some time during the course of their disease.

For an understanding of the rationale for radiation therapy, the biological behavior of cancer of the breast and its radiovulnerability must be considered.

BIOLOGICAL BEHAVIOR OF CARCINOMA OF THE BREAST

From a primary focus tumor extends through the walls of the regional mammary ducts, infiltrates the mammary fat, progresses along the fascial planes, and is transported through the periductal and perineural lymphatics to the retromammary lymphatic plexuses. Most primary carcinomas are in the upper, lateral quadrant of the breast (Figure 10-1). As the tumor progresses, it may at any time infiltrate directly through the walls of blood vessels.

The critical point in curability occurs when carcinoma extends beyond the breast proper, either by tumor embolism via the lymphatics into the regional lymph nodes (axillary, subclavicular, supraclavicular, and internal mammary nodes—Figure 10-2), or by embolic spread through the blood vessels. The relative five-year clinical cure rate drops from about 80 percent, when tumor cannot be found by careful examination of the axillary nodes, to about 40 percent when tumor can be found microscopically.

From the first relay in the axillary nodes, tumor may progress through lymphatics in the apex of the axilla, and along the subclavian vein to the supraclavicular and subclavicular nodes at the junction of the internal jugular and subclavian veins

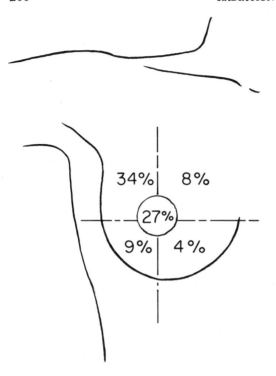

Fig. 10-1. Identified primary site (18% more than one quadrant) in 177 consecutive patients with breast cancer.[21]

(Figure 10-2). At least for primary tumors in the lateral half of the breast, supraclavicular and subclavicular node involvement is thus present only when coexistent with axillary lymph node tumor deposits and is less frequent than involvement of the internal mammary nodes,[7] probably because the supraclavicular and subclavicular nodes are a second relay, whereas extension into the internal mammary nodes occurs directly from the breast itself.

Involvement of the internal mammary nodes in the absence of axillary node involvement is infrequent.[7] If the primary tumor is in the lateral breast, the incidence is less than 5 percent, although, if medial or subareolar, it may be 10–15 percent. However, in the presence of tumor-bearing axillary nodes, involvement of internal mammary nodes has been found in about 25 percent of patients with tumors in the lateral breast and in 50 percent of those with subareolar or medial breast primaries.[5,10,23,33] There is no uniformity of opinion whether this difference in location of the primary tumor within the breast should influence therapy.

Carcinomas of the breast vary enormously in their rate of local growth and distant spread.[21,26,29] Some carcinomas remain localized in the breast for several years and do not seem to influence the life expectancy of patients, even if untreated. Other carcinomas, despite "early" and aggressive therapy, prove fatal within months. The course of the disease is influenced by a balance between the aggressive tendencies of the neoplasm and the resistance of the host. Reactivation of tumor foci many years after removal of the primary disease, for instance, can best be explained by growth of unrecognized metastatic foci, which had remained silent since the original treatment until the tumor-host balance changed.

Although malignant tumors of the breast are of a broad histological spectrum, correlation with specific tumor type has been of little value in formulating treatment or estimating prognosis for a specific patient. Most cancers of the breast are adeno-carcinomas which may be difficult to grade. Some infrequent types of tumors, such as mucoid carcinoma and medullary carcinoma with lymphoid infiltration, have a more favorable prognosis because of an indolent biological behavior. In contrast, inflammatory carcinoma, a clinical entity without correlation with tumor type, is a relentlessly progressive disease.

As in many other cancers, a clinical estimate of tumor extent (staging) has proved a better guide to treatment and prognosis than has any clinico-pathological correlation. Many such staging schemes have been proposed, each differing in rela-tively minor details. Typical is the "Columbia Clinical Classification" devised by Haagensen and Stout.[7]

Columbia Clinical Classification[7]

Stage A.

No skin edema, ulceration, or solid fixation of tumor to chest wall. Axillary nodes not clinically involved.

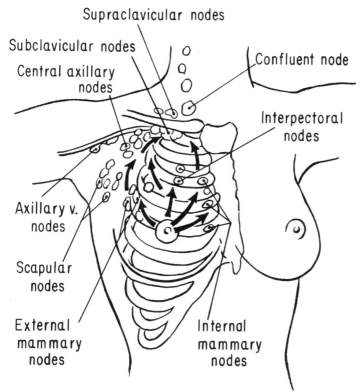

Fig. 10-2. Principal lymphatic drainage of breast.
1. Major node groups parallel major veins.
2. Most afferent lymphatics on deep layer of superficial fascia.
3. Supraclavicular nodes are a secondary station.
4. The drainage pattern may be disturbed by tumor in nodes.

Stage B.

No skin edema, ulceration, or solid fixation of tumor to chest wall. Clinically involved axillary nodes, but less than 2.5 cm in transverse diameter and not fixed to overlying skin or deeper structures of axilla.

Stage C.

Any one of five grave signs of comparatively advanced carcinoma.
1. Edema of skin of limited extent (involving less than one-third of the skin over the breast)
2. Skin ulceration
3. Solid fixation of tumor to chest wall
4. Massive involvement of axillary lymph nodes (measuring 2.5 cm or more in transverse diameter)
5. Fixation of the axillary nodes to overlying skin or deeper structures of axilla

Stage D.

All other patients with more advanced breast carcinoma, including:
1. A combination of any two or more of the five grave signs listed in Stage C
2. Extensive edema of skin (involving more than one-third of skin over the breast)
3. Satellite skin nodules
4. The inflammatory type of carcinoma
5. Supraclavicular metastases (clinically apparent)
6. Parasternal metastases (clinically apparent)
7. Edema of the arm
8. Distant metastases

In addition to extent of spread from the primary site (clinical staging), Mc-Whirter[25] considers size of the primary tumor at the time of diagnosis and treatment, natural rate of tumor growth, delay prior to treatment, age, sex, pregnancy, site of tumor within the breast, and treatment itself as factors influencing the prognosis in breast cancer.

In MacDonald's statistical studies,[21] about 25 percent of carcinomas progressed so slowly that the efficacy of treatment could not be evaluated; 50 percent progressed relentlessly, so that treatment had only a retarding effect, whereas for only 25 percent did "early" treatment possibly determine the final outcome. This study, although of great interest, should not influence therapeutic planning because there is no way to determine initially in which of the three groups an individual patient belongs. However, this study helps explain the contradictory conclusions drawn from evaluations of results following different methods of therapy.

Argument about the "best treatment" for patients with "early" (operable) carcinoma of the breast has not ceased since Halsted introduced the "radical mastectomy."[8] Innumerable statistics have been published by competent clinicians to demonstrate the superiority of one of several procedures: (a) radical mastectomy with or without pre- and/or postoperative irradiation; (b) supraradical surgery (including the removal of the internal mammary lymph nodes and/or supraclavicular lymph nodes); (c) total ("simple") or partial mastectomy alone or followed by irradiation; (d) irradiation alone. A review of the amassed evidence is as confusing to the beginning student as to the experienced physician.

RADIATION THERAPY

Radiovulnerability

In addition to the great variation in biological behavior, there are considerable differences in the radiovulnerability of cancers of the breast. These variations in radioresponsiveness have not been related to histological tumor type. The response of a small proportion (about 20 percent) of breast carcinomas is too slight to demonstrate by clinical examination. Even after the administration of 8,000 rads or more, persistent carcinoma has been histologically identified in specimens obtained at mastectomy many months following radiation therapy.[4,18] Another small proportion are markedly and sometimes rapidly responsive to irradiation. The largest number (about 60 percent) exhibit a moderate, but recognizable, response, manifested by a diminution in the size of the lesion. The average radiovulnerability is comparable to that of moderately differentiated epidermoid carcinomas.

Histological and clinical analyses have shown that, on the average, doses in the range of 4,500 to 6,500 rads in four to seven weeks are necessary for the eradication of the primary tumor[1,18] and that irradiation of the tumor involved lymph nodes is less effective than irradiation of the primary tumor.[4,18,20] (Fibrosis of lymph nodes following intensive irradiation, however, may encapsulate persistent tumor foci and thus inactivate them for long periods.)

Indications for Treatment

In the treatment of patients with carcinoma of the breast, radiation therapy has been used in the following clinical situations:

A. Operable cases:
    1. Radiation therapy alone
    2. Radiation therapy following total ("simple") or partial mastectomy
    3. Radiation therapy as an adjunct to radical mastectomy, either as pre- or postoperative irradiation
B. Inoperable cases:
    1. Radical radiation therapy in an attempt to retard progression of the tumor
    2. Palliative radiation therapy

A. Operable cases

1. *Radiation therapy alone,* in lieu of surgery, in "operable" cases has been used systematically by Baclesse.[2] Of 310 patients with histologically verified carcinoma of the breast (excluding Stage I), treated by radical radiation therapy between 1936 and 1951, 100 (32.2 percent) remained "clinically healed" (i.e., without demonstrable evidence of active disease) after five years. Of the 168 patients with Stage II tumor, 78 (46 percent) were clinically controlled after five years. Although

these results, obtained through meticulous personal attention to the details of daily treatments, compare favorably with surgical results, the method is not expected to supersede radical mastectomy because (1) the high doses (4,100 to 9,500 rads) to a large tissue volume to cover breast and chest wall, supraclavicular, subclavicular, axillary, and internal mammary nodes, administered over 16 to 18 weeks, caused greater morbidity than that from skillful radical mastectomy; (2) changes in the heavily irradiated tissues may cause later complications; and (3) most important, in almost 10 percent (5:54) of the patients who appeared "clinically cured," local recurrence developed 5 to 10 years following therapy.

2. *Radiation therapy following total ("simple") mastectomy:* McWhirter's[24] suggestion (1955) of replacing radical mastectomy with "simple" mastectomy, followed by irradiation of the chest wall, axilla, supraclavicular, subclavicular, and internal mammary nodes, has caused considerable controversy. From a total of 1,882 patients seen between 1941 and 1947, there was an absolute survival rate (not "clinical cure") of 42 percent. Haagensen[7] emphasized that the credit for this result belongs essentially to the roentgentherapy, since the "simple mastectomy," as performed in Edinburgh, consisted primarily of removal of the main neoplastic mass. Based on other experiences, a much lower survival rate (about 16 percent at three years) would be expected from simple mastectomy alone. In a possibly comparable, unselected group of patients treated by radical mastectomy with radiation therapy, Watson[34] reported a five-year survival rate of 52 percent in 1,055 patients seen between 1944 and 1952. The apparent difference may be due to a higher proportion of "earlier" cases in Watson's group.

Kaae and Johansen[12] compared groups treated either by "simple" mastectomy with postoperative radiation therapy (McWhirter method) or extended radical mastectomy with dissection of the lymph nodes in the supraclavicular region and the second to fourth intercostal spaces by the method of Dahl-Iversen.[5] Results did not differ as measured by survival or local "recurrence."

The proponents of "McWhirter's method" prefer it to radical mastectomy, not because of superiority of results, but because of a claimed lesser morbidity. However, this is not valid if the morbidity of radiation therapy is compared with that of radical mastectomy performed by skillful surgeons.

Recently, there has been an increased interest in operations of very limited extent. These wide local excisions of tumor (partial mastectomy, "lumpectomy") may be more appealing to many patients and even to some surgeons. However, any possible cosmetic, functional, and psychological benefits must be carefully related to an increased risk of less frequent local tumor control, even with adjuvant radiation therapy, and ultimately to less frequent survival.

3. *Radiation therapy as an adjunct to radical mastectomy:* Irradiation has been used preoperatively or postoperatively. The rationale and techniques differ fundamentally.

The alleged purpose of preoperative irradiation is to "devitalize" the presumably more aggressive and more radiovulnerable peripheral portions of the tumor, thus reducing the incidence of local recurrence after mastectomy and the risk of spread by surgical manipulation. Consequently, the irradiated volume must extend beyond the excision. The radiation doses tolerated by such large volumes of tissue are unlikely to be consistently "cancerocidal."

Postoperative irradiation has been used extensively for several decades in an attempt to eradicate unrecognized tumor foci in the regional lymphatics (supraclavicular, subclavicular, internal mammary) and chest wall, which are untreated by radical mastectomy.

Since the reason for failure in treatment of breast cancer is usually unrecognized distant tumor spread rather than tumor growth in regional nodes, the contribution of postoperative irradiation is difficult to evaluate because only those patients with tumor limited to regional nodes and responsive to irradiation will benefit. Statistical evidence is controversial, and a satisfactory answer is unlikely. Therefore, it is essential that "prophylactic" irradiation not cause significant morbidity inasmuch as its value is unproved.

Indications for treatment and treatment techniques must include recognition of the following:

1. Eradication of most carcinomas of the breast requires a high radiation dose.
2. Treatment that causes great patient morbidity may reduce the resistance of the host to the disease.
3. Reappearance of tumor in the surgical site (skin of the chest wall or axilla) is infrequent following a good radical mastectomy. For example, only 78 of 1,128 patients had chest wall recurrences and none had axillary recurrences after radical mastectomies performed by a small group of surgeons at the University of California (San Francisco).
4. If tumor cannot be demonstrated in the axillary nodes in a carefully examined surgical specimen, involvement of supraclavicular nodes is unlikely, and the incidence of involvement of the internal mammary nodes is low.

Based on these considerations, the following general policy (subject to individual variations) has been followed in our institutions for the last 12 years:

Radical mastectomy is advised in every "operable" case. Postoperative radiation therapy is based on the findings in the axillary nodes, the size, location and characteristics of the primary tumor, the adequacy of the surgical margins, and the condition of the patient.

Stage I or Columbia Stage A (no tumor in axillary nodes): Postoperative radiation therapy is not advised, except for large tumors arising in the central or medial breast.

Stage II or Columbia Stage B (tumor in axillary nodes): Postoperative radiation therapy is directed to the supraclavicular, subclavicular, apical axillary, and internal mammary lymphatics, but the chest wall is not treated unless the adequacy of the surgical removal is questionable.

Treatment to parasternal, supraclavicular, infraclavicular, and axillary fields does not appreciably affect the patient's general condition. In spite of doubts regarding the efficacy of the procedure, treatment adjusted to the individual tolerance probably causes no harm, and may devitalize tumor that has not passed the barrier of the regional lymphatics.

Stage III or Columbia Stage C (complete surgical removal unlikely because of local or regional tumor extension, particularly fixation of breast or axillary nodes): Radiation therapy, adjusted to the individual situation, is used without surgery or preoperatively.

Stage IV or Columbia Stage D (clinically demonstrable tumor extension beyond the volume resectable by radical mastectomy, i.e., supraclavicular adenopathy, distant spread): Treatment depends on the individual situation.

B. Inoperable cases

1. In some patients with inoperable breast cancer, radical radiation therapy may be used in an effort to retard tumor progression. Such treatment has occasionally resulted in apparent "cures."[1,11] However, tumor persistence and eventual clinical reactivation is the usual result.

2. Radiation therapy remains a most effective and reliable palliative agent when judiciously integrated into the entire plan of therapy (hormonal, surgical, chemical, psychological). Indications for treatment depend on the individual situation. The most important indications are:

a. With slowly progressing disease, it is possible to keep patients comfortable for years by treating individual *metastatic foci in bone* as they become symptomatic. With more rapidly progressing widespread skeletal involvement, radiation therapy may be used in conjunction with other methods, particularly hormonal therapy. In such situations, critical foci may be treated individually because the effects of radiation therapy are more predictable and more rapid than those of any other form of treatment. The involvement of weight-bearing bone is an urgent indication for treatment. In the presence of clinical evidence of compromise of the spinal cord, laminectomy must precede radiation therapy because the tumor response is too slow to avoid irreparable cord damage.

Irradiation of bone metastases relieves pain in over 90 percent of patients with breast cancer, even though radiographic reconstitution of bone follows in only 10 percent.[28] The dose necessary for adequate and sustained palliation and bone reconstruction often is considerably lower than that required for resolution of the primary tumor.

b. Radiation therapy may relieve symptoms and signs incident to *pressure on mediastinal structures* (trachea, esophagus, large vessels) by enlarged tumor-bearing nodes.

c. *Large, ulcerated, inoperable tumor masses* may heal following irradiation, thus relieving local discomfort. Large tumors, ulcerated but not fixed to the chest wall, may be better managed by simple "toilet" mastectomy.

d. Tumor growing on the chest wall after mastectomy rarely can be treated satisfactorily by radiation because often it is not possible to deliver an adequate dose to the large tissue volume microscopically involved, and more importantly, such *chest wall recurrence* heralds aggressive tumor activity. Frequently, even if there is regression at the treatment site, the disease will progress beyond the treatment fields. Occasionally, individual lesions, particularly implantation metastases in the surgical scar, can be adequately treated. For more extensive skin involvement, hormonal therapy is preferred.

e. *Intracranial metastases* are usually multiple, requiring treatment of the entire brain. Although such extensive irradiation may be profitable, indications for treatment must be reviewed in the overall perspective of the patient's care. Occasionally, a particular focus responsible for distressing clinical symptoms can be irradiated effectively.

f. Tumor involvement of the pleura may result in an *effusion in the pleural space*. This high protein fluid, which may contain blood, is a clinical problem when it rapidly recurs following removal. Radioactive colloids (^{198}Au, chromic phosphate) injected into the pleural space have effectively controlled this distressing problem. However, several nonradioactive materials (HN_2, atabrine) and even continuous drainage for several days have been equally effective and are cheaper, safer, and less cumbersome.

g. Radiation treatment of *pulmonary metastases* is not often useful. Clinical symptoms infrequently result until the tumor involves the pleural surface. Irradiation of large volumes of lung with adequate dose may produce changes in lung leading to greater discomfort than that caused by the tumor.

h. Similarly, *metastatic involvement of the liver* is not an indication for radiation therapy. In rare instances, when pain from tension on the capsule is the most distressing clinical symptom of a patient who is in good general condition, it is possible to reduce the size of the mass and relieve the pain.

Complications of Radiation Therapy

Whether used as an unproved adjunct to radical surgery in "curable" situations, as a "curative" method in lieu of surgery, or as a well-proved palliative agent, the complications of radiation therapy must be minimized by careful application. "Acute" complications of the late treatment and early post-treatment periods include transitory changes in the skin, occasional depression of the peripheral white blood cell count, and infrequent changes in small lung segments. "Late" changes, i.e., segmental pulmonary fibrosis, edema of the upper limb, significant skin change, or limitation of shoulder motion should be infrequent. Edema of the arm, often blamed on radiation therapy, is more frequently related to surgery or to progression of tumor. Particularly, it may be initiated by minor infections of the upper limb with resultant lymphangitis.

Inflammatory Carcinoma of the Breast

Inflammatory carcinoma of the breast requires special consideration. It is a clinical, not a pathological, entity, characterized by rapid development of a large tumor in the breast associated with reddening and edema of the overlying skin. This is caused by the rapid spread of carcinoma through the lymphatics of the dermis. The clinical picture of inflammatory carcinoma can be associated with any histological type and is not peculiar to any. The pathologist cannot diagnose inflammatory carcinoma because of infiltration with inflammatory cells, although he can suspect this clinical diagnosis if the lymphatics of the skin are diffusely filled with cancer. As expected, very radiovulnerable, as well as completely unresponsive, tumors are included in this clinical group.

Inflammatory carcinoma is incurable by present methods, surgery and radiation therapy being equally futile. Surgery is contraindicated because it is followed by rapid progression of satellite tumors in the surgical field. Intensive irradiation is used with little enthusiasm. Irradiation in moderate dose may reduce the primary tumor and the adenopathy, but it does not alter the prognosis because of the relentless distant spread of the disease.

SYSTEMIC TREATMENT

Two-thirds of all patients with carcinoma of the breast will not be **permanently** controlled by local treatment (surgery, radiation therapy) and will be **candidates** for systemic treatment. Institution of systemic treatment requires documentation of tumor dissemination which cannot be controlled better by judicious use of local treatment methods, i.e., local irradiation of a bony metastasis causing pain. This decision is a matter of judgment which may vary with the physician and the patient.

The availability of many potentially effective therapeutic agents has made selected sequential use necessary. These schemes (Figures 10-3, 10-4) often require the coordination of several physicians and depend upon the response of the patient to each agent.

Premenopausal and Menopausal Females

If the patient is judged to be a high estrogen producer (premenopausal, menopausal, questionable five to ten years postmenopausal), the initial therapy is castration. Oophorectomy is quick and certain, but carries a 4–6 percent operative mortality incidence[6,31] and is not possible with some patients. Ovarian radiation to adequate dosage is ultimately of comparable effectiveness and is applicable to all patients, but ovarian suppression may be delayed for as long as four to five months.[3]

Castration is followed by objective improvement for average periods of 10 to 14 months in one-fourth to one-third of premenopausal and menopausal women.[9, 19, 31] Remissions may not be accompanied by a measurable decrease in estrogen production, or may not occur in patients with marked estrogen suppression. The best responses are in bony and soft tissue metastases, and are most likely in females near the menopause[31] who have had a clinically tumor-free postmastectomy interval longer than two years.[6]

The debate whether castration should accompany the mastectomy ("prophylac-

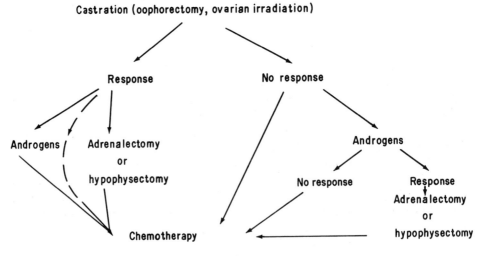

Fig. 10-3. Plan for patients with high estrogen production. (Premenopausal, Menopausal)*

*If any sequential therapy is effective, it is maintained until relapse and then discontinued. The next therapy is started after a short period of observation for a "rebound" response.

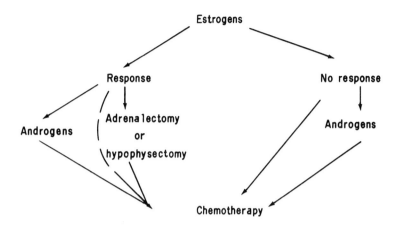

Fig. 10-4. Plan for patients with low estrogen production. (Post-menopausal)*

tic" or "early"), even in the absence of evidence of tumor dissemination, or should be reserved for initial treatment of patients with disseminated tumor ("therapeutic" or "late") has not abated. "Prophylactic" castration neither increases the probability of cure nor lengthens the survival, although it may slightly postpone the first clinical reactivation of tumor.[15] Therefore, "late" or "therapeutic" castration seems advisable because it not only eliminates many needless operations, but more importantly provides the best indicator for the next therapeutic procedure.

More than one-third of those women responding to castration will respond to adrenalectomy or hypophysectomy following clinical reactivation of tumor, although less than 10 percent of those nonresponsive to castration will be benefited.[22] The incidence and duration (12 to 16 months average) of favorable response, the specific sites influenced, and the postoperative mortality (12–14 percent[22]) are similar for both operations. Local irradiation is ineffective for adrenal suppression. Pituitary ablation may follow local irradiation with heavy particles (i.e., protons[17]) or isotope implantation.

Patients relapsing after a response to castration may not be considered candidates for adrenalectomy or hypophysectomy. Approximately 20 percent of these patients may respond to androgens.[6] Metastases in soft tissue are more likely to be responsive than are lesions in bone or viscera.[6] Some patients may convert testosterone to estrogen,[27] a possible explanation for the occasional exacerbation, especially noted in the young. Androgens have consequential side effects. Indeed, the hoarseness, voice lowering, hair loss, acne, and increased libido have been considered an inescapable accompaniment of adequate dosage. Of more importance is the substantial incidence of hypercalcemia (7.2 percent),[14] especially in those with osseous metastases. Other side effects, i.e., "a sense of well being," weight increase, and hematopoietic improvement may be welcome.

Since the introduction of effective chemotherapeutic agents, many physicians

*If any sequential therapy is effective, it is maintained until relapse and then discontinued. The next therapy is started after a short period of observation for a "rebound" response.

prefer to avoid the side effects of testosterone and the risks of adrenalectomy or hypophysectomy, and so proceed directly to the use of cytotoxic agents following postcastration relapse. These drugs are a heterogeneous group, including alkylating agents, antimetabolites, antibiotics, and alkaloids. The most frequently used are cyclophosphamide (Cytoxan), 5-fluorouracil, thioTEPA, and methotrexate.

5-FU will produce objective improvement for more than 6 months in 25 percent of patients treated.[16] However, remissions seldom exceed 12 months. A sizable toxicity (diarrhea, stomatitis, alopecia, nausea and vomiting, hematopoietic suppression, dermatitis) occasionally has led to drug-induced mortality.

Cyclophosphamide may have less serious toxicity and longer periods of remission than 5-FU.[16] Patients may respond to either 5-FU or cyclophosphamide despite lack of response to the other. However, either agent is more likely to be effective in patients with a long postmastectomy clinically tumor-free interval and in those previously responsive to hormone manipulation and other specific cytotoxins.

The premenopausal or menopausal female who does not respond to castration (allowing two to three months of observation if feasible) may be tried on exogenous androgens or cytotoxic agents. However, the incidence of response of this group to any therapy is less than that of the group responding to castration.

Postmenopausal Females

Initial treatment for those patients judged to be low estrogen producers is administration of estrogen. Objective improvement should follow in 35–40 percent of patients, a clear superiority over that produced by androgens (20 percent).[16] Estrogen is relatively ineffective for patients within five years of menopause. The incidence of favorable response is higher in patients with long tumor-free postmastectomy intervals. Metastases in bone, soft tissue, breast, and even viscera may respond favorably.

Estrogen use requires careful attention to a multitude of side effects. Some, such as mild anorexia, areolar pigmentation, breast engorgement, and even uterine bleeding, may be of little consequence. However, a few of these patients with osseous metastases (2.4 percent[14]), may develop hypercalcemia which requires early diagnosis and vigorous treatment to prevent death.

As many as one of ten postmenopausal patients responsive to estrogens may respond to its withdrawal.[13] They may then again respond to estrogens. Androgens are likely to be effective in at least 20 percent.[6] We have seen a patient responsive for several years to each move in a sequence of estrogen administration, withdrawal; androgen administration, withdrawal; estrogen administration. These postmenopausal estrogen responders also may benefit from adrenalectomy or hypophysectomy.

However, this group often is of advanced age and troubled by other serious medical disabilities. Thus, if neither surgical manipulation nor androgen administration is considered tolerable, cautious use of cytotoxic agents may be attempted.

For those postmenopausal patients not responsive to exogenous estrogens, androgens or cytotoxic agents occasionally may be effective, although this possibility is less than for estrogen responders.

Adrenal corticosteroids are capable of producing objective regressions in patients with mammary carcinoma. Remissions usually are brief (average three months[30]), although occasionally they may be long-term. The mechanism of action is unknown, although in part it may be anti-inflammatory. "Medical adrenalectomy" is an inappropriate term, for ACTH production is suppressed in contrast to its elevation after adrenalectomy. Neither response to castration nor age seems a reliable indicator of likelihood of response. About 75 percent of patients enjoy subjective improvement.[30] This is counterbalanced by a high incidence of bothersome and potentially serious sequelae, i.e., peptic ulcer, hypertension, diabetes, hypokalemia, edema, and Cushing's syndrome.

The Special Problem of the Male with Breast Cancer

Although males constitute only 1 percent of the breast cancer population, relatively few are controlled by primary local treatment. The hormonal indicators for castration are less overt in the male. Therefore, most males, even to advanced age, should be castrated as the initial therapy for disseminated breast cancer. Favorable objective responses to castration are of higher incidence than is expected for the female, being recorded in two of three patients.[32] These remissions average 29.6 months.[32] Like the female, longer postmastectomy, clinically tumor-free intervals make response to castration more probable. Data from use of estrogens, adrenalectomy, hypophysectomy, and cytotoxic agents are less plentiful and less reliable than for the female.

Students of clinical oncology soon realize that sequential therapy for patients with disseminated breast cancer is more art than science. After an initial judgment, based on menopausal status, each consequent therapy is an attempt to drastically change the tumor environment on the assumption that either the tumor cell population has adapted to the existing environment or that a new adapted tumor cell population has developed. Although the development of scientific bases of choice are desired, current empirical treatment can benefit a majority of the victims of breast cancer.

REVIEW QUESTIONS

1. Does the specific primary site in the breast have prognostic significance for patients with carcinoma of the breast? Which part of the female breast is host to most cancers?

2. By what routes does carcinoma, primary in the breast, extend beyond the breast? What are the clinical implications?

3. Is a patient still "curable" with metastases to regional lymph nodes? to distant nodes? to skin? via the blood vessels?

4. The clinical course of carcinoma of the breast is extremely variable. What is the longest clinical tumor-free interval between mastectomy and "recurrence" that you have seen? Would you estimate the prognosis to be better for a female with an untreated breast carcinoma 6.0 cm in greatest dimension known to be present for four years, or for a female with a carcinoma 2.0 cm in greatest dimension known to have become palpable and larger within two months?

5. What is the most frequent histological type of breast carcinoma? What limits the usefulness of clinico-histological tumor type correlation? Can you name any histological types of breast carcinoma which have a useful clinical correlation?

6. Which is the better guide to treatment and prognosis, clinical staging or tumor histology?

7. What are the basic components of clinical staging of breast carcinoma?

8. What are the grave signs of advanced breast carcinoma described by Haagensen? Have you seen a radical mastectomy attempted when these were present? Was it successful?

9. List prognostic indicators in addition to clinical staging.

10. What is the significance of histologically identifiable tumor in previously irradiated breast specimens? How does this correlate with your knowledge of cellular reproductive death?

11. Can irradiation control carcinoma at the primary site in the breast? in nodes? in parenchymal organs?

12. If simple mastectomy plus regional irradiation (McWhirter method) results in patient survival and local tumor control comparable to that produced by radical mastectomy, why may the latter method be preferable?

13. What are the objectives of preoperative irradiation? of postoperative irradiation? Are these objectives accomplished? If so, how frequently? If not, why use the method?

14. List four reasonable objectives of radiation therapy in the palliation of the patient with breast carcinoma.

15. Is inflammatory carcinoma of the breast a clinical or a pathological entity? How is the diagnosis established? What is the prognosis?

16. What is the first step in initiating sequential system therapy for the patient with disseminated breast carcinoma?

17. What are the indications for castration in the female with disseminated breast cancer? How often is castration followed by an objective favorable response? What is its duration?

18. What are the comparative advantages and disadvantages of oophorectomy and ovarian irradiation for castration?

19. What are the advantages of "therapeutic" or "late" castration compared with "prophylactic" or "early" castration?

20. When may exogenous estrogen be useful in treating females with disseminated breast cancer? What are the uses of androgens? of adrenal corticosteroids? What are the side effects of these agents?

21. Which cytotoxic agents have proved effective in treating females with disseminated breast carcinoma? What are their side effects?

22. When would you discontinue local irradiation in favor of systemic agents in the treatment of females with disseminated breast carcinoma? Can these agents be used simultaneously?

23. How does sequential systemic treatment vary for the male with disseminated breast carcinoma?

BIBLIOGRAPHY

1. BACLESSE, F. A method of preoperative roentgentherapy by high doses, followed by radical operation for carcinoma of the breast. *J Fac Radiol,* 6:145–163, 1955.
2. ———— Radiation therapy alone in cancer of the breast. *Acta Union Int contra Cancrum,* 15:1023–1026, 1959.
3. BLOCK, G. E., VIAL, A. B., and PULLEN, F. W. Estrogen excretion following operative and irradiation castration in cases of mammary cancer. *Surgery,* 43:415–422, 1958.
4. BUSCHKE, F., CANTRIL, S. T., and PARKER, H. M. In: *Supervoltage Roentgentherapy.* Charles C Thomas, Springfield, Ill., 1950, chap. VIII.
5. DAHL-IVERSON, E., and TOBIASSEN, T. Radical mastectomy with parasternal and supra-clavicular dissection for mammary carcinoma. *Ann Surg,* 157:170–173, 1963.
6. DONEGAN, W. L. Diagnosis of mammary cancer. In: *Cancer of the Breast,* Vol. V. In the series: *Major Problems in Clinical Surgery.* J. E. Dunphy, Ed, Saunders, Philadelphia, 1967.
7. HAAGENSEN, C. D. *Diseases of the Breast.* Saunders, Philadelphia, 1956.
8. HAAGENSEN, C. D., COOLEY, E., KENNEDY, C. S., MILLER, E., HANDLEY, R. S., THACKERAY, A. C., BUTCHER, H. R., JR., DAHL-IVERSON, E., TOBIASSEN, T., WILLIAMS, I. G., CURWEN, M. P., KAAE, S., and JOHNSON, H. Treatment of early mammary carcinoma: A cooperative international study. *Ann Surg,* 157:157–179, 1963.
9. HALL, T. C., DEDRICK, M. M., NEVINNY, H. B., and MUENCH, H. Prognostic value of response of patients with breast cancer to therapeutic castration. *Cancer Chemother Rep,* 31:47–48, 1963.
10. HANDLEY, R. S. Prognosis according to involvement of internal mammary lymph nodes. *Acta Union Int contra Cancrum,* 15:1030–1031, 1959.
11. HULTBORN, K. A., and TORNBERG, B. Mammary carcinoma: The biologic character of mammary carcinoma. Studies in 517 cases by a new form of malignancy grading. *Acta Radiol [Ther],* Suppl. 196, Stockholm, 1960.
12. KAAE, S., and JOHANSEN, H. Breast cancer. Five-year results: Two random series of simple mastectomy with postoperative irradiation versus extended radical mastectomy. *Amer J Roentgen,* 87:82–88, 1962.
13. KAUFMAN, R. J., and ESCHER, G. C. Rebound regression in advanced mammary carcinoma. *Surg Gynec Obstet,* 113:635–640, 1961.
14. KENNEDY, B. J., TIBBETTS, D. M., NATHANSON, I. T., and AUB, J. C. Hypercalcemia, a complication of hormone therapy of advanced breast cancer. *Cancer Res,* 13:445–459, 1953.
15. KENNEDY, B. J., MIELKE, P. W., JR., and FORTUNY, I. E. Therapeutic castration versus prophylactic castration in breast cancer. *Surg Gynec Obstet,* 118:524–540, 1964.
16. KENNEDY, B. J. Sequential therapies in breast cancer. *Bull Mason Clin,* 22:1–14, 1968.
17. LAWRENCE, J. H., TOBIAS, C. A., BORN, J. L., GOTTSCHALK, H., LINFOOT, J. A., and KLING, R. P. Alpha particle and proton beams in therapy. *JAMA,* 186:236–245, 1963.
18. LENZ, M. Radiotherapy of mammary cancer. In: *Progress in Radiation Therapy,* Vol. III. Buschke, Ed, Grune & Stratton, New York, 1965.
19. LEWISON, E. F. Castration in the treatment of advanced breast cancer. *Cancer,* 18:1558–1562, 1965.
20. LUMB, G. Changes in carcinoma of the breast following irradiation. *Brit J Surg,* 38:82–93, 1950.

21. MACDONALD, I. Indications of the fundamental biology of mammary carcinoma. Proc. Third National Cancer Conf., 1957.
22. MACDONALD, I. Endocrine ablation in disseminated mammary carcinoma. *Surg Gynec Obstet*, 115:215–22, 1962.
23. MARGOTTINI, M. Recent developments in the surgical treatment of breast carcinoma. *Acta Union Int contra Cancrum*, 8:176–178, 1952.
24. MCWHIRTER, R. Simple mastectomy and radiotherapy in the treatment of breast cancer. *Brit J Radiol*, 28:128–139, 1955.
25. ——— Some factors influencing prognosis in breast cancer. *J Fac Radiol*, 8:220–234, 1957.
26. NATHANSON, I. T., and WELCH, C. E. Life expectancy and incidence of malignant disease: Carcinoma of the breast. *Amer J Cancer*, 28:40–53, 1936.
27. NISSEN-MEYER, R. Prophylactic endocrine treatment in carcinoma of the breast. *Clin Radiol*, 15:152–160, 1964.
28. PARKER, R. G., and HARRIS, A. Unpublished data.
29. SHIMKIN, M., LUCIA, E., STONE, R., and BELL, H. G. Cancer of the breast. Analysis of frequency, distribution and mortality at the University of California Hospital, 1918–1947 inclusive. *Surg Gynec Obstet*, 94:645–661, 1952.
30. STOLL, B. A. Corticosteroids in therapy of advanced mammary cancer. *Brit Med J*, 2:210–214, 1963.
31. TAYLOR, S. G., III. Endocrine ablation in disseminated mammary carcinoma. *Surg Gynec Obstet*, 115:443–448, 1962.
32. TREVES, N. The treatment of cancer, especially inoperable cancer of the male breast by ablative surgery (orchiectomy, adrenalectomy and hypophysectomy) and hormone therapy (estrogens and corticosteroids): An analysis of 42 patients. *Cancer*, 12:820–832, 1959.
33. URBAN, J. A. What is the rationale for an extended radical procedure in early cases? *JAMA*, 199:742–743, 1967.
34. WATSON, T. Treatment of breast cancer. Comparison of results of simple mastectomy and radiotherapy with results of radical mastectomy and radiotherapy. *Lancet*, 1191–1194, 1959.

11

LYMPHOMAS

Primary, malignant tumors of lymphoid tissue are characterized by great cellular diversity and a broad spectrum of biological behavior. The general term *lymphoma* includes several well-defined clinicopathological entities: Hodgkin's disease; lymphosarcoma; giant follicular lymphoma; reticulum cell sarcoma; and an anaplastic variant (Hodgkin's sarcoma, lymphoblastic lymphoma, anaplastic reticulum cell sarcoma).

Classification

Although admittedly arbitrary, a workable clinical classification can be based on accepted concepts: (1) These are true tumors of lymphatic tissues, are interrelated, and have a link with leukemia. (2) The histological patterns can be reasonably well identified and can be correlated with clinical findings to form distinct, reproducible, useful clinicopathological entities. (3) The tumor cells arise from a common, primitive mesenchymal cell, even though the ultimate appearance is a diverse cellular pattern. (4) The cells of each tumor type become less differentiated as the tumor becomes more aggressive biologically.

Continuing difficulty of definition of the specific tumor types is acknowledged.[27] "The histologic classification of these tumors is not uniform, not only from institution to institution, but also from pathologist to pathologist within one institution and probably also for the same pathologist over a period of years."

Lumb[19] has designed a scheme relating the recognized clinical entities to three pathways of development: (1) lymphocytic, (2) reticulum cell, and (3) mixed cell. The approximate frequency of each tumor type in his series was:

1. No differentiation
   Hodgkin's sarcoma, lymphoblastic lymphoma, anaplastic reticulum cell
   sarcoma   15–20 percent
2. Lymphocytic differentiation
   Lymphosarcoma   20–25 percent
   Giant follicular lymphoma   5– 8 percent
3. Mixed cell differentiation
   Hodgkin's disease   45–50 percent
   Hodgkin's paragranuloma   5– 7 percent
4. Reticulum cell differentiation
   Reticulum cell sarcoma   5– 7 percent

Within each group of tumors, the histological appearance may vary from poorly differentiated to well differentiated. These variations may be present in a patient at any one time or consecutively over a long period. A specific tumor, if uncontrolled, becomes biologically more aggressive and histologically less differentiated. Such changing behavior of the different tumor types necessitates a flexible classification.

General Relationships

Lymphomas and leukemias are about one-quarter as frequent as cancer of the breast.[19] Each type of lymphoma is 2 to 2½ times as frequent in males as in females. The incidence of all lymphoid tumors, except Hodgkin's disease, continues to increase with increasing age. The peak incidence of Hodgkin's disease is between 20 and 40 years, but those under 20 years may be involved (12–14 percent).[19]

In discussing the biological behavior, treatment, and prognosis, it is useful to consider Hodgkin's disease separately from the other types of lymphoma. It is the most frequent, it has distinctive behavior patterns and histological appearance, and there is considerable agreement as to treatment and prognosis.

HODGKIN'S DISEASE

Since defined by Wilks[30] in 1856, Hodgkin's disease has been the subject of great interest and controversy. Many have considered it an infection or response to an unknown agent. By current concepts, Hodgkin's disease can be considered a mixed-cell malignant tumor of lymphoid tissue containing reticulum cell and lymphocytic derivatives.

Most patients, at the time of diagnosis, have been in excellent health until recent notice of a painless, enlarging, superficial mass (cervical 60–80 percent, axillary 10–20 percent, inguinal 10 percent). Infrequently, these patients may present with clinical findings indicative of extensive tumor, i.e., weight loss, fever, night sweats, pruritus, anemia, involvement of liver, spleen, bone, skin, marrow, or lung.

Patients with Hodgkin's disease have an immunological defect, as yet not understood. This defect changes with disease activity, apparently disappearing during complete clinical remissions. In early active disease, there may be a loss of delayed hypersensitivity, i.e., to tuberculin, and an inability to acquire contact sensitivity. With generalized disease these changes become intensified.[1]

Laboratory Findings

In patients with localized or controlled tumor, laboratory measurements usually are normal. In uncontrolled extensive disease, there may be anemia, secondary to gross blood loss or hemolysis; hypoferremia with increased uptake in the liver and spleen; platelet deficiency; elevated sedimentation rate; hypercalcemia; and serum abnormalities (lowered albumin, elevated globulins).

Pathologic Findings

Hodgkin's disease can be considered a morphologically diverse, malignant tumor of lymphoid tissue, composed of reticulum cell and lymphocytic derivatives, with an additional variable inflammatory cellular proliferation. This unique histological appearance has provoked the use of a variety of terms and raised the question whether Hodgkin's disease is truly a tumor. The hallmark of diagnosis is the Reed-Sternberg cell, a well-described[25] and usually identifiable reticulum cell of poorly understood function. The associated inflammatory cells and fibrosis may mirror host response.

Such pleomorphism and cellular diversity has led to subclassifications, such as that of Jackson and Parker,[16] in an attempt to correlate histological appearance and biological behavior. This particular grouping (Jackson and Parker) has been of minimal clinical value because the biologically aggressive Hodgkin's sarcoma and the indolent Hodgkin's paragranuloma include less than 10 percent of patients with Hodgkin's disease, whereas 90 percent of patients are diagnosed as having Hodgkin's granuloma.

In an effort to improve this histological-clinical correlation, Lukes[20] proposed a more elaborate scheme which correlates the relative cellularity and pattern of fibrosis and the biological behavior. In general, the prognosis is better with marked lymphocytic proliferation and nodular sclerosis, and deteriorates with lymphocytic depletion, reticulum cell proliferation, and diffuse fibrosis.

1. Lymphocytic and histiocytic
   a. nodular
   b. diffuse
2. Nodular sclerosis
3. Mixed
4. Diffuse fibrosis
5. Reticular

Biological correlations have established that most lymphocytic and histiocytic forms are clinically localized at the time of diagnosis, whereas most diffuse fibrotic or reticular patterns are associated with Stage II–III distributions; nodular sclerosis is an expression of regional disease in the upper mediastinum and lower neck; most patients surviving longer than 10 years had lymphocytic and histiocytic or nodular sclerosis types of tumor. For example, the nodular lymphocytic and histiocytic form had a mean survival of 16 years without any correlation with effective treatment, whereas the mean survival for the reticular type was 0.6 years.

Clinical Staging

The single most important prognostic indicator, with current knowledge, is the clinical stage of the disease. However, such an appraisal records but an instant in a panorama of progressive disease. In an effort to temper this inherent shortcoming, some[22] have advocated a short period of observation to attempt to measure the course of the tumor in a particular host. Recent diagnostic improvements (lymphography, isotopic liver scanning, direct inspection and biopsy at laparotomy, examination of the spleen) and increasingly thorough pretreatment evaluation have negated correlation between today's results and those only recently reported, for increasing diagnostic sensitivity has resulted in an increasing proportion of patients, who formerly would be classified Stage I, being correctly placed in Stages II and III.

For example, it has been documented by abdominal lymphography and findings at laparotomy that many patients with left supraclavicular adenopathy also have abdominal para-aortic adenopathy without apparent involvement of the intervening mediastinal nodes. The temporal sequence of involvement makes it likely that there was retrograde extension via the thoracic duct from the neck to the abdomen.[13]

Although clinical staging has long been advocated, widespread application has been recent. The staging most frequently used in the recent past, that of Peters and Middlemiss,[24] can be compared with Kaplan's[17] more recently proposed, more detailed plan, and an older, simplified plan of Craver[4] (Table 11-1).

In initially evaluating a patient, there are several other factors of prognostic importance, not accounted for in clinical staging: Young adults fare better than the elderly; females do better than males; those with a long history of localized disease are a preselected favorable group.

Treatment

"The presently increased interest in the treatment of Hodgkin's disease is mainly the result of the re-emphasis placed on the long recognized, but in general unheeded, observations of the better results of more radical treatment."[3]

For localized Hodgkin's disease, radiotherapy is unequivocally the treatment

Table 11-1.   Clinical Staging—Hodgkin's Disease

Stage	Craver (1947)[4]	Peters & Middlemiss (1958)[24]	Kaplan (1965)[17]
	(Used term "class" rather than "stage")		
0	—	—	No detectable tumor after biopsy
I	Localized	Single site or lymphatic region	Single node or contiguous structures without systemic symptoms
II	Regional (above or below diaphragm)	2–3 proximal lymphatic regions A—no systemic symptoms B—systemic symptoms	More than single site either above or below diaphragm A—no systemic symptoms B—systemic symptoms
III	Generalized with constitutional symptoms	2 or more distant lymphatic regions A—no systemic symptoms B—systemic symptoms	Tumor above and below diaphragm A—no systemic symptoms B—systemic symptoms
IV	—	—	Any of the following: Marrow, bone, lung, intestinal or multiple sites

Table 11-2. Hodgkin's Disease
Fraction of Lymph Node Groups Showing Recurrence at Any Time

Node Area Treated	Dose to Lymph Nodes (R)				
	100–600	601–1,000	1,001–2,000	2,001–3,000	> 3,000
Cervical	2/3	4/6	6/12	1/7	0/7
Supraclavicular	2/5	2/3	1/4	0/6	1/13
Axillary	4/10	–	1/4	0/4	0/6
Mediastinum	5/8	2/2	2/5	1/3	1/4
Other	3/4	0/1	1/5	0/1	0/1
Total	16/30	8/12	11/30	2/21	2/31

Noetzli and Sheline[21]

of choice. Surgery should be limited to biopsy and rare situations, i.e., gastric involvement with obstruction or hemorrhage, encroachment on the spinal cord, and splenectomy for uncontrollable hemolysis. This preference of radiotherapy over surgery is based on better local tumor control with less patient morbidity, widespread applicability without anatomical restrictions, and applicability to contiguous lymphatics, i.e., neck, mediastinum, and axillae. In more extensive disease, selective use of radiotherapy and chemotherapy depends on many factors, and treatment must be decided by radiotherapists and chemotherapists working together.

Local tumor control of high order (80–90 percent) follows adequate radiation dosage to sizable tissue volumes. Minimal tumor doses of 3,000 rads (orthovoltage x-ray), or 4,000 rads (supervoltage radiation), delivered in 3½ to 4½ weeks, now accepted as necessary and conventional,[29] have been advocated for 30 years.[3,10] A table relating dose to local recurrence in lymph nodes has been prepared by Noetzli and Sheline[21] (Table 11-2). Better local tumor control is reflected in increased patient survival.[8]

Enthusiasm for "prophylactic" or "complementary" treatment of clinically normal lymphatic tissue contiguous with clinically defined tumor has been recent. Studies championed by Peters[24] and Kaplan,[28] made possible by improved radiotherapy techniques, have not yet documented an advantage over treatment of liberal tissue volumes to adequate dosage. These techniques are still in the stage of clinical investigation.

Results

Although textbooks continue to describe Hodgkin's disease as "a progressive condition leading inevitably to death,"[19] many clinicians for many years have reported substantial numbers of clinically tumor-free survivors 15 to 20 years following "adequate" radiotherapy. Indeed, the tumor-free survival incidence 5 years after treatment far exceeds that of many forms of cancer considered "curable." Consequently, Easson and Russell[7] have suggested that, "After a period—usually a decade—those disease-free survivors whose progressive death rate from all causes is similar to that of a normal population of the same sex and age" may be considered cured.

Such results have been available prior to use of "supervoltage" equipment and current renewed enthusiasm. Gilbert and Babaiantz[12] reported the five-year

Table 11-3. Hodgkin's Disease
Generalized Adenopathy[6]

Years	No. Treated	Age—Corrected Survival Rate (%)		
		5 Years	10 Years	15 Years
1934–1949	216	19.6	13.4	12.6
1934–1954	466	18.4	11.3	—
1934–1959	689	18.9	—	—

survival of 13 of 46 patients (34.2 percent) irradiated between 1920–1934. Easson[6] recently reported results dating to 1934 from the Christie Hospital and Holt Radium Institute, Manchester, England (see Tables 11-3, 11-4, 11-5).

Crosbie[5] has listed post-treatment survival data from several sources dating from 1914 (Table 11-6).

Thus, it seems well documented that there are many patients answering Easson and Russell's[7] definition of "cure." These patients may increase in incidence and absolute numbers with improved treatment techniques and better ancillary care. Considering Hodgkin's disease to be of unicentric origin with a predictable pattern of spread, Kaplan[18] has predicted the "probability of cure" with adequate radiation therapy (Table 11-7).

In 1939, Gilbert[10] issued a challenge, still pertinent: "In this very special systemic disease, the therapeutic radiologist must act as a general physician; he should know well the manifestations of the disease and the regions involved by it, its modes of extension, its type of evolutionary caprices, and naturally, the mode of action of roentgen therapy as well as the reactions of the patient during treatment."

OTHER LYMPHOMAS

Giant follicular lymphoma, lymphosarcoma, reticulum cell sarcoma and anaplastic lymphoid tumors collectively account for about 50 percent of the lymphomas. In contrast to Hodgkin's disease, these entities increase in incidence with increasing age; have a broader spectrum of biological behavior, including certain specific organ forms and an association with leukemia; have a less certain response to treatment, and, consequently, a less predictable prognosis.

Table 11-4. Hodgkin's Disease
Localized Adenopathy[6]

Years	No. Treated	Age—Corrected Survival Rate (%)		
		5 Years	10 Years	15 Years
1934–1949	103	53.5	44.1	38.9
1934–1954	220	55.3	43.2	—
1934–1959	375	56.5	—	—

Table 11-5. Hodgkin's Disease
Localized Adenopathy[6]
(375 Cases Treated 1934–1959)

Age in Years at Treatment	No. of Patients Treated		Age—Corrected 5-Year Survival Rates (%)	
	Males	Females	Males	Females
under 35	100	47	57.5	77.2
35–54	100	36	53.9	68.3
55 and over	48	44	57.7	36.7

Pathologic Findings

These primary lymphoid tumors can be classified on the basis of predominant cell type, although boundaries between entities may be indistinct because of variations of cell type and maturity within a single mass or in a patient over a period of time. About one-fourth of all lymphomas are predominantly lymphocytic (giant follicular lymphoma—7 percent, lymphosarcoma—20 percent[19]), whereas less than one-fifth are anaplastic, and only about 5 percent are reticulum cell tumors.

Although some[14, 15] have considered such specific histological differentiation unnecessary for the therapeutic application of radiation, identification of the

Table 11-6. Hodgkin's Disease
Five-Year Survival (%)[5]

Source	No. Patients	Class I		Class II		Class III	
		Male	Female	Male	Female	Male	Female
Peters (Toronto) 1924–1942	113	82	100	68	77	12	0
Shimkin (San Francisco) 1914–1951	230	25	58.8	30.5	35	12.3	24
Swedish Hospital (Seattle) 1940–1960	74	77	71	14	61	8	12

Table 11-7. Hodgkin's Disease
Predicted Probability of Cure[18]

No. Fields At Risk	Clinical Stage	Theoretical Probability of Cure (%) If Each Field Receives:			
		1,000 Rads	2,000 Rads	3,000 Rads	4,000 Rads
1	I	40	65	83	96
2	II	16	42	69	92
3	II, III	6	27	57	88

predominant cell type allows gross correlation with expected biological behavior. Thus, giant follicular lymphoma tends to be benign, two of three patients surviving five years without correlation with effective treatment,[19] whereas the course of lymphosarcoma is generally more aggressive, and patients with reticulum cell sarcoma (except bone primary) or anaplastic lymphoid tumor infrequently survive.

Clinical Staging

The correlation between tumor extent, estimated by clinical appraisal, and prognosis is less certain for patients with lymphosarcoma, giant follicular lymphoma, reticulum cell sarcoma, and anaplastic lymphoma than for patients with Hodgkin's disease.

Peters[23] has proposed a staging system similar to that used for Hodgkin's disease.

Stage I

Involvement of single node region or single extranodal site

Stage II

Involvement of multiple lymph node regions or a single extranodal site plus an adjacent lymphatic region

Stage III

Evidence of systemic disease or involvement of liver, spleen, or marrow, or involvement of a single extranodal site plus a remote lymphatic region.

This clinical staging system, although used in recent reports,[9, 22] has not had widespread application.

Treatment

Evaluation of the treatment of patients with these lymphomas is difficult because of the infrequent occurrence and capricious biological behavior of the tumors, and lack of adequate controls in reported studies. Radical radiotherapy of clinically localized lymphoma would result in "cure" only if the tumor arose in a single site and spread predictably. These assumptions are valid for lymphomas arising in specific sites such as tonsil, nasopharynx, pharyngeal tongue, paranasal sinuses, and intestine, but they are not established for lymphomas limited to lymph nodes.

As with Hodgkin's disease, the total radiation dose, rather than a close dose-time relationship, seems the major influence. The radioresponsiveness may vary from lymphocytic tumors, which may respond to low doses (a few hundred rads) to reticulum cell tumors, i.e., those primary in bone, which may be only moderately radiation-responsive. Using doses of 3,000 rads (3 to 4 weeks) for lymphosarcoma, and 5,000 rads (5 to 6½ weeks) for reticulum cell sarcoma, local control rates have varied from 70–95 percent,[9] depending on the anatomical site involved.

The value of irradiating clinically normal lymphatics ("prophylactic" or "complementary" treatment) contiguous with tumor is unknown, and such a policy has received little encouragement,[23] although the necessity of irradiating regional lymphatics in lymphomas of specific sites (i.e., tonsil, pharyngeal tongue) has been established for a long time.

Chemotherapy has proved of value in the palliative treatment of those patients with widespread lymphoma. Its value in the treatment of patients with clinically localized tumor, or as an adjuvant to irradiation, is not established. Thus, experienced physicians such as Rosenberg, Diamond, and Craver[27] concluded (1961): "The therapeutic regime of choice for patients with lymphosarcoma (included all forms of lymphoma except Hodgkin's disease) is predominantly that of radiation therapy. This has been true for many years and has remained so despite the initial impression that alkylating agents, anti-metabolic drugs, and adrenal steroids might be more valuable in the control of the disease." Their conclusion was based on more frequent benefit and less frequent complications with radiation therapy in the management of 1,269 patients!

Inasmuch as radiation therapy can locally control lymphoma with greater certainty and less morbidity, surgery should be reserved for special problems: decompression of the spinal cord when cord viability is threatened; intestinal lesions, especially with obstruction. In these situations, postoperative radiotherapy usually is indicated.

Results

Most reported results of treatment of patients with lymphoma are actually post-treatment survival incidences in noncomparable patient populations. The effectiveness of controlling tumor locally is infrequently mentioned. Most available reports do not measure the potential of modern radiotherapy, for they antedate currently available techniques in which high doses can be delivered to large tissue volumes without serious sequelae.

Representative results are listed in Tables 11-8, 11-9, 11-10, 11-11, 11-12, and 11-13.

Table 11-8. Results of Treatment
Malignant Lymphoma (Exclusive of Hodgkin's Disease)

Authors	Years Inclusive	% 5-Year Survival Rate	No. of Patients	% 10-Year Survival Rate	No. of Patients
Rosenberg, Diamond, and Craver[27]	1928–1953	28.4	1,269	—	—
Peters[23]	1934–1952	26.0	415	16.0	415
Fuller and Fletcher[9]	1947–1959	38.4 ± 3.3 (age-corrected)	278	—	—

Table 11-9.   Results of Treatment
Lymphosarcoma—Localized Nodal

Authors	Inclusive Years	% 5-Year Survival Rate	No. of Patients
Holme and Kunkler[15]	1936–1953	43.8	21/48
Gilbert[11]	1940–1944	59.0	65/111
Boden[2]	1940–1944	50.0	25/50

Table 11-10.   Results of Treatment
Reticulum Cell Sarcoma—Localized Nodal

Authors	Inclusive Years	% 5-Year Survival Rate	No. of Patients
Holme and Kunkler[15]	1936–1953	30.2	26/86
Boden[2]	1940–1944	53.0	10/19

Table 11-11.   Results of Treatment
Malignant Lymphoma—Local Control

	Local Control	% 5-Year Survival Rate
Stage I		
Head and neck	20/25	44.8 ± 6.8
Neck nodes	30/42	
Axilla	15/16	
Inguinal	13/16	
Abdomen	9/22	
Stage II	31/53	51.6 ± 7.8
Data of Fuller and Fletcher[9]		

Table 11-12. Results of Treatment
Relationship of Tumor Type and Survival

Authors	Inclusive Years	Tumor Type	% 5-Year Survival Rate	% 10-Year Survival Rate	Median Survival (months)
Peters[23]	1934–1953	Lymphosarcoma	25.0	19.0	11.4
		Follicular lymphoma	46.0	24.0	42.0
		Reticulum cell sarcoma	16.0	15.0	7.9
Rosenberg, Diamond and Craver[27]	1928–1953	Lymphosarcoma	18.6	–	11.7
		Follicular lymphoma	33.9	–	48.0
		Reticulum cell sarcoma	13.9	–	8.2

Table 11-13. Results of Treatment
Lymphoma of Specific Organs
(Collective Data)

Site	Tumor Type	% 5-Year Survival Rate	No. of Patients
Nasopharynx	Lymphosarcoma	50	13/26
Tonsil	Lymphosarcoma	58	36/62
Maxillary sinus	Lymphosarcoma	75	3/4
Pharyngeal tongue	Lymphosarcoma	33	4/12

Lymphomas are biologically different in children in that they are more aggressive; are associated with leukemia twice as often; present more frequently in extranodal sites; more frequently involve the abdomen, retroperitoneum, and mediastinum. This biological difference is reflected in a lesser survival rate, as reported by Rosenberg et al.[26] in Table 11-14.

Table 11-14. Lymphoma
Relationship of Age and Survival[26]

	No. of Patients	% 5-Year Survival Rate	50% Tumor Death Rates (months)
Children	69	17.4	7.5
Adults	1,269	27.7	27.0

Although meager and outdated, such data establish that some patients with lymphoma, either nodal or organ specific, live for many years without tumor following treatment and thus answer Russell and Easson's[7] definition of "cure."

REVIEW QUESTIONS

1. Define lymphoma. What clinicopathological entities are included? Which is most frequent?

2. At what patient age is Hodgkin's disease most frequent? How does this compare with other lymphomas?

3. What is the most frequent clinical presentation of a patient with Hodgkin's disease?

4. Why is the Hodgkin's disease histological classification of Jackson and Parker of limited clinical value? How has Lukes attempted to improve this correlation?

5. What are some problems of histological diagnosis of the various types of lymphoma? How does this affect care of the patient?

6. What are the criteria for a histological diagnosis of Hodgkin's disease?

7. What is the best indicator of prognosis for the patient with Hodgkin's disease?

8. Why is radiotherapy the treatment of choice for the patient with localized Hodgkin's disease?

9. Do you believe Hodgkin's disease to be curable? What are your criteria? Is this concept new to you?

10. Have you seen a patient with lymphosarcoma grossly limited to a specific site, i.e., tonsil, nasopharynx? What is the significance of this anatomic localization compared to lymphosarcoma involving lymph nodes?

11. Do you believe that patients with lymphoma, other than Hodgkin's disease, grossly limited to lymph nodes can be "cured"? How does this concept influence patient care?

12. What is the place of surgery in the care of the patient with lymphoma?

13. How does lymphoma differ in children compared with that in adults?

BIBLIOGRAPHY

1. AISENBERG, A. C. Manifestations of immunologic unresponsiveness in Hodgkin's disease. *Cancer Res,* 26:1152–1160, 1966.
2. BODEN, G. Results of the x-ray treatment of the reticuloses. *Brit J Radiol,* 24:494–498, 1951.
3. BUSCHKE, F. Some reflections on the treatment and prognosis of Hodgkin's disease, *Radiol Clin (Basel),* 34:285–309, 1965.
4. CRAVER, L. F. Lymphoma and leukemias. *Bull NY Acad Med,* 23:79–100, 1947.
5. CROSBIE, J. A clinical study of Hodgkin's disease. *Progress in Radiation Therapy,* Vol. II, F. Buschke, Ed, Grune & Stratton, 1962.
6. EASSON, E. C. Long-term results of radical radiotherapy in Hodgkin's disease. *Cancer Res,* 26:1244–1247, 1966.
7. EASSON, E. C., and RUSSELL, M. H. The cure of Hodgkin's disease. *Brit J Med,* 1:1704–1707, 1963.

8. FAYOS, J., HENDRIX, R., MACDONALD, V., and LAMPE, I. Hodgkin's disease: A review of radiotherapeutic experience. *Amer J Roentgen*, 93:557–567, 1965.

9. FULLER, L. M., and FLETCHER, G. H. The radiotherapeutic management of the lymphomatous diseases. *Amer J Roentgen*, 88:909–923, 1962.

10. GILBERT, R. Radiotherapy in Hodgkin's disease. *Amer J Roentgen*, 41:198–241, 1939.

11. GILBERT, R. J. Lymphogranulome, Lymphosarcome, Reticulosarcoma. *Radiol Clin (Basel)*, 20:313–336, 1951.

12. GILBERT, R., and BABAIANTZ, L., Notre méthode de roentgentherapie de la lymphogranulomatose (Hodgkin); résultats iloignes. *Acta Radiol [Ther] (Stockholm)*, 12:523–529, 1931.

13. GLATSTEIN, E., GUERNSEY, J. M., ROSENBERG, S. A., and KAPLAN, H. S. The value of laparotomy and splenectomy in the staging of Hodgkin's disease. *Cancer*, 24:709–718, 1969.

14. HILTON, G., and SUTTON, P. M. Malignant lymphomas: Classification, prognsis and treatment. *Lancet*, 1:283–287, 1962.

15. HOLME, G. M., and KUNKLER, P. B. Treatment of reticuloses by chemotherapy and radiotherapy. *Brit J Radiol*, 34:569–573, 1961.

16. JACKSON, H., JR., and PARKER, F. Hodgkin's disease: II Pathology. *New Eng J Med*, 231:35–44, 1944.

17. KAPLAN, H. S. In: *Current Concepts in Cancer*, P. Rubin, Ed. No. 1. Hodgkin's Disease. *JAMA*, 190:910–911, 1964.

18. KAPLAN, H. S. Evidence for a tumoricidal dose level in the radiotherapy of Hodgkin's disease. *Cancer*, 26:1221–1224, 1966.

19. LUMB, G. *Tumors of Lymphatic Tissue*. Livingstone, Edinburgh, 1954.

20. LUKES, R. J. Relationship of histologic features to clinical stages in Hodgkin's disease. *Amer J Roentgen*, 90:944–955, 1963.

21. NOETZLI, M., and SHELINE, G. E. Local recurrence in lymph nodes irradiated for Hodgkin's disease. In: *Progress in Radiation Therapy*, Vol. II, F. Buschke, Ed, Grune & Stratton, New York, 1962.

22. PETERS, M. V. A study of survivals in Hodgkin's disease treated radiologically. *Amer J Roentgen*, 63:299–311, 1950.

23. PETERS, M. V. The contribution of radiation therapy in the control of lymphomas. *Amer J Roentgen*, 90:956–967, 1963.

24. PETERS, M. V., and MIDDLEMISS, K. C. H. Study of Hodgkin's disease treated by irradiation. *Amer J Roentgen*, 79:114–121, 1958.

25. REED, D. M. On the pathological changes in Hodgkin's disease with special reference to its relation to tuberculosis. *Johns Hopkins Hospital Report*, 10:133–196, 1902.

26. ROSENBERG, S. A., DIAMOND, H. D., DARGEON, H. W., and CRAVER, L. F. Lymphosarcoma in childhood. *New Eng J Med*, 259:505–512, 1958.

27. ROSENBERG, S. A., DIAMOND, H. D., and CRAVER, L. F. Lymphosarcoma: Survival and the effects of therapy. *Amer J Roentgen*, 85:521–532, 1961.

28. ROSENBERG, S. A., and KAPLAN, H. S. Evidence for an orderly progression in the spread of Hodgkin's disease. *Cancer Res*, 26:1225–1231, 1966.

29. SCOTT, R. M., and BRIZEL, H. E. Time-dose relationships in Hodgkin's disease. *Radiology*, 82:1043–1049, 1964.

30. WILKS, S. Cases of lardaceous disease and some allied affections. *Guy Hos Rep*, 2:103–132, 1856.

12
LEUKEMIA

The leukemias ("white blood"—a name proposed by Virchow) can be considered cancers of the hematopoietic tissues, characterized by widespread proliferation of leukocytes and their precursors.[23] In this group of diseases, immature leukocytes seem to be outside the control of normal mechanisms which regulate cell proliferation and maturation.[9]

Leukemias caused approximately 15,000 deaths in the United States in 1970.[2] Acute leukemia is the most frequent cancer of youngsters under 15 years.

The incidence of the leukemias is increasing in the United States.[1,2,23] In part, this may be related to more accurate diagnosis, but it also may be related to an aging population and an increase in leukemogenic influences in the environment.

Terminology and Classification

The leukemias generally have been described as acute or chronic, based on the rapidity of their course, exclusive of the influence of treatment. Wintrobe[23] noted that the term *acute leukemia* has been used for those types resulting in the death of the patient within 6 months of diagnosis, whereas the designation *chronic leukemia* has been used for those types with survivals exceeding one year. The term *subacute* has been used for those patients surviving 6 to 12 months, even though the biology is similar to acute leukemia.

The leukemias also are classified by predominant cell type, although occasionally, especially with immature forms, this may be difficult. The relative frequency of the common types is[23]: chronic lymphocytic leukemia, 30.9 percent; chronic myelocytic leukemia, 29.0 percent; acute lymphoblastic leukemia, 16.7 percent; acute myeloblastic leukemia, 16.4 percent; acute monocytic leukemia, 7.0 percent.

Clinical Manifestations

All types of leukemia occur more often in males than in females (3–4:1).[1,2,23]

Leukemia may be present at birth, in which case it usually is myeloblastic. A relatively high incidence occurs during the first 5 years of life. Up to the age of 20 years, most leukemias are of acute lymphoblastic type. From 20 to 45 years (peak in the fourth decade) chronic myelocytic leukemia is most frequent, but for

234

patients over 45 years the chronic lymphocytic type is most frequent. However, the acute types may occur in adults and the chronic forms in those under 20 years.[23]

The chronic leukemias usually start insidiously, and often are first noted as an unexplained leukocytosis in an asymptomatic person. When the patient seeks aid, there may be anemia, adenopathy, splenomegaly, hepatomegaly, or infiltrations of specific tissues and organs. Eventually, there is weight loss, ease of perspiration, fever, and general cachexia.

The acute leukemias are of sudden, rather violent onset and, without treatment, of short course. The patient usually appears gravely ill with fever, prostration, severe anemia, hemorrhagic incidents, oral and pharyngeal mucosal necrosis, adenopathy, hepatosplenomegaly, or bone and joint pain.

Although the diagnosis may be suspected because of the clinical findings, substantiation requires study of the bone marrow and/or peripheral blood. In this appraisal, the immaturity of the leukocytes is more important than the total leukocyte count.[23] The bone marrow characteristically is hyperplastic (diffuse or nodular). There often is thrombocytopenia with prolongation of the bleeding time, poor clot retraction, and a positive tourniquet test. The basal metabolic rate (BMR) may be elevated, and there may be evidence of metabolic abnormalities (increased blood uric acid, altered purine, and pyrimidine metabolism).[23]

Patients with aleukemic or subleukemic forms may have normal or even subnormal leukocyte counts in the peripheral blood. However, a few telltale immature cells can be identified.

Differential diagnosis may be difficult at times because of similarity to such conditions as leukemoid reactions, infectious mononucleosis, and myelofibrosis with extramedullary hematopoiesis.[1]

Pathologic Findings

All hematopoietic sites may be involved. In the chronic lymphocytic form the architecture of the hyperplastic nodes, spleen, and marrow is disturbed. Frequent infiltration of various tissues and organs, i.e., kidneys, liver, lungs, skin, gastrointestinal tract, and CNS, is the basis for the protean clinical findings.

A curious localized tumor, termed a *chloroma,* may be a problem, particularly in children and young adults with acute myeloblastic leukemia.[1,23] These masses, usually involving the bones of the orbit, skull, sinuses, ribs, or spine,[23] are characterized by green pigmentation from the breakdown of hemoglobin.

Histologically, the leukemias are characterized by the dominant cell, as previously discussed.

Treatment

The first step in treatment is to make certain that the diagnosis is correct.[23] Although an occasional patient has been "cured," the reasonable objectives with current treatment methods are palliative.

Wintrobe[23] lists the somatic therapeutic problems as: (1) suppression of the leukemic cells in the marrow, blood, and tissues; (2) prevention and control of hemorrhage; (3) control of infections; (4) relief of anemia; and (5) maintenance of well-being of the patient.

The comfort and length of survival of patients with the acute leukemias can be directly correlated with ever-improving, aggressively applied systemic therapy. Although available treatment has improved the quality of life for patients with the chronic leukemias, it has not convincingly increased survival time, nor even frequently resulted in complete hematological remissions.[13] Many of these patients do very well for many years with little, if any, treatment. Johnson[13] has noted that, in contrast to most other forms of cancer, current therapeutic ineffectiveness has discouraged extension of treatment to the patient with early, asymptomatic leukemia. Disagreement persists whether asymptomatic or minimally symptomatic patients should be treated on the basis of an established diagnosis with abnormal laboratory findings,[12,19] or whether therapeutic efforts should be reserved for relief of bothersome symptoms and signs.[4,12,22]

It is appropriate that the leukemias, which can be considered systemic diseases, be treated predominantly by systemic methods. Thus, hematologists, who are primarily responsible for the management of these patients, have used *cytotoxic agents, antimetabolities, corticosteroids,* and *supportive* measures to good advantage. A discussion of the selection and use of these agents is not appropriate here.

For many years, *ionizing radiation* was the major effective therapeutic agent for patients with the chronic leukemias. Moss (1969)[17] states: "Radiotherapy quite justifiably remains the modality preferred by many in the treatment of the chronic forms of both granulocytic and lymphocytic leukemia." Johnson et al.[13] have recently documented that radiotherapy remains "one of the most effective therapies yet reported for induction of remission in this disease (chronic lymphocytic leukemia)."

Radiation therapy, available in several forms, can be used effectively for selective local or total body treatment. Its advantages are flexibility and more immediate control of application than is possible with systemic agents.

Local irradiation is the most effective treatment for local problems, i.e., discomfort from enlarged nodes in the axilla, groin, or neck; discomfort from a massively enlarged spleen; dysfunction and disfigurement from a retro-orbital chloroma; or meningeal involvement in a patient doing well otherwise. Response usually is rapid and complete following small doses. Such local treatment may quickly solve isolated problems without interfering with systemic treatment.

Total body radiation may be done with teletherapy or ^{32}P. ^{32}P is incorporated in newly fabricated cells. Thus, all types of cells may be affected, although the influence should be greatest in cells with the shortest turnover times (i.e., certain tumor cells, intestinal mucosa, and bone marrow). In patients with the chronic leukemias, the white cell response has an inverse exponential relationship to dose.[7] Administration of ^{32}P, either orally or intravenously, is convenient but less under immediate physician control than teletherapy. It has been estimated[7] that 1 mc injected intravenously gives a "total body" dose of approximately 6 rads, although the distribution differs from the nearly homogeneous dose from teletherapy. Leading advocates of carefully titrated ^{32}P treatment of patients with the chronic leukemias have been Osgood,[19] Reinhard,[20] and Lawrence.[15] Enthusiasm for this technique has diminished concurrently with increasing interest in systemic chemotherapy.

Total body radiation from a teletherapy source has been used effectively for many years. In a recent study,[13] a few patients with chronic lymphocytic leukemia received small, fractionated doses protracted over many weeks, with relief of constitutional symptoms and return of the absolute lymphocyte count to normal in all patients and reversal of the neutrophil:lymphocyte ratio, and correction of the anemia in a majority, thus documenting this often overlooked therapy to be as effective as any reported.

Destruction of circulating leukemic cells has been attempted by irradiation of the patient's blood as it flows through an extravascular arteriovenous shunt *(extracorporeal irradiation)*. This treatment, which is currently being investigated,[5,21] has reduced the peripheral leukocyte count and improved the associated anemia and thrombocytopenia without causing systemic or local (i.e., marrow) radiation effects.

Local irradiation of the spleen may result in both local and systemic benefit to a patient.[14] An enlarged spleen, causing local discomfort, may be quickly reduced in size with small doses (i.e., 25–50 rads per day to large fields and 100 rads per day to small fields to a total of a few hundred rads). Such treatment must be administered with caution, for there may be marked indirect effects (i.e., rapid reduction of WBCs in peripheral blood). Granulopoietic cells may be damaged as they cycle through the spleen,[10] resulting in a reduction in the number of myeloid cells in the peripheral blood and marrow. Erythropoiesis may improve secondary to a decrease in erythroclastic activity in the spleen,[3,17] and erythropoietic activity may shift back to the marrow from extramedullary sites.[3] Hemolysis may be suppressed.[3] Such effects may be reflected in a clinical remission, which although perhaps less long-lasting than that produced by total body radiation, may be less dangerous for patients with compromised marrow.[17] Such systemic benefits of local splenic irradiation do not result from splenectomy in these patients.[17]

The use of radiation therapy can be correlated with specific problems caused by particular types of leukemia.

Patients with the *acute leukemias* are not helped by total body or splenic irradiation.[6,17] However, local irradiation with small doses (less than 400 rads), probably through direct cell lysis, can relieve problems caused by infiltration of such structures as the CNS (headache, irritability, somnolence), bones and joints (pain), urinary bladder (hematuria), and skin and mucous membranes (sore mouth) without significant hematologic insult.[6]

Approximately 80 percent[17] of patients with *chronic lymphocytic leukemia* may be benefited by a reduction of bothersome adenopathy or splenomegaly; hematological improvement, such as lessening of the anemia secondary to "crowding" of the marrow by leukemic cells, lowering of the elevated peripheral white cell count, and increase in the percentage of granulocytes; or relief of the systemic complaints of fever, weight loss, and malaise.

Approximately 90 percent[17] of patients with *chronic myelocytic leukemia* may benefit from reduction of a massively enlarged spleen; hematological improvement manifested by a decrease in total white cells and immature granulocytes in the peripheral blood, an increase in the percentage of mature granulocytes in the peripheral blood and marrow, and a lessening of anemia; or relief of systemic toxicity.

Radiation therapy must be closely supervised by an experienced and interested physician. Treatment can be futile and even dangerous. Patients with a high percentage of blast cells (greater than 50 percent) in the peripheral blood usually are not helped.[17] Rapid dissolution of cellular masses may result in a rapid rise of the blood uric acid in patients with impaired renal function. Patients with leukopenia and thrombocytopenia related to a compromised bone marrow may be made worse.

Results and Prognosis

The role of radiation therapy is to improve the quality of the life of patients with leukemia by relieving specific somatic problems. There is no convincing evidence that treatment prolongs the lives of patients with the chronic leukemias, except on rare occasions through relief of an immediately life-threatening complication. However, 80–90 percent of these patients may enjoy nearly normal activity if carefully managed.[17]

Variations in reported survival data more likely relate to differences in the composition of the material than to "effectiveness" of treatment.[11]

In a recent report from the Ontario Cancer Foundation Clinics,[16] the post-diagnosis median survival for patients with chronic lymphocytic leukemia was 24 months and for patients with chronic myelocytic leukemia it was 21 months. Two-thirds of each group were alive one year after diagnosis, although at 5 years, only 25 percent of those with chronic lymphocytic leukemia and 10 percent of those with chronic myelocytic leukemia survived.

For groups in which patients with chronic lymphocytic or chronic myelocytic leukemia have been combined, the median survival from onset of symptoms or signs has varied little for many years, (Tivey, 1954,[22]—2.65 years; Osgood, Seaman, and Koler, 1957,[18]—4.3 years; Feinleib and MacMahon, 1960,[8]—1.53 years); those patients with chronic lymphocytic leukemia fared slightly better.

REVIEW QUESTIONS

1. What are the frequent types of leukemia? What are the gross correlations of various cell types with the clinical course?

2. Cancer is the most frequent disease killer of children under 15 years. What proportion of these deaths is from leukemia? What type of leukemia is most frequent?

3. Can you correlate age and type of leukemia?

4. How do the clinical presentations of the acute and chronic leukemias differ?

5. How is the diagnosis of leukemia established? What are the pitfalls?

6. What is a chloroma? Which patients usually are involved?

7. What somatic problems are frequent objectives of treatment?

8. What radiation therapy techniques may be useful for patients with leukemia? What are the advantages of each technique?

9. What are some contraindications to radiation therapy for patients with leukemia?

BIBLIOGRAPHY

1. ACKERMAN, L. V., and DEL REGATO, J. A. *Cancer*, 4th ed. Mosby, St. Louis, 1970.
2. American Cancer Society. 1970 Facts and Figures.

3. AWWAD, H. K., BADEEB, A. O., MASSOUD, G. E., and SOLAH, M. The effect of splenic x-irradiation on the ferrokinetics of chronic leukemia with a clinical study. *Blood*, 29:242–256, 1967.

4. BOGGS, D. R., SOFFERMAN, S. A., WINTROBE, M. M., and CARTWRIGHT, G. E. Factors influencing the duration of survival of patients with chronic lymphosytic leukemia. *Amer J Med*, 40:243–254, 1966.

5. CRONKITE, E. P. Extracorporeal irradiation of blood and lymph in treatment of leukemia and for immunosuppression. *Ann Intern Med*, 67:415–423, 1967.

6. D'ANGIO, G. J., EVANS, A. E., and MITUS, A. Roentgen therapy of certain complications of acute leukemia in childhood. *Amer J Roentgen*, 82:541–553, 1959.

7. EASSON, E. C. A quantitative study of the radiosensitivity of chronic leukemia. *Brit J Radiol*, 30:35–39, 1957.

8. FEINLEIB, M., and MACMAHON, B. Variation in the duration of survival of patients with the chronic leukemias. *Blood*, 15:332–349, 1960.

9. FURTH, J. Recent studies on the etiology and nature of leukemia. *Blood*, 6:964–975, 1951.

10. GALBRAITH, P. R. Mechanism of action of splenic irradiation in chronic myelogenous leukemia. *Canad Med Ass J*, 96:1636–1641, 1967.

11. GREEN, R. A., and DIXON, H. Expectancy for life in chronic lymphocytic leukemia. *Blood*, 25:23–30, 1965.

12. HUGULEY, C. M. Survey of current therapy and of problems in chronic leukemia in *Leukemia-Lymphoma*, Year Book, Chicago, 1970.

13. JOHNSON, R. E., KAGAN, A. R., GRALNICK, H. R., and FARS, L. Radiation-induced remissions in chronic lymphocytic leukemia. *Cancer*, 20:1382–1387, 1967.

14. KING, D. Radiotherapy in management of leukemia. *Canad Med Ass J*, 96:1621–1625, 1967.

15. LAWRENCE, J. H. The clinical use of radioactive isotopes. *Bull NY Acad Med*, 26:639–669, 1950.

16. MACKAY, E. N., and SELLERS, A. H. Statistical survey of leukemia in Ontario and at the Ontario Cancer Foundation Clinics. *Canad Med Ass J*, 96:1626–1635, 1967.

17. MOSS, W. T. *Therapeutic Radiology*, 3rd ed., Mosby, St. Louis, 1969.

18. OSGOOD, E. E., SEAMAN, A. J., and KOLER, R. D. Natural history and course of the leukemias. *Proc. 3rd Natl. Cancer Conf.*, 366–382, 1957.

19. OSGOOD, E. E. Treatment of chronic leukemias. *J Nucl Med*, 5:139–153, 1964.

20. REINHARD, E. H., NEELY, C. L., and SAMPLES, D. Radioactive phosphorus in the treatment of chronic leukemias. *Ann Intern Med*, 50:942–958, 1959.

21. THOMAS, E. D., EPSTEIN, R. B., ESCHBACH, J. W., JR., PRAGER, D., BUCKNER, C. D., and MARSAGLIA, G. Treatment of leukemia by extracorporeal irradiation. *New Eng J Med*, 273:6–12, 1965.

22. TIVEY, H. The prognosis for survival in chronic granulocytic and lymphocytic leukemia. *Amer J Roentgen*, 72:68–93, 1954.

23. WINTROBE, M. M. *Clinical Hematology*, 5th ed., Lea & Febiger, Philadelphia, 1961.

13

INTRATHORACIC TUMORS

CARCINOMA OF THE BRONCHUS

Carcinomas arising from the bronchial epithelium kill more men in the United States than do any other malignant tumors, or all other respiratory diseases combined. Women are afflicted 10–20 percent as often as men.[26] The rapid and continuing increase in incidence of bronchial carcinoma is real and not the result of improved diagnosis.[1]

Continued failure to establish the diagnosis prior to dissemination of tumor and consequent ineffectiveness of available treatment for most patients make preventive measures of prime importance.

Noting the statistical relationship between the inhalation of tobacco smoke and the development of squamous cell and undifferentiated bronchial carcinomas, Doll[15] has estimated that discontinuation of smoking would reduce the mortality 80–90 percent in males and 50 percent in females.

An increased incidence of bronchial carcinoma has been documented in those with prolonged exposures to inhaled radioactive substances, asbestos, arsenic, chromium, nickel, petroleum oil mists and coal tar fumes,[21] and in those with chronic pulmonary diseases, i.e., bronchiectasis and tuberculosis.[26]

Pathologic Findings

Most lung cancers arise from bronchial epithelium, but a few arise from bronchiolar epithelium. Transitions from atypical epithelial change to carcinoma in situ to invasive carcinoma have been documented.[26] Two-thirds of all bronchial carcinomas arise in the main stem or first division bronchi, whereas one-quarter arise in segmental bronchi, and one-tenth arise in small peripheral bronchi.[26] Slightly more than one-half of these neoplasms may be visualized at bronchoscopy.[25] Koletsky[23] found that tumors proximal to the bifurcation of the main-stem bronchi were likely to be anaplastic carcinomas, whereas epidermoid carcinomas often arose peripheral to the first bronchial bifurcation, and adenocarcinomas also were peripheral.

Bronchial carcinomas may extend submucosally for considerable distance; may occlude the bronchial lumen with consequent peripheral atelectasis and infection;

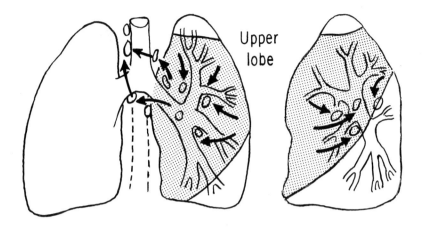

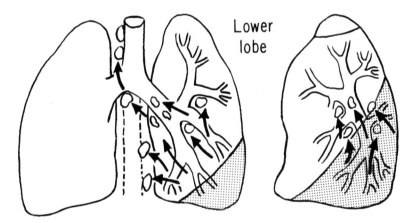

Fig. 13-1. Lymphatic drainage of left lung. (after Nohl[30]).

may invade cartilage, bone, pleura, pericardium, chest wall, and vessels; and may compress vessels, i.e., superior vena cava.

Extrathoracic metastases are most frequent with anaplastic carcinomas and adenocarcinomas and least frequent with differentiated epidermoid carcinomas.[23]

Lymphatic metastases are frequent (75 percent in operative series[31] and 94 percent in autopsy series[43]) through abundant pathways[31, 37] (Figures 13-1, 13-2). At surgical exploration, mediastinal nodes were found involved by tumor in 60 percent of those patients with undifferentiated carcinoma and in 34 percent of those with squamous cell carcinoma.[31]

Hematogenous metastases usually involve brain, bone, and liver. Resulting symptoms and signs occasionally may be the first produced, and often may become the major clinical problem.

The biological behavior and consequently the diagnosis, management, and prognosis vary with histological tumor type. In 4,000 patients with bronchial

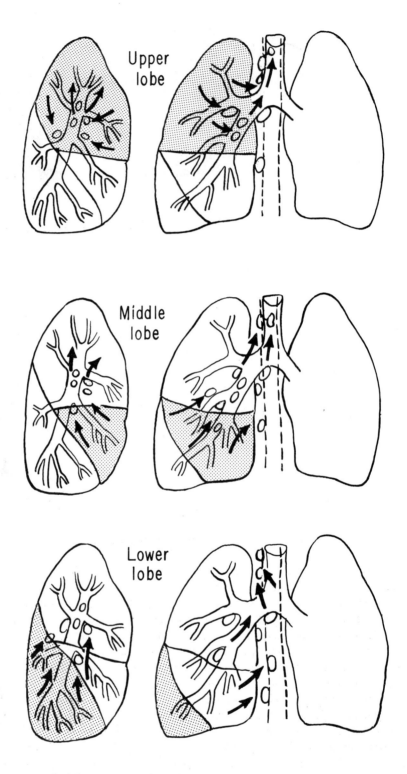

Upper
lobe

Middle
lobe

Lower
lobe

Fig. 13-2. Lymphatic drainage of right lung. (after Nohl[30]).

cancer studied in the Thoracic Surgical Unit in Edinburgh,[25] the frequency of the predominant cell type was: squamous cell carcinoma, 47.5 percent; undifferentiated carcinoma, 39.8 percent; adenocarcinoma, 5.1 percent; alveolar cell carcinoma, 0.4 percent; mixed cell type, 1.4 percent; unknown, 5.8 percent.

Bronchial adenomas, which constitute 6–10 percent of all primary lung tumors,[26] arise from the mucous glands of bronchial epithelium. These slow-growing, very vascular neoplasms usually involve proximal bronchi. Males and females, usually less than 50 years of age, are equally afflicted. Although initially circumscribed, by the time of diagnosis only 25 percent are exclusively intrabronchial.[26] The dominant clinical problems of hemoptysis and bronchial obstruction are related to the primary neoplasm, rather than to the biologically "late-appearing" and sluggish metastases. Generally it is not realized that some bronchial adenomas are radio-vulnerable to a clinically useful degree. Although the primary treatment of choice is surgery, the proximal position of most of these lesions may preclude complete removal. In such instances radiation therapy may be of considerable help.

Bronchiolar or alveolar cell carcinomas constitute 3–4 percent of malignant lung tumors.[26] These peripheral neoplasms usually ultimately involve both lungs, whether by metastases or multicentric origin, but they are slow to metastasize beyond the lungs. The clinical findings usually are related to extensive parenchymal involvement rather than to bronchial ulceration or obstruction or to distant metastases.

Pleural mesothelioma is a poorly defined tumor which may be more rare than the few cases reported, inasmuch as other primary sources of tumor often are difficult to exclude. These neoplasms apparently can extend locally and may metastasize to regional nodes and distant sites.[1] They may respond to irradiation but are not curable because of their anatomical extent. In selected situations substantial regression of tumor has provided palliation.

Clinical Presentation of Bronchial Carcinoma

Bronchial carcinoma may produce symptoms and signs by (1) local extension; (2) metastases; or (3) systemic effects. Most patients (68 percent[25]) present with nonspecific respiratory findings of cough, increased sputum, hemoptysis, chest pain, dyspnea, or wheezing. Fewer patients present with findings specifically related to tumor extension or metastases (13 percent[25]), i.e., superior vena cava compression, hoarseness, bone pain, or jaundice, or with nonspecific findings (12 percent[25]), i.e., loss of appetite and weight. An interesting, but small (2 percent[25]) group presents with manifestations associated with the presence of tumor. These may be[40] (1) metabolic, i.e., wasting, hypercalcemia, secretion of excessive antidiuretic substance, carcinoid syndrome, adrenal cortical hypersecretion; (2) neuromuscular, i.e., peripheral neuropathy, cortical cerebellar degeneration, and myopathy; (3) dermatological, i.e., acanthosis nigricans or dermatomyositis; (4) skeletal, i.e., osteoarthropathy, clubbing; (5) vascular, i.e., migratory thrombophlebitis, verrucal endocarditis; or (6) hematological, i.e., anemia, purpura.

When bronchial cancer compresses the superior vena cava, a characteristic clinical presentation includes (1) venous hypertension in the upper extremities with normal pressure in the lower limbs; (2) development of collateral circulation, visible on the chest wall and demonstrable by x-rays with contrast material in the vessels or by infrared photography; (3) edema and cyanosis of the face and neck aggravated by reclining.

About 5 percent of patients[25] may be asymptomatic, but have bronchial carcinomas that are discovered on chest x-rays requested for other purposes. Two-thirds of these patients have "peripheral" tumors not visible by bronchoscopy. These usually are histologically more differentiated and more often surgically removable and "curable."

Malignant tumors, usually well-differentiated epidermoid carcinomas, which arise at the thoracic inlet may (1) invade the lymphatics of the endothoracic fascia; (2) involve the roots of the brachial plexus, the sympathetic chain, the stellate ganglion, and the intercostal nerves; and (3) invade ribs, chest wall, and vertebrae, thus producing severe pain and Horner's syndrome. These patients with *superior pulmonary sulcus syndrome* or *Pancoast's tumor* are a special problem because of a protracted morbidity.

Diagnostic Methods

"The most available, least expensive and simplest method for the detection of a malignant lesion in the lung, when it is small, is roentgen examination."[33] Rigler[35] has described the "earliest roentgen signs" of carcinoma of the lung, but, even under these optimal conditions, in most patients the cancer has already spread at the time of diagnosis.

Bronchoscopy with biopsy is the best available method of establishing the diagnosis of bronchial carcinoma. There are few false positive diagnoses, but the method results in a diagnosis in only one-half of the patients with lung cancer.[41]

Carefully collected sputum specimens may be diagnostic for a good cytologist in 75 percent of patients with less than 1 percent false positives.[41] Selective bronchial aspirates may increase the diagnostic accuracy of bronchoscopy.

The diagnostic accuracy of scalene node biopsy increases with palpable adenopathy, upper lobe tumors, experienced surgeons, and plentiful biopsy material for study.

Umiker[41] has estimated that selective use of all of these diagnostic methods should result in a correct diagnosis in three of four patients.

Treatment and Results

Local treatment methods are infrequently curative for patients with bronchial carcinoma because in most patients tumor dissemination precedes diagnosis. This unfavorable situation has not been improving despite refinement of diagnostic methods and improvement of surgical and radiotherapeutic techniques.

Surgery

When applicable, resection of the primary tumor has been considered the most effective "curative" treatment. However, in a general hospital, of every 100 patients in whom the diagnosis of bronchial carcinoma is established, only 50 to 60 are operable, tumors in 25 to 35 are surgically removable, and 5 to 10 patients are "cured."[1] Although the incidence of operability (patient expected to survive the procedure) and "resectability" has increased, this may not be synonymous with an increased benefit to the patient.[10]

Surgical removal (lobectomy or pneumonectomy) with an objective of "cure" is contraindicated when there is extrathoracic spread of tumor, spread of tumor to the other lung, tumor extension causing paralysis of the recurrent laryngeal or phrenic nerves, or tumor involvement of the pulmonary artery close to the bifurcation. Attempted surgical removal is of doubtful value for patients with oat cell carcinoma, when tumor encroaches on the carina, when there is tumor-produced pleural effusion, when tumor invades the chest wall, and possibly even when the mediastinal nodes contain tumor.[10]

Even limited surgery may be contraindicated in 5–10 percent of patients[25] for medical reasons, i.e., poor respiratory function, cardiovascular disease, serious systemic illness, and age.

Lobectomy may be preferable for "peripheral" neoplasms which do not extend across interlobar fissures or to the chest wall. These patients were half as frequent as those subjected to pneumonectomy in the Edinburgh study, and suffered half the operative mortality (7 percent[25]).

Pneumonectomy, first performed by Graham in 1933,[16] may be preferable for patients with "central" tumors and for peripheral tumors which transcend the boundaries of a lobe.

Surgery may be of palliative value for patients with lung infection and abscess peripheral to bronchial obstruction, hemorrhage, and pulmonary osteoarthropathy. However, in this group, even more than in those patients potentially "curable," the morbidity and mortality of exploratory thoractomy (6 percent[25]) and resection (up to 20 percent[25]) must be considered.

Radiation Therapy

The indiscriminate use of radiation therapy for every patient with bronchial carcinoma not treated by surgery is to be condemned. Indications for treatment must be related to the specific clinical problem, the condition of the patient, and an estimate of the biology of the tumor. Most patients with bronchial carcinoma have been referred to the radiotherapist because (1) the patient is inoperable or the tumor is not removable because of extent or biological type (oat cell carcinoma); (2) the patient is inoperable for medical reasons even though the tumor may be localized. In our experience, few patients refuse surgery if offered.

The radiotherapist must estimate whether all tumor definable by available diagnostic methods is limited to a small volume, for these patients are potentially "curable," or whether because of tumor extent the initial objective should be palliation. A current dilemma is that most patients with apparently grossly localized tumor will prove incurable because of occult tumor dissemination. Therefore, radical radiotherapy will merely add needless morbidity to most of these patients, although withholding of treatment occasionally may deprive a patient of a chance for "cure."

Biological Correlation. 1. *Oat cell or small cell carcinoma* progresses rapidly, usually causing the patient's death within 12 months. The cancer locally invades lung parenchyma; spreads to the mediastinum, often causing mediastinal embarassment, and metastasizes via the lymphatics and the blood stream to brain, bone, liver, and other sites. Many surgeons consider this tumor type a contraindication to attempted removal. Therefore, the radiotherapist may see a few patients with "localized tumor" at the time of diagnosis. However, treatment is usually palliative from the onset with objectives of relieving mediastinal compression, bronchial obstruction, pain from bony metastases, and neurological change from intracranial metastases. Such treatment can be limited to modest dosage, and should be delivered rapidly and with minimal morbidity.

2. *Keratinizing epidermoid carcinomas* and *adenocarcinomas* may grow slowly and remain localized for many years.[34] These lesions have been considered best treated surgically. The radiotherapist usually sees those patients with regional adenopathy after resection or those denied surgery for medical reasons. Irradiation of a small tissue volume containing the tumor to a high dose may be "curative." However, most of these patients have tumor extension or metastases, and radiation therapy should be used to relieve specific tumor-created problems.[8]

3. The majority of bronchial cancers are *epidermoid carcinomas of poor to moderate histological differentiation*. The biology of these tumors is less predictable than either of the above. The usual place of radiotherapy is as a surgical adjunct to treat regional adenopathy or as a palliative agent with specific purpose.

Morrison, Deeley, and Cleland[30] randomized 58 patients considered operable between surgery and radical supervoltage radiotherapy and concluded that "surgery is the better method of treatment for operable cases of squamous carcinoma of the lung," whereas "in anaplastic tumours it appeared that neither method of treatment showed a preference" (Table 13-1).

In a planned study of the treatment of 144 patients with oat cell carcinoma of the bronchus,[28] it was concluded that those irradiated survived longer with less treatment-produced mortality than those treated surgically (Table 13-2).

Therefore, surgery seems preferable to radiotherapy for patients with squamous cell carcinoma (and probably adenocarcinoma) of the bronchus, which is removable, while radiotherapy is preferable for patients with oat cell carcinoma. For patients with less than well-differentiated carcinomas, the choice of treatment depends on specific conditions for each patient.

Preoperative Radiation Therapy. The potential advantages of preoperative irradiation are[6]: (1) conversion of some tumors from being not removable to being removable; (2) control of regional lymph node metastases inaccessible to surgical

Table 13-1. Treatment of Patients with "Operable" Bronchial Carcinoma

	Entire Group		Squamous Cell Carcinoma		Anaplastic Carcinoma	
	No. Pts. Treated	4-Year Survival Rate	No. Pts. Treated	4-Year Survival Rate	No. Pts. Treated	4-Year Survival Rate
Surgery	30	23%	20	30%	10	10%
Radiation therapy	28	7%	17	5%	9	11%

From Morrison, Deeley and Cleland.[30]

Table 13-2.   Treatment of Patients with Oat Cell Bronchial Carcinoma[28]

	No. Pts. Treated	Mean Survival
Surgery	71	190 days
Radiation therapy	73	256 days

removal; (3) decrease in local and systemic tumor seeding at the time of operation; (4) occasional reduction of the necessary extent of surgery.

In several studies,[4,7,19,24] patients judged inoperable because of tumor extent became technically operable after local irradiaton. Tumor was not found in up to 40 percent of postradiation surgical specimens.[24] Possibly of greatest significance was the finding of an increased incidence of "tumor-free" mediastinal nodes.[4] However, such preliminary reports must await documentation that patient survival has been lengthened or improved qualitatively.

Presurgical irradiation (without biopsy) has been advocated[27] for superior sulcus cancers, for these tumors usually are well-differentiated, grow slowly with invasion of surrounding structures, and metastasize "late."

Postoperative Radiation Therapy.   Irradiation of regional nodes (bronchial, mediastinal, supraclavicular Figures 13-1, 13-2), following surgical removal of the primary tumor might be attempted in two situations: (1) when the nodes are at risk, but are not known to be tumor-bearing; and (2) when there is biopsy proof of metastases. Such treatment for patients with squamous cell bronchial carcinomas would seem more logical than similar treatment for patients with cancer of the breast, inasmuch as persistent local tumor without widespread dissemination may be more frequent in the former.

However, despite the abundance of available patients, little useful data have been accumulated. Thus, De Jong and Renner[14] stated that "routine" postoperative radiation therapy improved their results, whereas Paterson and Russell[32] found no difference. When attempted removal of tumor was grossly incomplete, Guttmann[17] stated that local irradiation relieved related symptoms and signs, but did not alter life expectancy. Deeley[11] noted 4 of 30 patients surviving more than three years when irradiated for residual neoplasm.

The University of Michigan Group[22] recently has reported on 231 patients with bronchogenic carcinoma in whom mediastinal lymph node dissection was performed in conjunction with pulmonary resection. Forty-eight patients were found to have mediastinal metastases, 36 of these patients underwent mediastinal irradiation in the immediate postoperative period, and 12 patients did not. The absolute 5-year survival rate of the patients receiving irradiation was 19.5 percent. In 17 patients with squamous cell carcinoma and mediastinal metastases, the 5-year survival rate was 29.5 percent. In 17 patients with adenocarcinoma and mediastinal metastases it was 5.9 percent. Of 12 patients who did not receive postoperative irradiation to the mediastinum (including 5 squamous cell carcinoma, 5 adenocarcinomas, and 2 undifferentiated carcinomas) none survived 5 years. This would suggest that the finding of mediastinal node involvement during mediastinoscopy or exploratory thoractomy in patients with squamous cell carcinoma is not a contraindication to resection, and that a significant percentage of these patients can still be saved by this combined treatment

Radiation Therapy as a Primary Treatment   Inasmuch as radiotherapy usually has been used for patients inoperable because of tumor extent or because of severe medical disability, comparison with surgery as a primary treatment method has not been legitimate. Smart and Hilton[39] selected 40 patients without clinical, x-ray, or bronchoscopic evidence of node involvement and treated them by radiation methods. Eight patients had oat cell tumors, 27 had squamous cell tumors, and in 5, the diagnosis was established by cytology. Nine of the 40 patients (22.5 percent) survived five years, and most who survived longer than six months returned to work.

Palliative Radiotherapy.   Local irradiation is the most effective palliative treatment and can be delivered rapidly and with little morbidity. Objectives and likelihood of accomplishment are:

1.   Suppression of hemoptysis—75[38]–94 percent[29]
2.   Relief of mediastinal compression syndrome—75 percent[38]
3.   Relief of bronchial obstruction and atelectasis—over 50 percent[18]
4.   Relief of dyspnea secondary to bronchial obstruction—50 percent[3,38]
5.   Relief of symptoms from intracranial metastases—vast majority[9] with 7 percent living for more than three years and 47 percent returning to functional life[13]
6.   Relief of cough—less than 50 percent[38]
7.   Relief of pain—(a)   from bony metastasis—frequent[38]
     (b)   from nerve invasion—infrequent[38]
8.   Relief of dysphagia from adenopathy—frequent[3]
9.   Improvement in patient's general well-being—over 50 percent[38]

Chemotherapy

Inasmuch as widespread dissemination of tumor is frequent at the time of diagnosis, the potential advantage of systemic treatment is apparent. Various agents have been used as adjuvants with surgery and radiation therapy without improvement in duration of survival, but with the added burden of toxicity.[20,36] Any palliative effects usually are short-lived,[20] although various nonradioactive agents have been valuable in controlling tumor-stimulated pleural effusion.

Prognostic Factors

The following factors have been correlated with the prognosis of patients with bronchial carcinoma:

1.   Histology—Well-differentiated epidermoid carcinoma has the best prognosis, oat cell carcinoma the worst, with other types intermediate.[12] The prognosis for patients with adenocarcinoma varies widely in various reports.[11]
2.   Site—Tumors primary in the upper and middle lobes are less ominous than those in the lower lobes, whether treated by surgery[2] or irradiation.[12]
3.   Age and sex—Perhaps females and patients less than 50 years fare better.[11]

4. Growth rate—Patients with tumor known to develop over a long period, as expected, do better after the diagnosis.[42]
5. "Incomplete" removal—If tumors are not grossly removable, partial removal may be worse than no surgery prior to irradiation.[17]
6. General condition—Patients with concurrent weight loss and asthenia do worse.[5]

REVIEW QUESTIONS

1. What is the site of origin of most bronchial carcinomas? How should this affect diagnostic effort?

2. What is your understanding of the etiological relationship of tobacco smoking and bronchial cancer?

3. What are the most frequent types of cancer arising from bronchial epithelium? Which type of bronchial carcinoma has the highest incidence of regional and distant metastases?

4. What is the most frequent clinical presentation of patients with bronchial carcinoma?

5. If a 50-year-old male has a mediastinal mass associated with paralysis of one vocal cord, which is the likely diagnosis—Hodgkin's disease or bronchial carcinoma? Why?

6. What manifestations may be associated with bronchial carcinoma? Have you seen a patient with any of these?

7. What clinical findings are characteristic of tumor compression of the superior vena cava?

8. What clinical findings are associated with malignant tumors arising near the thoracic inlet?

9. What available diagnostic method is likely to first detect bronchial carcinoma? How often may these patients be asymptomatic? How often is the tumor still localized?

10. What are the diagnostic advantages and limitations of bronchoscopy? sputum cytology? scalene node biopsy? chest x-ray?

11. What is the biological basis for failure of currently available treatment for patients with bronchial carcinoma?

12. How often is surgical resection applicable for patients with bronchial carcinoma? What percentage of all patients diagnosed are "cured" by resection? What is the mortality of thoracotomy? of pulmonary resection?

13. What biological characteristics of oat cell carcinoma make cure by resection unlikely? Do these characteristics pertain to radiotherapy? What is the basis of selection of therapy?

14. What are the usual uses of radiotherapy for patients with regionally limited bronchial carcinoma?

15. Can patients with bronchial carcinoma be "cured" by irradiation?

16. What are the objectives of preoperative radiotherapy for patients with bronchial carcinoma? What have been the accomplishments?

17. What are the palliative indications and accomplishments of radiotherapy for the patient with bronchial carcinoma?

18. List and discuss five prognostic factors for patients with bronchial carcinoma?

BIBLIOGRAPHY

1. ACKERMAN, L. V., and DEL REGATO, J. A. *Cancer: Diagnosis, Treatment, Prognosis,* 4th ed. Mosby, St. Louis, 1970.
2. BIGNALL, J. R., and MOON, A. J. Survival after lung resection for bronchial carcinoma. *Thorax,* 10:183–190, 1955.
3. BLANSHARD, G. The palliation of bronchial carcinoma by radiotherapy. *Lancet,* 2:897–901, 1955.
4. BLOEDORN, F. G., COWLEY, R. A., CUCCIA, C. A., and MERCADO, R. J. Combined therapy: Irradiation and surgery in the treatment of bronchogenic carcinoma. *Amer J Roentgen,* 85:875–885, 1961
5. BLOEDORN, F. G., COWLEY, R. A., CUCCIA, C. A., MERCADO, R., WIZENBERG, M. J., and LINDBERG, E. J. Preoperative irradiation in bronchogenic carcinoma. *Amer J Roentgen,* 92:77–87, 1964.
6. BLOEDORN, F. G. Rationale and benefit of preoperative irradiation in lung cancer. *JAMA,* 196:21–22, 1966.
7. BROMLEY, L. L., and SZUR, L. Combined radiotherapy and resection for carcinoma of bronchus: Experiences with 66 patients. *Lancet,* 2:937–941, 1955.
8. BUSCHKE, F. Roentgen therapy of carcinoma of the lung. *Radiology,* 69:489–493, 1957.
9. CHU, F. C. H., and HILARIS, B. B. Value of radiation therapy in the management of intracranial metastases. *Cancer,* 14:577–581, 1961.
10. CLIFTON, E. E. The criteria for operability and resectability in lung cancer. *JAMA,* 195:13–14, 1966.
11. DEELEY, T. J. The treatment of carcinoma of the bronchus. *Brit J Radiol,* 40:801–822, 1967.
12. DEELEY, T. J., and SINGH, S. P. Treatment of inoperable carcinoma of the bronchus. *Thorax,* 22:562–566, 1967.
13. DEELEY, T. J., and RICE-EDWARDS, J. M. (quoted in reference 11).
14. DE JONG, K., and RENNER, K. Zur Behandlung des Bronchialkarzinoms. *Strahlentherapie,* 129:348–359, 1966.
15. DOLL, R. Present knowledge of causation of carcinoma of the lung. In: *Neoplastic Disease at Various Sites,* Vol. 1. D. W. Smithers, Ed, Livingstone, Edinburgh, 43–111, 1958.
16. GRAHAM, E. A., and SINGER, J. J. Successful removal of entire lung for carcinoma of bronchus. *JAMA,* 101:1371–1374, 1933.
17. GUTTMANN, R. J. Results of radiation therapy in patients with inoperable carcinoma of the lung. *Amer J Roentgen,* 93:99–103, 1965.
18. HACKENTHAL, P. Zur palliativbestrahlung des Bronchialkarzinoms. *Strahlentherapie,* 111:190–196, 1960.
19. HELLMAN, S., KLIGERMAN, M. M., VON ESSEN, C. F., and SEIBETTA, M. P. Sequelae of radical radiotherapy of carcinoma of the lung. *Radiology,* 82:1055–1061, 1964.
20. HIGGINS, G., and BEEBE, G. W. Present status of surgical adjuvant lung cancer chemotherapy. *JAMA,* 196:24–25, 1966.
21. HUEPNER, W. C. Epidemiologic experimental and histological studies on metal cancers of the lung. *Acta Union int contra Cancrum,* 15:424–436, 1959.
22. KIRSH, M. M., KAHN, D. R., GAGO, OTTO, LAMPE, I., and SLOAN, H. Treatment of bronchogenic carcinoma with mediastinal metastases. *Ann Thorac Surg,* 1971 (in press).

23. KOLETSKY, S. Primary carcinoma of the lung: A clinical and pathological study of 100 cases. *Arch Intern Med* (Chicago), 62:636–651, 1938.

24. LAWTON, R. L., ROSSI, N. P., LATOURETTE, H. B., and FLYNN, J. R. Preoperative irradiation in the treatment of clinically operable lung cancers. *J Thorac Cardiovasc Surg*, 51:745–750, 1966.

25. LE ROUX, B. T. *Bronchial Carcinoma*. Livingstone, Edinburgh, 1968.

26. LIEBOW, A. A. Tumors of the lower respiratory tract. *Atlas of Tumor Pathology*, Section V, Fascicle 17, Washington, D.C., 1952.

27. MALLAMS, J. T., PAULSON, D. L., COLLIER, R. E., and SHAW, R. R. Presurgical irradiation in bronchogenic carcinoma, superior sulcus type. *Radiology*, 82:1050–1054, 1964.

28. Medical Research Council. Comparative trial of surgery and radiotherapy for primary treatment of small cell or oat cell carcinoma of the bronchus. *Lancet*, 2:979–986, 1966.

29. MORRISON, R., and DEELEY, T. J. Inoperable cancer of the bronchus treated by megavoltage x-ray therapy. *Lancet*, 2:618–620, 1960.

30. MORRISON, R., DEELEY, T. J., and CLELAND, W. P. Treatment of carcinoma of the bronchus: A clinical trial to compare surgery and supervoltage radiation therapy. *Lancet*, 1:683–684, 1963.

31. NOHL, H. C. An investigation into the lymphatic and vascular spread of carcinoma of the bronchus. *Thorax*, 11:172–185, 1956.

32. PATERSON, R., and RUSSELL, M. H. Clinical trials in malignant disease: IV. Lung cancer. *Clin Radiol*, 13:141–144, 1962.

33. RIGLER, L. G. The detection of cancer of the lung. In: *Proceedings of the Third National Cancer Conference*. Lippincott, Philadelphia, 1956.

34. RIGLER, L. G. A roentgen study of the evolution of carcinoma of the lung. *J Thorac Cardiovasc Surg*, 34:283–297, 1957.

35. RIGLER, L. G. The earliest roentgenographic signs of carcinoma of the lung. *JAMA*, 195:3–5, 1966.

36. ROSWIT, B. Present state of chemotherapy of bronchial cancer. *Radiology*, 69:499–506, 1957.

37. ROUVIERE, H. Anatomie des lymphatiques de l'homme. Masson, Paris, 1932. English translation: Edwards, Ann Arbor, Michigan.

38. SCHULZ, M. D. Palliation by radiotherapy. *JAMA*, 196:33–34, 1966.

39. SMART, J., and HILTON, G. Radiotherapy of cancer of the lung. *Lancet*, 6:880–881, 1956.

40. SMITH, L. H. What are the extrapulmonary manifestations of bronchogenic carcinoma? *JAMA*, 195:8–9, 1966.

41. UMIKER, W. O. Diagnosis of bronchogenic carcinoma: An evaluation of pulmonary cytology, bronchoscopy and scalene lymph node biopsy. *Dis Chest*, 37:82–90, 1960.

42. WEISS, W., BOUCOT, K. R., and COOPER, D. A. Growth rate in the detection and prognosis of bronchogenic carcinoma. *JAMA*, 198:1246–1252, 1966.

43. WILLIS, R. A. *Pathology of Tumours*, 2nd ed., Butterworth, London, 1953.

CARCINOMA OF THE ESOPHAGUS

Carcinoma of the esophagus occurs more frequently than does cancer arising in the tongue, larynx, kidney, or bone. This cancer has a peak incidence in patients in their seventh decade of life, more often affects males than females (3–4 to 1), and usually is an epidermoid carcinoma[1,6,19] (epidermoid carcinoma: 80–90 percent, adenocarcinoma: 10–20 percent).

The diagnosis rarely is established until the tumor is extensive. Obstructive dysphagia, the most frequent symptom, is noted by 60–90 percent[1,25] of these patients. Clinically recognized obstruction may not result until after two-thirds of the lumen of the thoracic esophagus is compromised.[25] Symptoms and signs of obstruction may be caused by smaller tumors at sites of anatomic narrowing of the lumen, i.e., at the cricopharyngeal sphincter, the diaphragm, or where the aorta and left main stem bronchus cross the esophagus. Obstruction is more likely to be caused by bulky, exophytic tumors than by surface-spreading or deeply infiltrative neoplasms, although the latter may be associated with ill-defined symptoms, i.e., retrosternal discomfort and pain with swallowing. Persistent retrosternal or midback pain, independent of swallowing or aggravated by swallowing, is most suggestive of a penetrating ulceration or imminent perforation. Once obstruction interferes with ingestion, weight loss is rapid.

Other clinical findings, usually indicative of extension of tumor beyond the esophagus—hemiparalysis of the larynx secondary to involvement of the recurrent laryngeal nerve, cough, and pulmonary problems from tracheo-esophageal fistula, or mediastinitis from esophageal perforation—can be anticipated from a knowledge

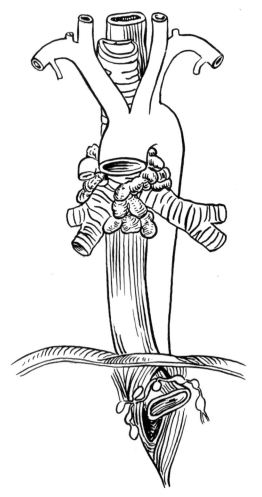

Fig. 13-3. Spread of carcinoma of esophagus.
1. Along the long axis in mucosa, submucosal lymphatics, and intermuscular spaces.
2. Direct extension to adjacent structures depending on the level.
3. Lymph node involvement generally downward from primary lesion with metastases to subdiaphragmatic nodes in over 30 percent.
4. Distant metastases, i.e., to liver, lung, and bones.

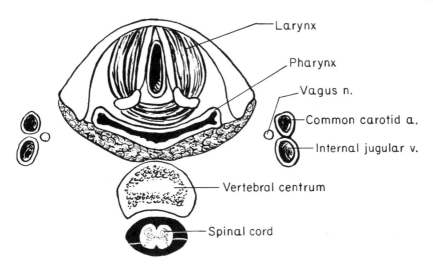

Fig. 13-4.   Postlaryngeal pharynx, level of C₅.

of the intimate relationship of the esophagus to many important structures (Figs. 13-3–13-8).

Even when the symptoms and signs indicate extensive tumor, there is considerable delay in establishment of the diagnosis and institution of treatment (Table 13-3). The mean interval between clinical indication of obstruction and initiation of treatment was 4 months in Smither's series[19] and 3.9 months in ours (Table 13-4). In 14 of our 70 patients (20 percent), the diagnosis was not established at the time of initial medical consultation, and in 11 percent the delay between initial consultation and establishment of diagnosis was 2 to 6 months.

This poor diagnostic performance adversely affects prognosis, for regional barriers to the spread of tumor are relatively ineffective, and extensive cancers involving adjacent structures and lymph nodes rarely are controlled by any treat-

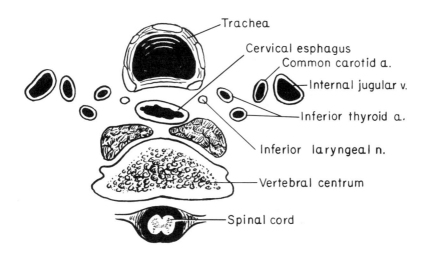

Fig. 13-5.   Cervical Esophagus, Level of C₇.

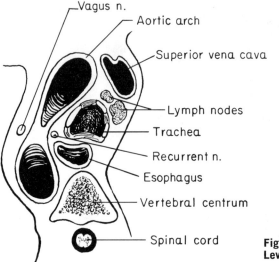

Fig. 13-6. Intrathoracic Esophagus Level of T₄.

ment method. The incidence of tumor involvement of regional lymph nodes increases with the duration of symptoms and signs, as noted by Helsley[10] who found that in patients with a history exceeding five months, the incidence of adenopathy was 43 percent as compared with an incidence of 18 percent in those with shorter histories. Fleming[6] found that tumor had extended outside the thoracic esophagus in 88 percent of patients when the primary lesion measured more than 5.1 cm along the esophageal axis.

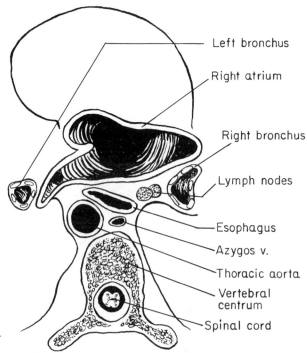

Fig. 13-7. Mid-thoracic Esophagus, Level of T₇.

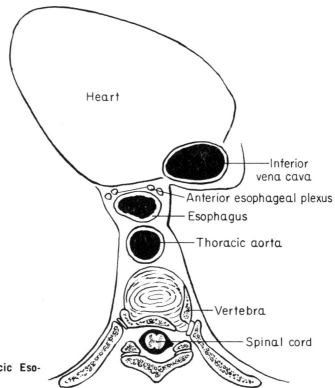

Fig. 13-8. Lower Thoracic Esophagus, Level of T9-10.

Heart

Inferior vena cava

Anterior esophageal plexus

Esophagus

Thoracic aorta

Vertebra

Spinal cord

Table 13-3. Carcinoma of the Esophagus
Duration of Symptoms Before Treatment

Royal Marsden Hospital 356 Patients	
3 mo.	28.2%
3–5 mo.	36.8%
6–11 mo.	22.1%
1 yr.	12.9%

Smithers & Payne[19]

Table 13-4. Carcinoma of the Esophagus
Delay in diagnosis

UCSF 1957–1961 70 Patients		
Symptoms to first consultation	2–6 mo.	48%
No diagnosis at first consultation	14/70	20%
First consultation to diagnosis	2–6 mo.	11%
Average delay, symptoms to diagnosis	3.9 mo.	

Pathologic Findings

The biology of esophageal cancer and, consequently, optimal treatment and prognosis vary with the anatomic site of involvement. Several arbitrary anatomic divisions have been proposed, although each has separated cervical and lower thoracic segments and related the intrathoracic esophagus to the aortic arch, a site of concern to the surgeon. Lederman[11] proposed a division into three segments: an upper third including cricopharyngeal, pharyngo-esophageal, cervical, and supra-aortic mediastinal components; a middle third related to the aortic arch and left main stem bronchus, and a lower third including the esophagus extending from the left main stem bronchus to the stomach. Sweet[21] and Buschke[4] suggested division into four segments: a cervical segment extending from the lower margin of the cricoid cartilage to the thoracic inlet; and a thoracic segment subdivided into upper fourth, lower fourth, and middle half.

Incidence of involvement naturally varies with the system of designation of segments. Buschke[4] noted the frequency of involvement by epidermoid carcinoma to be cervical, 10 percent; lower fourth of thoracic segment, 13 percent; upper fourth of thoracic segment, 7 percent; and middle half of thoracic segment, 70 percent. Marcial et al.[12] also noted the highest incidence in the middle third (upper one-third, 17 percent; middle one-third, 54 percent; lower one-third, 27 percent).

Grossly, cancers of the esophagus can be exophytic and bulky, flat and surface-spreading, or deeply infiltrating. They usually spread extensively in the submucosa along the long axis, through the wall and into adjacent tissues, and via lymphatics and blood vessels.

The standard lymphatic drainage pathways are from the upper third to the lower cervical and supraclavicular fossa nodes; from the lower third to the upper abdominal nodes; and from the middle third to the mediastinal and subdiaphragmatic nodes.[1] Thus, nodal metastases from any segment of the thoracic esophagus may be outside the thorax, placing those lesions beyond cure by available treatment.

Hematogenous metastases frequently involve liver, lung, and brain. Such lesions occasionally are the basis of the initial clinical presentation.

Fleming[6] documented that, at autopsy, 41 of 52 untreated patients (79 percent) had spread beyond the esophagus, the incidence of spread being 88 percent in those with primary lesions longer than 5.1 cm.

Most malignant tumors arising in the esophagus are epidermoid carcinomas (Geschickter,[7] 87 percent epidermoid carcinoma and 13 percent, adenocarcinoma), Farrell,[5] 78 percent epidermoid carcinoma and 18 percent adenocarcinoma), often rather poorly differentiated.[1]

The incidence of adenocarcinoma varies with the inclusion of lesions involving both lower esophagus and stomach, for these may also be considered primary in the stomach, with extension to the esophagus.

Treatment

Patterns of patient management have changed as better surgical and radio-therapeutic methods have become available, as noted by Pearson[18] at the Royal Infirmary, Edinburgh, Scotland, where until 1947 radiotherapy was the only effective treatment, and between 1948 and 1955 surgery superseded radical irradiation as "curative" treatment; since then, radical irradiation has again become the "preferable" initial treatment.

In any consideration of treatment, initial objectives of "cure," no matter how unlikely, or palliation need be defined. Pearson[18] has noted that an initial treatment objective of "cure" has become more frequent over the past 40 years, although there has been only a very modest increase in tumor control during this same interval. Conversely, palliation has become more frequent with the availability of better radiotherapy equipment, and consequently more frequent adequacy of radiation dose and better radiation tolerance.

In this large clinical material,[18] at the time of initial evaluation more than one-third of all patients continue to have evidence of hematogenous metastases, remote lymphatic spread, tracheo-esophageal fistula, or a primary tumor longer than 10.0 cm and, therefore, are excluded from an attempt at curative treatment.

Inasmuch as most patients die with their tumor uncontrolled, treatment-produced morbidity and mortality would seem of disproportionate importance. Likewise, quality of life for a short survival period is very important. Thus, retention of the larynx, retention of a functional esophagus, and avoidance of permanent intubation or gastrostomy are important.

Any comparison of treatment methods requires attention to several details often ignored: competence in use of the method; discussion of the same disease, i.e., epidermoid carcinoma; comparison by stages and by various anatomic levels; assessment of a large and meaningful clinical material.[4]

Radiation Therapy

Epidermoid carcinoma of the esophagus illustrates that inherent tumor "radiovulnerability" is but one of many factors determining radiocurability. Anatomic location of tumor, local tumor extent, and condition of the tumor bed influence the ultimate accomplishment of radiation therapy more than does the "radiovulnerability" of the tumor.

Although gross tumor regression follows vigorous irradiation in 50–80 percent[4, 12, 24] of treated patients, cure is the exception.

Obstacles to control of tumor by radiation therapy are frequent extension of tumor through the thin esophageal wall with fixation to vital mediastinal structures, i.e., large vessels and trachea, with the consequent threat of perforation; frequent spread of tumor through submucosal lymphatics, with ultimate involvement of nearly the entire length of the esophagus; spread of tumor to regional lymph nodes; poor nutritional status and general condition of the frequently elderly patients, with consequent reduction of their tolerance to the treatment.

Although adequate dosage may be delivered with orthovoltage x-ray through the use of elaborate techniques, i.e., multiple fields or rotation, as documented by Nielsen[15] (Table 13-5), potentially effective radical radiation therapy has been possible only since the introduction of "supervoltage" teletherapy equipment.

Adequate doses, i.e., 6,000–6,500 rads in 6½ to 7½ weeks can be accurately delivered with opposing anterior-posterior or three-field techniques. Rotation therapy, attractive in principle, is hampered by the curvature of the thoracic esophagus, irregularity of tumor extensions, and variations in thoracic contours.

Table 13-5. Carcinoma of the Esophagus
Medium Voltage X-ray Rotation Therapy
(4,000 R in 5 to 6 weeks)

Number treated	96
Alive 3 years	10
Alive 5 years	5
Died 2 to 5 years without local recurrence	8
Benefited	13/96

Nielsen[16] 1949 (personal communication)

Early therapeutic attempts using local radiation methods (intracavitary or interstitial radium) were doomed to failure for both biological and physical reasons.

Technical improvements have facilitated radiation therapy for both the patient and the radiotherapist, thus improving palliative treatment. However, even if the control of the primary tumor has improved, there has been no significant increase in the overall frequency of "cure", which remains 3–8 percent at five years for large unselected groups of patients (Tables 13-6, 13-7), although as expected, control of tumor is better for selective groups of patients.

Treatment performance for both radiation therapy and surgery varies with the anatomical level of involvement. The effectiveness of radiation therapy may decrease slightly from cervical to lower thoracic segments, and the effectiveness of surgery may increase (Tables 13-8, 13-9). The operative morbidity and mortality clearly decrease for patients with tumors below the aortic arch. Therefore, radiation therapy usually is preferred for carcinomas of the cervical, upper, and mid thoracic esophagus, whereas surgery is preferred for tumors of the lower thoracic esophagus and esophago-cardiac junction, although there are objectors, i.e., Nakayama[14] and Adams,[3] who believe that resection is preferable at all levels, and Pearson,[18] who

Table 13-6. Carcinoma of the Esophagus
800 kv X-ray Therapy
Swedish Hospital, Seattle 1940–1953

Patients seen in consultation	77
Patients accepted for treatment	43
Patients completely treated	34
Patients well to date (1963)	3*
Histology negative at autopsy	3†
Primary tumor controlled	6
Esophagus grossly normal until patient's death	11
Number of patients benefited by complete treatment	17:34 (50 percent)
Number of patients benefited of all seen	17:77 (22 percent)

(Buschke[4])
*15, 13, 12 years.
†10 years, 4½ years, 8 months.

Table 13-7. Carcinoma of the Esophagus
Compilation of Radiation Therapy Results
From Centers Reporting All Patients Seen

	Years	No. Seen	% Irrad.	5-Year Survivals
Royal Marsden Hospital	1936/1954	382	73	10
Radiumhemmet	1940/1950	691	58.9	10
Swedish Hospital	1940/1950	59	52.5	3
University Lund	1944/1952	249	86.7	12
Total		1,381		35 (2.5%)

Tanner, N. C. and Smithers, D. W.[23]

notes that in his hospital radiation therapy has proved more effective than surgery for carcinomas at all levels, including the lower thoracic esophagus.

During recent years it has been our policy to treat lesions in the upper third of the esophagus by radiation therapy, those in the lower third by primary surgery, and those in the midthoracic segment, in selected instances, by radical preoperative irradiation (5,000 to 5,500 rads to the entire esophagus with a weekly tumor dose of 800 or at most 900 rads) followed by resection of the esophagus within the treated volume and primary esophago-gastric anastomosis.

When with current methods of treatment, 95 percent of patients die with uncontrolled tumor, palliation must be a primary treatment objective. The most frequent objective of such treatment, the re-establishment of esophageal patency and function for the remainder of the patient's life, must be accomplished with the least morbidity possible. Relief of esophageal obstruction alters the mechanism of dying by avoiding starvation (and gastrostomy) and by allowing the patient to control his saliva. There are few clinical situations in which palliation can be assessed so accurately. Fifty to 75 percent[4,12,24] of those patients irradiated adequately can be helped, and many become symptom-free (Table 13-10).

Table 13-8. Carcinoma of the Esophagus
5-Year Survival by Site

	Surgery 1948–1962	Radiation Therapy 1956–1962
Cervical	3/14 (21%)	7/31 (23%)
Upper half Thoracic	11/128 (9%)	8/39 (20%)
Lower half Thoracic	27/221 (12%)	5/29 (17%)
Total	41/363 (11%)	20/99 (20%)
Of total patients seen (429) 1956–1962 with all methods of treatment	34/429 (8%)	
Of total patients radically irradiated (99) plus those patients treated for palliation or not treated (156)		20/255 (8%)

Pearson[18]

Table 13-9.   Carcinoma of the Esophagus
5-Year Survival by Site
Surgical Treatment

	Esophagus Mid-thoracic	Esophagus Lower Thoracic	Total
Number of patients treated	40	100	140
Number of patients "sufficiently treated"	30	74	104
Number of patients well at 5 years	1	11	12
Frequency of control of all patients treated	1/40 (2.5%)	11/100 (11%)	12/140 (8.6%)
Frequency of control of patients "sufficiently treated"	1/30 (3.3%)	11/74 (14.8%)	12/104 (11.5%)

Sweet[21]—up to 1949

Technically, the major difference between radical "curative" and palliative radiation therapy is the length of esophagus and volume of tissue treated, for the necessary dose is comparable in either situation. Sometimes it is not possible at the onset of treatment to determine whether radiation therapy should be radical or palliative. Frequent re-evaluation during treatment may resolve this difficulty.

Radiation therapy of carcinoma of the esophagus, whether with curative or palliative intent, is a major procedure, requiring the patient to be in reasonably good condition. It may be necessary to provide nutrition through a small intra-esophageal tube. During this critical phase of management, hospitalization is advisable.

Carefully directed radiation therapy should result in few serious sequelae. The tumor-narrowed lumen should not be closed by radiation-induced edema. Esophageal perforation occurs with uncontrolled, progressing cancer, whether irradiated or not. Therefore, any implication of superimposed irradiation is difficult to establish. The

Table 13-10.   Carcinoma of the Thoracic Esophagus
Percentage of Patients Symptom-Free After Treatment

	Of All Patients Treated		Of Patients "Sufficiently" Treated	
	Surgery	Radiotherapy	Surgery	Radiotherapy
1 year	36.8 (46:125)	33 (20:60)	48.5 (46:95)	42.5 (20:47)
2 years	13.1 (15:114)	13.3 (8:60)	17.2 (15:87)	17.2 (15:87)
3 years	9.7 (9:92)	6.8 (18:262)	12.9 (9:70)	10.4 (18:173)
5 years	2.5 (1:40)	3.6 (8:218)	3.3 (1:30)	6.2 (8:128)

Buschke[4]

presence of a fistula is a contraindication to treatment. Perforation with fistula occurring during therapy calls for its discontinuation. With careful selection of patients and proper fractionation (not more than 800 rads per week) perforation rarely occurs during therapy. Imminent perforation can be recognized either radio-graphically (penetrating, deep ulceration) or clinically (retrosternal or back pain) and treatment can be avoided. However, perforations one to two months following therapy have occurred in about 10 percent of our patients due to the progressing, uncontrolled carcinoma. The potential of long-term sequelae, i.e., pulmonary fibrosis or spinal cord damage, is practically eliminated by the short survival of most patients, but should be considered in treatment planning.

Surgery

Improvements of surgical technique, endotracheal anesthesia, blood transfusions, and pre- and postoperative care have made increasingly aggressive resections possible. Thus, the surgical treatment of patients with carcinoma of the esophagus has become dependent on the philosophy of the surgeon (less frequently on that of the patient).

Some surgeons[3, 14] continue to advocate resection as the preferable initial treatment of cancers at all levels of the esophagus. Extensive resections with immediate restoration of the continuity of the upper gastrointestinal tract are performed for palliation in the face of certain failure of control of tumor.

As with radiation therapy, there has been no significant increase in overall survival with more frequent application of improved surgical methods, and thus it is not hopeful that further improvements of the method will favorably influence the incidence of tumor control.

Reasons for surgical failure are biological and thus similar to the reasons for the failure of radiation therapy. Although control of tumor in the esophagus should be better with resection, extra-esophageal extensions may be less controllable.

The morbidity and mortality of surgery are less for cancers below the level of the aortic arch. Thus Sweet[22] (1960) reported an operative mortality of 24 percent for tumors of the midthoracic esophagus and 12 percent for tumors of the lower esophagus and junction with the stomach; Adams[2] (1958) reported a 39 percent operative mortality for patients with lesions above the aortic arch requiring pharyngeal anastamosis compared with a mortality of 16.7 percent for patients with tumors below the arch.

This variation in operative mortality related to anatomic level has prompted use of radiation therapy for lesions at the level of, or above, the aortic arch, until a superiority in tumor control can be documented for surgery. To date, the results of surgery have been similar to the unsatisfactory results of radiation therapy (Tables 13-8, 13-9, 13-10).

Combined Treatment

Recently, surgery and radiation therapy have been used in combination.[8, 9, 14, 17] Although the addition of one ineffective procedure to another in general is not likely to result in great improvement in tumor control, certain potential advantages are worth investigation: (1) Control of tumor in the esophagus may be more frequent because radiation therapy may reduce the incidence of persistent tumor at and beyond the line of anastamosis, and removal of the esophagus should increase the incidence of local control beyond that possible with irradiation alone. This assumes that resection and anastamosis are within the irradiated tissue volume, a feat possible with optimal surgical and radiotherapeutic techniques. Our limited experience documents the safeness of this procedure, if careful radical irradiation is followed by the simplest surgical procedure possible, i.e., resection and primary anastamosis. Likewise, it would seem advisable that the radiation therapy be preoperative and carried to the maximal tolerable dose short of causing increased surgical problems. (2) Limited regional extension of tumor and adenopathy may be controlled more frequently. The surgeon is likely to remove the largest tumor-containing nodes, which are least frequently controlled by irradiation. Also, it is possible that preoperative irradiation might convert a few nonremovable tumors to removable ones if there is regression of tumor initially fixed to nonremovable structures, i.e., the aortic arch.

Goodner,[8] in a series of 85 patients preoperatively irradiated, found that although the incidence of surgical removal increased, the five-year survival was not influenced. Parker and Gregorie,[17] in a study of 135 patients compared in retrospect with those treated by either surgery or radiation therapy, found that the incidence of surgical removal increased, and the survival improved slightly. Guernsey et al.[9] found that, in a group of 40 patients, only 23 completed preoperative radiation therapy followed by esophagectomy. Only three of this group were alive and well at three years, but in three others, death was attributed to the irradiation.

The most extensive experience is that of Nakayama.[14] Since 1960, he has treated patients with carcinomas of the upper and middle thoracic esophagus by a multiple-stage surgical procedure following 2,000–2,500 rads delivered in four to five days with 250 kv x-ray. For this group, the operative mortality is said to be 2.5 percent, and the survival at one year (38 of 64, 59.3 percent) and five years (3 of 8, 37.5 percent) exceeds that previously obtained by surgery alone. It is difficult to extrapolate these unequaled results reported by this most experienced surgeon to clinics in this country.

Prognosis

There has been discouragingly little change since 1944 when Steele[20] stated: "The outlook for a patient with carcinoma of the esophagus is indeed gloomy because we are dealing in the majority of cases with a poor, half-starved, old man with a growth which has already spread to his vitals."

Merendino and Mark,[13] allowing an operative mortality of 20 percent and an incidence of death from intercurrent disease of 20 percent, calculated a theoretical curabiltiy of 20 percent. This level of therapeutic performance has been reached only in very selected patient groups.

Any assessment of treatment must include all patients seen, the fraction eligible for treatment, the number adequately treated, and the survival related to both the number of patients seen as well as treated. These numerical results need be tempered by treatment-produced mortality and morbidity and by the quality of life of the survivors.

Generally, a greater proportion of the total patients seen are treated by radiation than by surgical methods, and more patients with extensive tumor are included in the radiotherapy series. This does not negate the advisability of rigid selection of patients for surgery, but it invalidates direct comparisons of the number of survivors following treatment.

Nevertheless, comparisons of all patients treated and patients "sufficiently" treated are remarkably similar (Tables 13-8, 13-9, 13-10). Tumor-free survival results from a single institution where nearly all patients in a geographic area are treated have been reported recently by Pearson[18] (Table 13-8).

As noted previously, up to 80 percent[4,12,24] of those patients irradiated adequately are usefully palliated (Tables 13-9, 13-10).

The quality of life following treatment (irradiation) has been assessed by Pearson.[18] Twenty-two of 157 patients (14 percent) not "cured" died within 3 months of treatment and are considered initial management failures. Seventy-three of the 157 deaths (46 percent) were attributed to lack of local tumor control. Half of these "local recurrences" occurred within 6 months, 47 (64 percent) within 12 months, 68 (93 percent) within 24 months, and all within 3 years. Half of these patients ate a normal diet for a "worthwhile period." Eight of these 73 (11 percent) developed a tracheo-esophogeal fistula, and 7 (10 percent) died of massive hemorrhage.

Thirty-six of the 157 (23 percent) died from distant metastases, 27 within 12 months and 34 within 24 months. Nearly all ate a normal diet until death.

Twenty-six patients (16 percent) died of causes not related to their esophageal cancer, 14 within 12 months and 20 within 24 months. Nearly all ate a normal diet until death.

Seventeen of 20 patients (85 percent) surviving more than five years continue to eat a normal diet, although nine have had esophageal dilatation at least once. Two of these patients had dietary restrictions attributed to strictures at the site of the treated tumor.

With currently available treatment methods, a major improvement in prognosis rests on diagnosis of tumors of lesser extent. There is little reason to be encouraged that such improved detection is likely. However, very gratifying palliation is obtainable by currently available treatment, and these unfortunate patients should be helped with the least treatment-produced morbidity.

REVIEW QUESTIONS

1. What are the most frequent symptoms and signs caused by carcinoma of the esophagus? Relate these findings to tumor size, location, and extent.

2. What factors delay the diagnosis of carcinoma of the esophagus? What is the mean interval between clinical onset and treatment? How does this delay affect prognosis? Why?

3. If your patient has an epidermoid carcinoma of the thoracic esophagus exceeding 5.1 cm in the long axis, what is the chance that tumor remains localized to the esophagus? How many tumors smaller than this have you seen?

4. Why is the esophagus arbitrarily divided into anatomical segments for evaluation of carcinomas? What is the basis of this segmental division? Which segment is involved most frequently?

5. How do the anatomical site of involvement and tumor extent influence treatment of patients with carcinoma of the esophagus?

6. What is the normal lymphatic drainage of the esophagus? How does this affect treatment planning and execution and prognosis?

7. What are the frequencies of histological tumor types in the esophagus? Can these be related to anatomical site? to selection of treatment? to prognosis?

8. What factors limit control of carcinoma of the thoracic esophagus in patients treated by irradiation?

9. How frequently does cancer of the esophagus regress following radiation therapy? Can you relate this gross tumor regression to "cure"? to palliation?

10. If technical improvements in radiation therapy have not significantly improved the incidence of cure of patients with epidermoid carcinoma of the thoracic esophagus, what is the implication? Have these technical improvements been of value in treating these patients? Why?

11. What are the reasons for the failure of surgery for these patients? How do these compare with the reasons for failure of radiation therapy? What are the comparative treatment-related morbidity and mortality of surgery and radiotherapy?

12. Why might combined radiation therapy and surgery be slightly more effective than either method alone? Should the irradiation be pre- or postoperative? Why? How would you expect the morbidity of such combined treatment to compare with that of either surgery or radiotherapy alone?

13. Relate the frequency of "cure" to all patients seen, to those patients adequately treated, to anatomical level of tumor involvement, to treatment method. How does this compare to the theoretical maximal curability?

14. Why is palliation an important objective in treating patients with cancer of the esophagus? What is the most frequent objective of such treatment? How often is this objective achieved?

15. Why is the "quality of survival" important for patients with cancer of the esophagus? How would you measure this?

BIBLIOGRAPHY

1. ACKERMAN, C. V., and DEL REGATO, J. A. *Cancer: Diagnosis-Treatment-Prognosis*, 4th ed., Mosby, St. Louis, 1970.
2. ADAMS, H. D. The treatment of esophageal carcinoma. *Spectrum*, 6:430–433, 1958.
3. ADAMS, H. D., and SALZMAN, F. A. Present management of carcinoma of the esophagus and cardia, *S Clin N Amer*, 39:691–698, 1959.
4. BUSCHKE, F. Surgical and radiological results in the treatment of esophageal carcinoma. *Amer J Roentgen*, 71:9–21, 1954.

5. FARRELL, J. T., JR. Integration of clinical and roentgenologic findings in the diagnosis of carcinoma of the esophagus. *Radiology,* 30:412–416, 1938.

6. FLEMING, J. A. C. Radiotherapy in cancer of thoracic oesophagus. *Thorax,* 2:206–215, 1947.

7. GESCHICKTER, C. F. Tumors of the digestive tract. *Amer J Cancer,* 25:130–161, 1935.

8. GOODNER, J. T. Surgical and radiation treatment of cancer of the thoracic esophagus. *Amer J Roentgen,* 105:523–528, 1969.

9. GUERNSEY, J. M., DOGGETT, R. L. S., MASON, G. R., KOHATSU, S., and OBERHELMAN, W. A. Combined treatment of cancer of the esophagus. *Amer J Surg,* 117:157–161, 1969.

10. HELSLEY, G. F. Metastasizing tendency of esophagus carcinoma. *Ann Surg,* 77:272–275, 1923.

11. LEDERMAN, M. Carcinoma of esophagus, with special reference to upper third: I. Clinical considerations. *Brit J Radiol,* 39:193–197, 1966.

12. MARCIAL, V. A., TOME, J. M., UBINAS, J., BOSCH, A., and CORREA, J. N. Role of radiation therapy in esophageal cancer. *Radiology,* 87:231–239, 1966.

13. MERENDINO, K. A., and MARK, V. H. An analysis of one hundred cases of squamous cell carcinoma of the esophagus. Part II. With special reference to its theoretical curability. *Surg Gynec Obstet,* 94:110–114, 1952.

14. NAKAYAMA, K., ORIHATA, H., and YAMAGUCHI, K. Surgical treatment combined with preoperative concentrated irradiation for esophageal cancer. *Cancer,* 20:778–788, 1967.

15. NIELSEN, J. Clinical results with rotation therapy in cancer of the esophagus. *Acta Radiol* [Ther] (Stockholm), 26:361, 1945.

16. NIELSEN, J. personal communication, 1949.

17. PARKER, E. F., and GREGORIE, H. B., JR. Combined radiation and surgical treatment of carcinoma of esophagus. *Ann Surg,* 161:710–722, 1965.

18. PEARSON, J. G. The value of radiotherapy in the management of esophageal cancer. *Amer J Roentgen,* 105:500–513, 1969.

19. SMITHERS, D., and PAYNE, P. M. Analysis of the patients with carcinoma of the oesophagus seen at the Royal Marsden Hospital, 1936–1954. In: *Tumours of the Esophagus.* N. Tanner and D. Smithers, Eds, Livingstone, Edinburgh, 1961.

20. STEELE, G. H. Discussion on the treatment of carcinoma of the esophagus. *Proc R Soc Med,* 37:331–340, 1944.

21. SWEET, R. H. Late results of surgical treatment of carcinoma of the esophagus. *JAMA* 155:422–425, 1954.

22. SWEET, R. H. In: *Treatment of Cancer and Allied Diseases,* G. T. Pack, and I. M. Ariel, Eds, Hoeber-Harper, New York, 1960.

23. TANNER, N. C., and SMITHERS, D. W. Survey of published work on survival following treatment for carcinoma of the oesophagus. In: *Tumours of the Esophagus.* N. Tanner and D. Smithers, Eds, Livingston, Edinburgh, 1961, pp. 282–284 (Table XIX).

24. WATSON, T. A. Radiation treatment of cancer of the esophagus. *Surg Gynec Obstet,* 117: 346–354, 1963.

25. ZUPPINGER, A. Die Behandlung der Oesophagus Karzinom. *Ergebn Med Strahlenforsch,* 7:389–456, 1936.

THYMOMA

A continuing lack of understanding of the behavior of malignant tumors of the thymus interferes with proper treatment, which can be effective and even occasionally control extensive tumors for many years.

This is an extension of our inadequate understanding of the variations in structure and function of the normal thymus. These variations, especially of size, shape, and position, have been noted at all ages, and may in part be related to very sensitive reactive atrophy to varying stresses such as starvation, fatigue, and fever.[2] Ordinarily, the thymus is maximally developed in adolescence and involutes after puberty, fat replacing the parenchyma. However, malignant tumors of the thymus usually occur in adults (average age, 46 years,[8] those with myasthenia gravis averaging 31 years[6]).

The thymus is a duplex organ, rather than a single organ with two lobes. In the adult, the greater portion is situated in the anterior, superior mediastinum behind the sternum and in front of the trachea, great vessels, and pericardium, although the cranial extremities of the two "lobes" may extend through the upper thoracic aperture, ventral to the trachea, as high as the lower border of the thyroid gland.[5]

Pathologic Findings

The thymus is an entodermal derivative with a basic framework of epithelial cells invaded by lymphocytes.[5] Thus, tumors of the thymus may vary from an almost exclusive composition of lymphocytes ("thymocytes"), often resulting in an interpretation of small cell lymphosarcoma, to a preponderance of epithelial cells, resulting in a diagnosis of carcinoma.[13] As with other tumors, the histological appearance may vary in different parts of the tumor and change throughout the course of the tumor.

Hillenius and Mosetitsch[7] classified tumors of the thymus by predominant cell type: lymphocytic, 30 percent; epithelial, 15 percent; mixed, 30 percent; and spindle cell, 25 percent. A definition of malignancy by histological criteria may be very difficult. Thus, the diagnosis of malignancy is likely to be based on the gross findings of direct extension of the tumor through the capsule, implantation of tumor within the thorax, distant metastases, and perhaps active regrowth after treatment.[4]

Although it had been doubted (Castleman, 1955)[3] that thymomas generate embolic metastases, several patients with distant metastases now have been reported (including a patient of ours reviewed by Castleman). Such embolic spread may be hematogenous or lymphatic into the regional (anterior mediastinal) nodes.

The often discussed entity, *granulomatous thymoma* probably represents a special form of Hodgkin's disease[9] and will be discussed with other lymphomas.

The pathogenesis of the rare "seminoma-like" tumors of the thymus[10] remains a matter of speculation.

Clinical Manifestations

The most important symptoms and signs appear in that group of patients who suffer coexistent thymoma and myasthenia gravis. Thirty to 45 percent of those patients with thymoma may have myasthenia gravis, and 8–15 percent of those patients with myasthenia gravis may have thymic tumors.[13] In those patients with thymomas without myasthenia gravis, complaints such as pressure in the chest or lassitude are not characteristic.

Rubin, Straus, and Allen[15] have noted an association of thymic tumors and such diverse entities as acquired idiopathic hypogammaglobulinemia and erythroid hypoplastic anemia. They question whether the common denominator may be an autoimmune disorder.

Treatment

Management of patients with thymomas should be based on the type and extent of neoplasm and on the presence of myasthenia gravis.

If *myasthenia gravis is not detectable*, direct surgical removal of the tumor seems preferable. If complete removal is not possible because of local extension, vigorous radiation therapy is advisable. This implies tumor doses of 5,000–6,000 rads in five to seven weeks to a tissue volume including the neoplasm and its potential local extensions (from the isthmus of the thyroid to the fourth intercostal space). It has been our experience that such treatment can control locally extensive tumors (including that of a patient with invasion of the pericardium).[13]

Review of available data[12, 13] indicates that all *patients with thymoma and myasthenia gravis* should be irradiated preoperatively. These tumors are grossly and histologically indistinguishable from neoplasms in patients without coexistent myasthenia gravis and so require the same radiation dose to the same anatomical volume. Those patients who are poor operable risks or have tumors which cannot be completely removed surgically, may be managed with some success by radiation therapy alone.

About 50 percent of those patients with myasthenia gravis without detectable thymic tumors may improve following local irradiation to doses as low as 3,000 rads in four to five weeks.[13] Such a remission may lessen the risk of thymectomy.

For patients with myasthenia gravis, it has been customary to initiate local irradiation with low doses (50–100 rads per day)[11, 13] because of fear of precipitating a "crisis."

Experience with chemotherapy has been even less than the limited surgical and radiotherapeutic experience. However, responses varying with the lymphocytic and epithelial components might be expected to resemble those noted for other tumors.

Prognosis

The results of treatment are less dependent on the tumor type than on the tumor extent and the coexistence of myasthenia gravis.

Bernatz, Harrison, and Claggett,[1] using surgery selectively followed by radiation therapy, reported a 5-year survival of 63 percent and a 10-year survival of 50 percent. The frequency of survival was similar for patients with or without myasthenia gravis. Variations in 5-year survival according to tumor type (lymphocytic, 78 percent; epithelial, 44 percent; mixed cell, 55 percent; and spindle cell, 77 percent) may have been related to variations in local tumor extent. Wilkins, Edmunds, and Castleman[17] reported that 17 of 22 patients survived 5 years and 11 of 15 patients survived 10 years after surgery. All 12 patients with encapsulated tumors survived 5 years and 7 of 8 survived 10 years. Only 3 of 10 patients with locally invasive tumors survived 10 years, although one died of a pulmonary embolus at 5 years, and no tumor was found at autopsy. These 3 survivors received supervoltage radiation therapy. Two are apparently free of tumor at 15 and 18 years after treatment, but the third is alive with detectable neoplasm 13 years following treatment.

There are no good data bearing on the likelihood of local tumor control by radiation therapy. Although very extensive neoplasms have been controlled, local response may be expected to be better for tumors of minimal extent and for those which are predominantly lymphocytic. As with other malignant tumors, clinical evidence of tumor regrowth may not be noted until many years (5 to 10) after apparently successful treatment.[14]

The myasthenia gravis present in 6 of Effler and McCormack's 16 patients[4] was not benefited by treatment of the tumor. Although Schwab and Leland[16] concluded that most patients with myasthenia gravis with or without thymic tumors were not benefited by local treatment, remissions resulted in 68 percent of those females under 30 years.

REVIEW QUESTIONS

1. What histologic types of tumors arise in the thymus?

2. If the thymus is of maximal size and cellularity in the adolescent, why are most thymic tumors found in adults?

3. What are the criteria of malignancy for tumors of the thymus?

4. Why is coexistent myasthenia gravis so important in patients with malignant thymic tumors? Has myasthenia gravis been related to any particular type of malignant thymic tumor?

5. Would you treat the thymic tumor differently in the patient with myasthenia gravis compared with the patient without?

6. Does the coexistence of myasthenia gravis alter the prognosis? If so, how?

BIBLIOGRAPHY

1. BERNATZ, P. E., HARRISON, E. G., and CLAGETT, O. T. Thymoma—a clinicopathologic study. *Thorac Cardiovasc Surg*, 42:424–444, 1961.

2. CAFFEY, J. P. *Pediatric X-ray Diagnosis*. A textbook for students and practioners of pediatrics, surgery and radiology. 5th ed. Year Book, Chicago, 1967.

3. CASTLEMAN, B. Tumors of the thymus gland. Section V, Fascicle 19, *Armed Forces Institute of Pathology*, Washington, D.C., 1955.

4. EFFLER, D. B., and MC CORMACK, L. J. Thymic neoplasms, *J Thorac Cardiovasc Surg*, 31:60–82, 1956.

5. GUDERNATSCH, J. F. In: *Morris' Human Anatomy*, 11th ed. Schaeffer, J. P., McGraw-Hill, New York, 1953.

6. HARPER, R. A. K. Investigation of thymic tumours in myasthenia gravis. *J Fac Radiol*, 3:164–175, 1952.

7. HILLENIUS, C., and MOSETITSCH, W. On the diagnosis of "thymoma". *Fortschr Roentgenstr*, 99:28–35, 1963.

8. JONES, A., KEYNES, G., and HARPER, R. A. K. Tumours of the thymus. In: *Practice in Radiotherapy* by E. R. Carling, B. W. Windeyer, and D. W. Smithers, Eds, Mosby, St. Louis, 1955.

9. KATZ, A., and LATTES, R. Granulomatous thymoma or Hodgkin's disease of thymus, *Cancer*, 23:1–15, 1969.

10. LATTES, R. Thymoma and other tumors of the thymus. *Cancer*, 15:1224–1260, 1962.

11. MURPHY, W. T. *Radiation Therapy*, 2nd ed. Saunders, Philadelphia, 1967.

12. PERLO, V. P., SCHWAB, R. S., and CASTLEMAN, B. Myasthenia gravis and thymoma. In: *Remote Effects of Cancer on the Nervous System*, L. Brain, and F. H. Norris, Jr., Eds, Grims and Shattos, New York, 1965, pp. 55–66.

13. PHILLIPS, T. L., and BUSCHKE, F. The role of radiation therapy in myasthenia gravis. *Calif Med*, 106:282–289, 1967.

14. POOL, J. L. Discussion to Wilkins et al. (4)

15. RUBIN, M., STRAUSS, B., and ALLEN, L. Clinical disorder associated with thymic tumors. *Arch Intern Med* (Chicago), 114:389–398, 1964.

16. SCHWAB, R. S., and LELAND, C. C. Sex and age in myasthenia gravis as critical factors in incidence and remission. *JAMA*, 153:1270–1273, 1953.

17. WILKINS, E. W., JR., EDMUNDS, L. H., and CASTLEMAN, B. Cases of thymoma at Massachusetts General Hospital, *J Thorac Cardiovasc Surg*, 52:322–328, 1966.

14

CANCER
OF THE FEMALE GENITALIA

Malignant tumors of the female genital tract exhibit a great variation in response to ionizing radiation. Ovarian dysgerminoma is one of the most radiovulnerable malignant tumors, comparable to seminoma and lymphosarcoma. At the other end of the scale, malignant teratomas contain elements too unresponsive to irradiation to be controlled without intolerable damage to other pelvic structures. Between these extremes are the epidermoid carcinomas of the cervix, vagina, and vulva, the adenocarcinomas of the cervix and endometrium, and certain malignant ovarian tumors. These tumors are sufficiently radiovulnerable for permanent control, but the margin between the dose necessary to destroy tumor and the dose tolerated by the normal pelvic structures, particularly the rectum, intestinal mucosa, bladder, and vasculoconnective tissue, is small. Radiation treatment technique can be adjusted so that many of these tumors can be controlled without production of clinically significant damage to normal structures.

CARCINOMA OF THE CERVIX

One of the most important malignant neoplasms amenable to curative radiation therapy, usually in preference to surgery, is invasive carcinoma of the cervix. Increasingly widespread use of cytological examination has resulted in more frequent diagnoses of cancer of the cervix of minimal extent. In our experience, 10 to 15 years ago, a large percentage of untreated patients had Stage III tumor on admission, while now most patients have Stage I–II tumor, and Stage III tumor is less frequent.[22] However, cancer of the cervix killed approximately 10,000 females in the U.S. in 1968, being second in incidence only to cancer of the breast.[2]

Many interesting and perhaps important relationships have been observed with this tumor. The incidence of neoplasm increases with increasing sexual activity, with a comparatively higher "risk" in those frequently childbearing, with minimal risk in sexually inactive groups (i.e., nuns). Jewish females, particularly those with circumcised husbands, rarely are victims of cancer of the cervix, thus prompting speculation about a relationship to hygiene.

Cancer of the cervix is easy to diagnose, being available for visualization, palpation, and biopsy. The major deterrent to diagnosis is patient and physician

lethargy, often prompted by lack of symptoms or signs even with moderately extensive tumor. Delay in diagnosis has direct, measurable impact, for cancer arising from
the epithelium of the cervix may remain localized to the cervix for long periods,
usually spreads progressively to involve adjacent pelvic structures, and infrequently
spreads outside the pelvis until the tumor is extensive within the pelvis. Thus,
carcinoma of the cervix, during much of its frequently prolonged course, is curable
by currently available local treatment methods and the results of adequate treatment
can be correlated with local tumor extent.

Pathology

Primary tumors of the cervix usually originate at the squamo-columnar junction
and may assume any of several gross forms: (1) an ulceration of the mucosa of the
anterior or posterior lip; (2) an exophytic growth which may fill much of the upper
vagina before infiltrating the fornices; or (3) a nodular enlargement usually associated with involvement of the endocervix.

Five to 10 percent of these primary tumors will be adenocarcinomas (arising
from endocervical mucosa) while the remainder will be squamous cell carcinomas
of varying histologic differentiation.

Spread of Tumor

Carcinoma primary in the mucosa of the cervix extends predominantly by
direct invasion of the cervix, vaginal fornices, parametria, uterine corpus, rectovaginal and vesicovaginal septa and by metastases to lymph nodes within the pelvis
(Figs. 14-1, 14-2, 14-3). Hematogenous and distant lymph nodes metastases are
comparably infrequent.

Three main lymphatic routes drain the cervix: (1) The principal route is the
external iliac (anterior, preureteral) trunk which follows the uterine artery in the
broad ligament, passes anterior to the ureter and terminates in nodes of the external
iliac group; (2) The internal iliac (hypogastric, retroureteral) trunk follows the
uterine vein to terminate in hypogastric nodes near the origin of the uterine artery;
(3) The sacral (posterior) trunk passes along either side of the rectum in the utero-
sacral folds to nodes in the concavity of the sacrum, connecting above with the para-
aortic trunks (Fig. 14-3).

Clinical Evaluation

Careful appraisal of tumor extent is essential for the choice of the best therapeutic approach and for necessary evaluation of results. This appraisal is based on
symptoms and signs and examination of the patient, inclusive of general physical
examination, careful pelvic and abdominal palpation, cystoscopy, sigmoidoscopy,
intravenous pyelography, and chest x-ray.

The most frequent related complaint is vaginal bleeding, often intermenstrual
or post-coital, frequently antedated by an abnormal vaginal discharge. However,
patient-recognized symptoms and signs may be absent even with extensive tumor.
Pain is a late-appearing symptom usually indicative of invasion of extrauterine
pelvic structures by tumor. Pain over the distribution of the sciatic nerve results

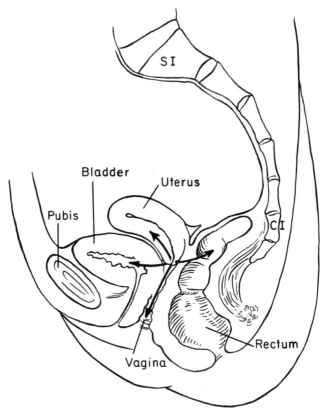

Fig. 14-1.   Female pelvis (sagittal view).   Routes of regional spread of cancer of the cervix.   1.   Uterine corpus   2. Bladder   3.   Vagina   4.   Rectum.

from involvement of the sacral plexus and often is the first clinical indication of reactivation of tumor after radiation therapy. Dull backache may result from invasion of the uterine supporting structures. Pain radiating into the groin is associated with invasion of the broad ligament or occlusion of the ureter. The latter may be accompanied by flank pain secondary to hydronephrosis and urinary tract infection. Pertinent bladder or rectal symptoms or signs are indicative of extensive intrapelvic tumor.

Clinical Staging

Pre- and post-treatment evaluation, appropriate therapeutic application and evaluation of results have profited from worldwide adherence to rules for clinical assessment of tumor extent dating to 1929 (Subcommittee on Radiotherapy of Cancer of the League of Nations[39]). These rules have been revised periodically and recently have been reissued by the American Joint Committee for Cancer Staging and End Results Reporting[7] (Fig. 14-4).

Pre-invasive Carcinoma of the Cervix

Stage O

Carcinoma-in-situ or intra-epithelial carcinoma.

272

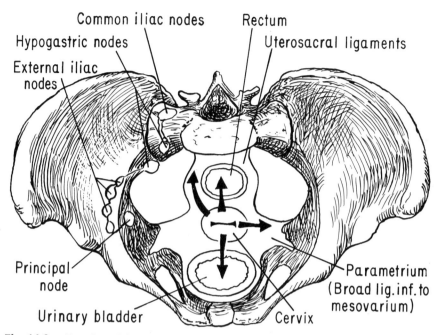

Fig. 14-2. Female pelvis (from above). Routes of regional spread of cancer of the cervix. 1. Bladder 2. Parametrium 3. Rectum 4. Rectovaginal septum 5. Regional lymph nodes.

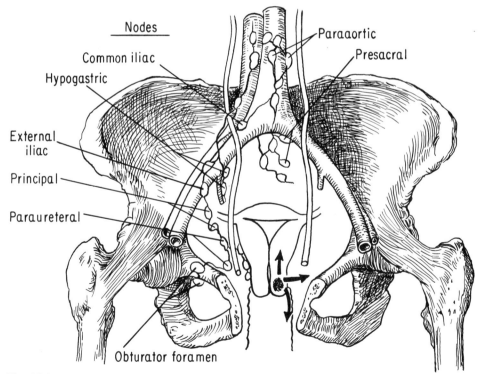

Fig. 14-3. Female Pelvis (frontal view). Routes of regional spread of cancer of the cervix. 1. Paracervical extension 2. Regional lymph nodes 3. Uterine corpus 4. Vagina.

Invasive Carcinoma of the Cervix

Stage I

Carcinoma confined to the cervix.

Stage II

Carcinoma extending beyond the cervix, but not reaching the pelvic wall or the lower third of the vagina.

Stage III

Carcinoma reaching the pelvic wall (on rectal examination no cancer-free space between tumor and pelvic wall) or the lower third of the vagina or both.

Stage IV

Carcinoma involving the mucosa of the urinary bladder or rectum, or both, or extending outside the true pelvis.

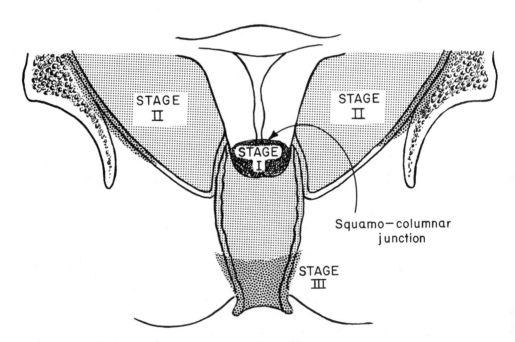

Fig. 14-4. Clinical staging of carcinoma of the cervix.
  I.   Tumor limited to the cervix
 II.   Tumor extending beyond the cervix, but not reaching the pelvic wall or lower one-third of the vagina, or both
III.   Tumor reaching the pelvic wall or the lower one-third of the vagina or both
IV.   Tumor involving the mucosa of the bladder or rectum, or both, or extending outside the true pelvis

It must be emphasized that except for a requirement for histological confirmation of the primary tumor site (and recently for histological confirmation of invasion of the mucosa of the urinary bladder), this estimate of tumor extent is based on clinical examination. Evidence for distant spread, i.e., to intrathoracic structures or bone, may be roentgenologic.

Pelvic palpation does not permit unequivocal differentiation of tumor extension from inflammatory or reactive fibroblastic induration. Thus, the tumor extent may be "overstaged" and treatment results exaggerated. Nonpalpable pelvic adenopathy results in "understaging" and penalization of treatment results. These inherent difficulties apparently counterbalance each other and dictate against unfounded judgments that palpable pelvic abnormalities can be discounted because they "don't feel like cancer."

Unfortunately, clinical staging does not account for tumor-produced ureteral obstruction as demonstrable on pyelography. Such obstruction is associated with a poorer prognosis in all clinical stages (32.8 percent vs. 55.6 percent 5-year survival rate for all stages[21]). Thus, ureteral obstruction by tumor is a grave sign, perhaps equivalent in prognostic significance to infiltration of the bladder or rectum (Stage IV) and more ominous than unilateral parametrial extension to the pelvic wall (Stage III). Yet ureteral obstruction may be present in "early" Stage II carcinoma of the cervix because of the close anatomical relationship of the lower ureter to the cervix.

Clinical staging does not clearly define another ominous development, extension of tumor to involve the uterine corpus. Although this extension is infrequently documented, it is not adequately treated by standard radiation techniques and may account for some treatment failures.

Recent introduction of a requirement for biopsy proof in a clinical classification has introduced unwelcome difficulties. Thus, proof of tumor invasion of the bladder requires substantiation by a biopsy which is not always possible or reasonable. In the presence of bullous edema without ulceration, biopsy through the intact bladder epithelium for staging purposes only is, in our opinion, contraindicated.

In contrast, tumor invasion of the recto-vaginal septum can be claimed on the basis of clinical examination. Needle biopsies within the pelvis can very usefully document the presence of tumor, but failure to identify tumor by such biopsy must not be considered synonymous with absence of tumor.

While clinical staging is most important, it is not completely sufficient for prognostication. For example: limited Stage II tumor, based on extension to the fornices, does not differ significantly in prognosis from Stage I tumor; Stage II tumor, based on extensive parametrial infiltration, may be comparable prognostically to Stage III tumor, based on parametrial extension; Stage II tumor based on extensive bilateral parametrial infiltration may be more ominous than Stage III tumor with unilateral involvement of the parametrium; Stage II or III tumor based on vaginal extension may be less foreboding than comparable Stages II–III based on parametrial extension.

The influence of minor variations in staging, due to interpretation, on results of treatment is shown in Figure 14-5.

In spite of these shortcomings, clinical staging, used throughout the world for four decades, has proved of great value both for prognostic appraisal and comparative evaluation of results of treatment.

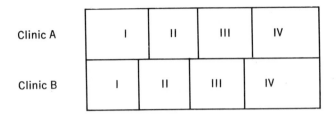

Fig. 14-5.   Influence of variation in staging on results of treatment. For the same group of patients and the same treatment, the results from Clinic B will be better for each stage, because of more rigid interpretation of criteria for each stage.

Histological Grading

Compared to clinical staging of tumor extent, histological grading has been of little clinical significance for patients with carcinoma of the cervix. Although undifferentiated tumors may spread to lymph nodes "earlier" and more frequently and may be more radioresponsive, such behavior has not influenced radiation treatment planning nor its outcome. The very few failures of destruction of the primary tumor focus (3–5 percent[3,5,23]), attributed to radioresistance, have not been synonymous with the well-differentiated lesions.

Adenoacanthoma and adenocarcinoma, in our experience, do not differ significantly from epidermoid carcinoma as measured by local tumor control by irradiation.

The myth of radioresistance of carcinoma-in-situ need be confronted. Carcinoma-in-situ, correctly diagnosed, can be effectively treated by transvaginal x-ray or intracavitary radium with results comparable to those reported by surgeons.[11] The dominant use of hysterectomy, rather than local irradiation, in this group, has been based on the desirability of a specimen for study and the preservation of ovarian function.

Treatment

The improvement of treatment of patients with carcinoma of the cervix during the last 70 years is a dramatic chapter in medical progress. In 1850, Dr. Charles D. Meigs[25] described a diagnosis of cancer of the cervix as "ipso facto, a prognostic of death." This formerly relentlessly fatal disease now can be controlled in at least 5 to 6 of 10 patients overall and in 8 to 9 of 10 patients when anatomically limited disease is thoroughly treated.

Curative treatment first became available about 1898 with the introduction of an extensive surgical procedure by Wertheim.[41] During the next two decades, rapid improvement of surgical techniques resulted in a 20–40 percent curability of patients with anatomically limited tumor.

Concurrently, radiation treatment techniques were being developed, following initial use of intracavitary radium (radium bromide in a sealed glass water jacket of a roentgen tube) by Margaret Cleaves in New York in 1903.[6] Major techniques were developed by Forssell[13] in Stockholm at the Radiumhemmet about 1911 and by Regaud[30] in Paris at the Institut du Radium about 1922. Both techniques initially emphasized the use of radium in the vagina and corpus and later incorporated supplementary pelvic irradiation from external x-ray sources.

The Manchester Technique as developed by a group (Paterson, Parker, Tod, Meredith) at the Holt Radium Institute, Manchester, England, is an adaptation of the Paris technique with delivery of a predetermined "maximum permissible dose" measured in the paracervical tissues and at the lateral pelvic wall.

In May, 1932 at the meeting of the Academy of Medicine in Paris, Regaud[10,31] compared the results of his radiation therapy with the surgical results of Faure, an outstanding gynecologic surgeon. The evidence was that: (1) In the operable stages (I and II), tumor control, measured statistically, was superior with radiation therapy; (2) Radiation treatment-produced morbidity was much less and there was only a 2 percent treatment mortality (due to pelvic infection in the pre-antibiotic era) compared with a 19 percent surgical mortality; (3) Many patients untreatable by surgery, because of tumor extent (Stages III–IV) or other serious illness, were salvable by radiation therapy. This comparison was followed by an almost universal acceptance of radiation therapy as the treatment of choice. In the early 1940s, Meigs[26] reopened the question in an attempt to investigate the accomplishments of surgery under modern conditions. In a large pilot study he demonstrated that for the operable stages (I and II) the surgical results now obtainable were comparable to the radiotherapeutic results, which had remained little changed since Regaud's time. Both the radiological and surgical mortality rates had become negligible. However, there still is considerable morbidity associated with radical hysterectomy and pelvic lymphadenectomy (mainly urinary tract complications because of interference with the vascularization of the ureters), while radiotherapy for these early operable stages has minimal morbidity. In addition, a large number of inoperable patients with advanced tumor (Stages III and IV) still can be salvaged by radiation therapy (Tables 14-1 and 14-2). For these reasons, radiation therapy remains the preferable primary procedure while surgery is reserved for radiation failures and selected circumstances.

The current relationship between use of radiotherapy and surgery for patients with limited tumor is summarized by the gynecological surgeon, Graham[15]: "There is no significant difference in the cure rate following surgery or radiation. The applicability of radiation is superior to surgery, for about one-fifth of the patients are inoperable. The mortality of the two procedures does not differ significantly. However, the morbidity of surgery is at least twice as great as that following radiotherapy. For these reasons, radiotherapy is the obvious treatment of choice and must remain so until unequivocal evidence to the contrary is presented."

Radiation Therapy

The major difficulty for surgeon and radiotherapist is control of tumor extension into pelvic structures rather than control of the primary lesion of the cervix.

Until recent presentation of evidence, surgeons and radiotherapists doubted that irradiation often destroyed epidermoid carcinoma metastatic in lymph nodes, even though there was ample evidence that extensive tumor infiltration of the parametria, vagina, and cervix could be controlled rather consistently. This therapeutic faintheartedness flourished for several reasons: (1) The radiation doses that could be introduced with standard radium and medium voltage x-ray techniques often did not destroy such metastatic tumor deposits; (2) Clinical reactivation of tumor was often first evident in nodes; and (3) The finding of a 15 to 20 percent incidence of pelvic adenopathy in surgical specimens from patients with Stage I disease and a 15 to 20 percent incidence of treatment failure in this same group was considered as evidence of a cause and effect relationship between these two factors. (A similar coincidence exists for Stages II and III.)

A more current appraisal has been stated by Rutledge,[34] a gynecological surgeon: "That irradiation is ineffective in the control of nodal metastases from cervical carcinoma is a cherished belief of some authorities, particularly those who prefer surgical treatment. This belief, however, is largely based on experience with the older methods of x-ray treatment, methods which are inadequate by modern standards. Today, an increasing amount of evidence indicates that, with apparatus now available, a cancerocidal dose of irradiation can indeed be delivered to the pelvic nodes." This includes indirect evidence that results for patients with Stage II–III–IV tumor improved with use of vigorous pelvic irradiation and direct evidence from planned studies. Rutledge and Fletcher[32] found that three months following vigorous pelvic irradiation of patients with Stage III carcinoma of the cervix, the surgically identified nodes with tumor (? viable) were reduced threefold from an expected 66 percent to 22 percent. In another group of 142 patients with adenectomies after pelvic irradiation,[35] only 16 of 142 (11.3 percent) had microscopically identified tumor as follows:

Table 14-1.

Extent of Tumor	Post-Irradiation Incidence	Expected Incidence
Stage I	3.3% (1 of 30)	15%
Stage II	14.1% (9 of 64)	27%
Stage III	12.5% (6 of 48)	66%

Guttmann[17] added the following evidence:

Table 14-2.

Extent of Tumor	Number of Patients	Number of + Nodes	Percent of + Nodes	Expected Percent + Nodes
Stage I	28	0	0%	11.3%
Stage II	23	1	3.8%	35.2%
Stage III	4	2	50%	—

Thus, there is accumulating evidence that vigorous radiation therapy can control tumor metastatic to pelvic lymph nodes from primary carcinomas of the cervix. It is likely that this level of performance exceeds that possible with pelvic lymphadenectomy, where the removal is anatomically incomplete. It is reasonable to assume that difficulty in controlling extensive well-differentiated epidermoid carcinoma in lymph nodes is related to interference with the blood supply and cellular oxygenation. In contrast, tumor control is possible with minimal tumor involvement that does not interfere with the circulation.

Treatment Techniques

Radiation treatment of carcinoma of the cervix includes two distinct components, each with different purpose.

The primary tumor site and immediate paracervical and vaginal extensions are treated by intracavitary irradiation. This consists of radiation sources (usually ^{226}Ra, occasionally ^{60}Co, ^{137}Cs) placed in the endocervical canal and vaginal vaults or transvaginal x-ray directed through a vaginal cone placed against the cervix. The anatomy is uniquely favorable for intracavitary radium therapy. The thick walls of the corpus and endocervix and the pliability of the vaginal vaults permit adequate separation between the radiation sources and the most vulnerable pelvic structures (rectum, bladder). Thus, it is possible to safely deliver doses far in excess of those used for treating epidermoid carcinomas in other locations. The surface dose to the primary tumor in the cervix from adequate intracavitary radium is 20,000–30,000 rads,[37] but because of rapid "fall-off," a cancerocidal dose does not extend more than 2–3 cm from the radium source. Therefore, although such local treatment controls at least 95 percent of the primary tumors[3,5,23] (measured in Stage I disease), it is effective only for patients with Stage I and minimal Stage II tumor.

The time-tested methods of intracavitary radium therapy are the so-called Paris and Stockholm techniques, or minor variations of these procedures (Manchester technique). The difference between these two methods is mainly in dose/time relationship. With the technique developed at the Institut du Curie in Paris, weaker sources are left in position over a longer period of time (100 hours for a single application in uterus and vault, or two times 100 hours with an interval of a few days if the intracervical and vaginal therapy are applied separately). With the method developed at the Radiumhemmet in Stockholm, applicators with larger amounts of radium are introduced for short periods (about 30 hours in two or three applications, one to three weeks apart). The specific type of applicator used, particularly for the treatment of the vaginal vault (different types of colpostats, ovoids) is not critical as long as the radiation therapist is thoroughly aware of the distribution of the radiation. The total necessary hospitalization varies between five and ten days.

It is not possible by transvaginal roentgentherapy to raise the local doses to the same high level as obtained with intracavitary radium. The main advantage of transvaginal roentgentherapy is an economic one since hospitalization is not necessary. When there is marked infection or bleeding, transvaginal roentgentherapy may be preferable. However, because of the lower dose level, control of the primary tumor is less frequent. Therefore, with this method the results in Stage I and early Stage II disease are inferior to those obtained by good intracavitary radium.

Interstitial irradiation of the primary tumor and its immediate extensions is more traumatic to the tissue and the distribution of radiation is less favorable. Therefore, the incidence of damage to the rectum and bladder is higher while the results are no better than obtainable with intracavitary radium.

External irradiation is directed against extension of tumor into the extra-uterine pelvic soft tissues where the influence of intracavitary radiation is minimal. The externally introduced dose must increase as the contribution from the intracavitary sources decreases with distance. With adequate intracavitary irradiation of the central pelvic structures, the rectum and bladder must be indirectly shielded from the external treatment beam.

The sequence of intracavitary and external irradiation is determined by the extent and distribution of tumor, the anatomical arrangement of the host and the prejudices of the therapist. Prior to the availability of antibiotics, initial external irradiation often promoted necessary clearing of infection prior to the intracavitary insertion of radium. Such initial treatment also may usefully stop bleeding prior to insertion of intracavitary applicators.

However, when the tumor is of limited extent (Stage I and early Stage II) and the anatomy is not compromised, initial intracavitary irradiation, the basic component of treatment, should be completed prior to the appearance of any rectal reaction which might prove a deterrent to completion of treatment. However, if tumor has made the anatomy unfavorable for good intracavitary placement, this situation may improve as the tumor regresses during initial external irradiation. Inasmuch as external irradiation is the mainstay of the treatment of extensive intrapelvic tumor, intracavitary irradiation is used only as a supplement when appropriate.

Megavoltage x-ray has prompted use of techniques in which the entire pelvis is irradiated to homogeneous dose. Whether this is preferable to selective inhomogeneity of dosage is doubtful.

Regardless of technique, tumor above the pelvic brim is not irradiated routinely and thus, is synonymous with incurability by current treatment methods. This restriction of treatment volume is based on limits of intestinal tolerance to radiation.

Even with guiding principles and standard techniques, treatment should be adjusted to each individual situation with consideration of gross and histological tumor type, tumor extent, condition and tolerance of the patient. Changes can be made in response to the reaction of the tumor and evidence of bowel or bladder intolerance. This necessary close observation enabling integration of all phases of treatment is possible only if the entire procedure is controlled by a single physician. If the intracavitary treatment is divorced from the external irradiation, the risks of accident and the proportion of failures increase.

Results of Radiation Therapy

"The results of radiotherapy in the treatment of carcinoma of the cervix are the best ever obtained by any treatment of any major form of cancer and the possibilities of that form of treatment extend well beyond the operable cases."[1] A clinical-tumor-free survival incidence five years post treatment is a satisfactory measurement of treatment performance, for few tumor-related problems occur after that interval. Representative results dating 30 years are presented in Table 14-3. These data appear even more impressive when adjusted for age and death from intercurrent diseases (Table 14-4). Based on treatment performances in many institutions throughout the world, it is apparent that the results of adequate radiation therapy of comparable clinical stages of tumor are similar regardless of varying technical details. The survival incidence, reported from many selected institutions, has been progressively improving over the years and even for patients with extensive tumor (Stages III–IV) exceeds the survival currently achievable for patients with

Table 14-3. Carcinoma of the Cervix
Results of Radiation Therapy (Uncorrected data)
Tumor Institute of Swedish Hospital Seattle (1954)

Stage	Number	L&W 5 yrs.	% 5-year Survival Rate
I	97	78	80
II	143	71	49
III	84	24	28
IV	26	3	11
Total	350	176	50

cancers of the stomach or lung. More widespread optimum application of currently available treatment methods would represent substantial medical progress.

Improvement in overall curability can, in part, be attributed to an increase in the relative proportion of patients with limited cancer at the time of initial treatment. In our experience, Stage III carcinoma of the cervix has become infrequent, while 20 years ago this was the most frequent clinical stage.[22] This favorable change results from physician and patient awareness of the disease, regular gynecologic examination inclusive of Pap smear, and consequent attention to carcinoma-in-situ and invasive carcinoma of limited extent.

Surgery

Coexistent with improvements in anesthesia, blood replacement and antibiotics, the use of surgery for patients with carcinoma of the cervix has been reevaluated.

Table 14-4. Carcinoma of the Cervix
Results of Radiation Therapy
(Corrected for intercurrent deaths*)

Stage	Number Treated	% 5-year Survival
Squamous Carcinoma, Uterus Intact		
I (all treated)	271	90.3 ± 1.8
IIA (7 not treated)	340	81.1 ± 2.1
IIB (7 not treated)	307	63.3 ± 2.8
II (total) (14 not treated)	647	72.6 ± 1.8
III (55 not treated)	615	43.6 ± 2.0
IV (115 not treated)	71	13.4 ± 11.1
Total All Stages (184 not treated)	1604	61.8 ± 1.2
Adenocarcinoma of Cervix		
All Stages (6 not treated)	62	63.0 ± 6.3
Cancer of Cervical Stump (including 7 adenocarcinomas)		
All Stages (13 not treated)	145	68.8 ± 3.9

M. D. Anderson Hospital, 1964[12]
*Berkson-Gage Method

This has resulted in a broad spectrum of opinion among gynecological surgeons ranging from proposals that surgery be the dominant treatment to tempered statements that the optimum use of surgery requires restriction to selected problems. Reasons frequently offered for a preference for surgery as primary treatment do not withstand close scrutiny: (1) Surgery safeguards against recurrence and new growth. (Tumor-free survival incidence no better even for highly selected patient groups.); (2) The prognosis is bad in the young. (If this is so, it applies to all treatment methods.); (3) Epidermoid carcinoma is sometimes radioresistant. (In Stage I, failure to control the primary tumor should be less than 5 percent.); (4) Adenocarcinoma and adenoacanthoma are unsuitable for radiotherapy. (There is no substantiating evidence.); (5) Radiotherapy is impossible in patients with salpingitis. (This is a statement of history, accurate prior to antibiotics. Even then radiotherapy was effective following salpingectomy.); (6) Radiotherapy is unsuitable for carcinoma of the cervix associated with pregnancy. (There is refuting evidence, see page 289.); (7) Lymph node metastases can be controlled by surgery, but not by radiotherapy. (See previous discussion, page 278.); (8) There is less injury with surgery. (This is in violent contradiction to abundant, long-standing evidence.)

Rutledge[33] has proposed that optimum use of surgery, with current knowledge, requires highly specific indications. His indications for radical hysterectomy plus pelvic lymph node dissection would include: (1) extension of the tumor to involve the corpus; (2) a poor response to a thorough trial of radiation therapy; (3) an unsatisfactory application of radiation; (4) "barrel shape" lower uterine segment secondary to extensive tumor; (5) adenocarcinoma of the cervix; (6) carcinoma of the cervix associated with pregnancy.

Two different operations are used currently: (1) The radical hysterectomy (Wertheim operation) requires meticulous dissection of the entire pelvis with removal of the uterus, ovaries, tubes, and uterine supporting structures to the pelvic wall and resection of the upper third of the vagina. This extensive operation should be accompanied by a pelvic lymphadenectomy. This procedure requires careful patient selection and great surgical skill. Used as a primary treatment method or as a "rescue" procedure following radiation failure in a patient with centrally persistent tumor, such surgery can be curative and life-saving. Applied as primary treatment to a select patient population (nonobese, not old, no serious illness) with limited tumor, the results have been comparable to those resulting from good radiotherapy applied to a nonselected population. Despite continued improvement of technique, complications from surgery far exceed those from radiotherapy, comparing patients with similar stages of tumor as reported by Parsons,[29] a gynecological surgeon. "The operative mortality is low, but the complications occur immediately and appear more frequently than they do following irradiation. Primarily they are fistulae, bladder atony, and pelvic sepsis. When meticulous dissections are done around the bladder, the surgeon runs the risk of interrupting the blood supply to both bladder and lower end of ureter. The incidence of vesicovaginal and ureterovaginal fistula varies widely in the literature, but it is usually recorded in the region of 10 percent. This is too high. Serious attempts are constantly being made to reduce the incidence, but we should constantly keep in mind that the problem is inherent in any operation designed to remove all the cancer. We cannot do less and leave potential disease behind."

The proposal that "radical hysterectomy" is advisable because an ovary can be conserved in a young female ignores the anatomic fact that potential tumor-bearing lymphatics are likewise spared and fails to credit currently available endocrine replacement therapy.

(2) Pelvic exenteration requires removal of all intrapelvic soft tissues including bladder and rectum. Anterior and posterior exenteration have been tried, but generally found unsatisfactory. Such mutilating surgery is justified only as a heroic "curative" effort, usually following failure of radiation therapy. It is not justified as a palliative measure. It is to be considered only in patients with centrally located tumors without spread to the pelvic wall. In well-selected cases this procedure has been life-saving and patients have become adjusted to the defects and able to lead reasonably normal lives.

Although radical surgery occasionally can salvage patients following failure of initial radiation therapy, and radiotherapy infrequently can salvage patients after failure of initial surgery, the planed combination of both modalities does not result in more frequent tumor control than is possible following either procedure alone. Rather it inflicts a markedly increased incidence of complications.

Complications of Radiation Therapy

Morbidity resulting from properly conducted radiation therapy of patients with carcinoma of the cervix is minimal, being only a fraction of that resulting from the surgical treatment of selected patients with limited tumor. Frequent unfortunate misconceptions about this small radiation morbidity have several origins: (1) failure to distinguish that unnecessary, adverse effects resulting from bad techniques should not be extrapolated to use of proper techniques (2) failure to recognize that much of the radiation morbidity is related to the often compromised treatment of patients with extensive tumor, where surgery is not applicable, and that these results cannot be extrapolated to the use of optimum techniques in the treatment of patients with limited tumor; (3) failure to recognize that much of the morbidity attributed to irradiation results from uncontrolled tumor (i.e. rectovaginal and vesico-vaginal fistulae).

As with surgery, although treatment-related morbidity can be minimized by good application, it cannot be eliminated. Thus, each complication need not be the result of improper treatment application. This unavoidable minimal risk must be tolerated in the attempt to control lethal disease.

Early treatment complications, occurring during and shortly following irradiation include irritation of the rectum, small intestine, and bladder, reactions in skin folds and mild hematopoietic depression.

A transitory reaction in a previously normal rectum may be manifest by tenesmus and the passage of mucus and even blood. The most frequent offending agent is the vaginal radium, particularly if physical separation from the rectovaginal septum is substandard because of inadequate packing, inelastic narrowing of the vaginal apex or misplacement of the applicator. With proper treatment of uncomplicated cases, significant rectal reactions rarely occur. A bloody rectal discharge should not be accepted as unavoidable, but should lead to investigation of the details of treatment.

Diarrhea and abdominal cramping characterize small intestinal irritation. Such morbidity is more frequent when a portion of intestine is fixed in the pelvis by post-surgical adhesions or other pathology. The usual offending agent is the external irradiation.

Dysuria and frequency may result from bladder irritation secondary to a localized high radiation dose from radium or irradiation of the entire organ from an external source. This morbidity is more likely with pre-existing abnormality, i.e., infection and inadequate drainage with residual urine.

Considerable pelvic marrow is irradiated with a consequent mild, transitory depression of circulating white blood cells. These changes should not be severe enough to interfere with treatment. Anemia is not a consequence of properly conducted pelvic irradiation. Anemia due to bleeding or infection should improve during irradiation. Anemia which develops, persists, or worsens during treatment is an unfavorable prognostic sign, usually indicative of widespread tumor.

Although systemic "radiation sickness" should not result from proper radiation therapy of patients with cancer of the cervix, patients occasionally notice fatigability during the 6 to 8 weeks of daily pelvic irradiation.

Late radiation sequelae include damage to the rectum, bladder, bone, and pelvic vasculoconnective tissue. The incidence and severity of late sequelae are proportional to the early morbidity.

The symptoms of radiation proctitis may follow an asymptomatic interval of many months dating from treatment. The changes most often are localized to the anterior rectal wall, at the site of maximum dosage from radium, and range from a thickened, fragile mucosa to a thinned atrophic mucosa or mucosal ulceration. The upper rectal-vaginal septum often is thickened, but pliable. These changes usually heal with conservative management, but occasionally a diverting colostomy is necessary, particularly if there is marked fibrosis of the rectal wall. It is important that these characteristic late changes be recognized and not confused with tumor, either as primary carcinoma of the rectum or extension from the cervix, for the latter concern prompts biopsy which interferes with already inadequate healing processes.

Fibrosed, stenotic changes in the remainder of an irradiated intestine (sigmoid colon, cecum, parts of small intestine) should be sufficiently rare to require a thorough search for another cause.

Late bladder reactions may occur many years following treatment. Bleeding, sufficient to cause gross hematuria, may originate from a small telangiectatic vessel under an atrophic mucosa in the lower posterior bladder, where the radium dosage was maximal. Occasionally such focal damage may progress to necrosis and ulceration. These changes are best managed conservatively and should not be confused with tumor with resultant ill-considered biopsy.

Rectovaginal and vesicovaginal fistulae should be only exceptional radiation sequelae. Such fistulae, following good radiation therapy, usually are secondary to uncontrolled tumor.

Fibrotic changes are common in the uterine supporting structures. When these changes are marked, the differential diagnosis from persistent carcinoma is difficult and may only follow prolonged observation. Lower ureteral obstruction, pain radiating along the sciatic nerve, or obstructive edema of the lower limb do not result from such pelvic fibrosis and consequently are indicative of progressive, intrapelvic tumor. Standard radiation therapy techniques do not result in fibrosis of the wall of the ureter. Therefore, the appearance of lower ureteral obstruction following good

Table 14-5.   Carcinoma of the Cervix
Serious Rectal and Bladder Injuries in 3,376 Cases
(all cases 1936–1947)

	Number	Fistula
Bladder/ureter	26	7
Rectum	34	11
Total	60 (1.8%)	18 (0.5%)

Radiumhemmet[20]

treatment application is synonymous with progression of tumor even in the absence of palpable change on pelvic exam.

Bone damage, of clinical consequence, is limited to avascular change in the femoral neck associated with poorly healing fractures. These fractures have been associated with techniques no longer used (orthovoltage pelvic irradiation including lateral fields, multiple split courses of treatment) and today have not been seen in many institutions where thousands of patients have been treated.

Although considerable bone marrow is irradiated, careful studies[18] have documented that there is no increased incidence of leukemia in long-term survivors.

The low incidence of significant late sequelae following properly conducted radiation therapy is listed in Tables 14-5, 14-6, and 14-7. Table 14-8 documents the importance of adequate protraction of treatment in the avoidance of injuries to normal structures. There is a lower incidence of rectal injury when the same dose from radium is extended to 24–30 hours compared to 15–22 hours.

Table 14-6.   Carcinoma of the Cervix
Treated at Tumor Institute of the Swedish Hospital, Seattle
1939–1956
583 Cases

	Major Complications of Irradiation
Stage I	1–Bladder ulceration for one year. Healed. Well 8 years.
Stage II	1–Bladder ulceration for one year. Healed. Well 13 years. 1–Small bowel obstruction 4 years post-irradiation. Resected. Well 9 years. 1–Rectal ulceration and stenosis. Permanent colostomy. R-V fistula 4 years post-irradiation. Well 8 years with colostomy. Fistula closed.
Stage III	1–Temporary colostomy for sigmoidal obstruction. Temporary colostomy. Well 8 years.
Stage IV	3–Temporary colostomy. 1–Permanent colostomy. Well 3 years.

Table 14-7. Carcinoma of the Cervix
Rectal Reactions and Late Rectal Injuries
in 3,392 Cases

	Number	% of all cases treated
Subjective symptoms only	28	0.8
Slight local lesions	178	5.2
Ulceration	91	2.7
Rectovaginal fistulas	16	0.5
Total	313	9.2

Ingelman-Sundberg[19]
Radiumhemmet

**Table 14-8. Correlation of Rectal Injuries
with Intesity of Treatment[16]**

	Duration of Treatment	
Gamma R per Single Treatment	24–30 hours	15–22 hours
2500–2999	6.0%	16.6%
3000+	12.1%	30.0%

CARCINOMA OF THE STUMP OF THE CERVIX

For an accurate assessment, it is necessary to separate carcinoma arising in the cervical stump from carcinoma of the cervix which was overlooked at the time of subtotal hysterectomy, for the latter group ("coincident cases") may compare unfavorably. An arbitrary interval of two years between subtotal hysterectomy for benign disease and symptoms leading to a diagnosis of invasive carcinoma of the cervix has been proposed to minimize "coincident cases," although some workers[36] suggest a three year symptom-free interval as minimal.

Patients with carcinoma of the cervical stump must be evaluated like those with intact uteri and clinical staging serves the same valuable role. In many institutions, there are proportionately fewer patients with invasive carcinoma of the cervical stump in Stages III–IV compared to those with intact uteri.

Treatment

The absence of the uterine fundus and the shortened endocervical canal eliminate or severely handicap the use of radium in an intrauterine applicator, the single most important component of treatment of limited carcinoma of the cervix. Thus, there is greater emphasis on vaginal radium, transvaginal x-ray, and external pelvic irradiation.

Results

The tumor-free survival incidence following use of modern radiation techniques in the treatment of adequately defined carcinoma of the cervical stump equals or exceeds that for treatment of carcinoma of the cervix in an intact uterus (Table 14-9).

In contrast, when the subtotal hysterectomy was performed less than two years before the onset of pertinent symptoms, the control rate is much less (Fricke and Decker,[14] 4 of 13 patients living 5 years; Moss,[27] 2 of 42 patients living 5 years; Sala and Leon,[36] 4 of 16 patients living 5 years).

ADENOCARCINOMA OF THE CERVIX

There is considerable controversy regarding the preferable treatment of patients with adenocarcinoma primary in the cervix. This uncertainty is based on: relative infrequency of the tumor (5 percent of cancer of the cervix); possible biological variation as compared to squamous cell carcinoma (i.e., different incidence of pelvic adenopathy); possible variation in radiation responsiveness (less responsive or slower to disappear after treatment than squamous cell carcinoma); and diagnostic confusion with adenocarcinomas involving both the cervix and the corpus. In a recent study, Cuccia, Bloedorn, and Onal[9] concluded: (1) there is no evidence that adenocarcinoma of the cervix is more resistant to radiation than squamous cell carcinoma; (2) a high incidence of identifiable tumor in the uterus six weeks after irradiation may reflect a slower response, but there is no correlation with prognosis; (3) hysterectomy after radical irradiation did not modify the survival, but did increase the complications; (4) the results for radiation therapy of adenocarcinoma and squamous cell carcinoma of the cervix are similar. Definitive answers about optimum treatment await planned studies. At present, there is no substantial evidence that primary radiation therapy is excelled by radical surgery or is aided by its routine co-application.

Table 14-9. Carcinoma of the Cervical Stump
5-year survival (Uncorrected data)

Stage	Fricke and[14] Decker (traced pts.)	Sala and[36] Leon
I	7/7 (100%)	7/7 (100%)
II	25/28 (89.3%)	4/6 (66%)
III	14/24 (58.3%)	3/7 (43%)
IV	4/14 (28.6%)	1/3 (33%)
Unknown	0/1 0	
Total	50/74 (67.6%)	15/23 (65%)

CARCINOMA OF THE CERVIX ASSOCIATED WITH PREGNANCY

Carcinoma of the cervix and pregnancy coexist in approximately 0.024 percent of pregnancies and 1.8 percent of patients with cancer of the cervix.[38] Each entity seriously affects the other with a threat to two lives. This important clinical association includes postpartum patients (up to 12 months) because of suggestive evidence that in most, the carcinoma of the cervix was present during the pregnancy.

These patients usually are multiparous with an average age 10–15 years less than that of all patients with carcinoma of the cervix (45–50 years). The most frequent clinical findings, vaginal bleeding and discharge, in these circumstances may be attributed erroneously to the pregnancy.

There is divergent medical opinion regarding the reciprocal interrelationships between invasive carcinoma of the cervix and pregnancy and the development of either entity, the effect on biological behavior of the tumor, the choice of treatment and ultimately the prognosis.

In the past, an apparent poorer prognosis for pregnant patients with cancer of the cervix raised questions whether the changes of pregnancy unfavorably altered the biological behavior of the carcinoma by acceleration of tumor growth and increased incidence of spread. Such possibilities are difficult to substantiate.

The histological diagnosis of carcinoma of the cervix may be difficult because of the coexistent changes of pregnancy. However, the diagnosis must be unequivocal prior to the institution of treatment which disrupts the existing pregnancy and permanently destroys child-bearing potential.

The enlarged and altered uterus may make clinical staging more difficult. However, the same criteria apply. Many[4,38,40] report that carcinoma of the cervix coexistent with pregnancy usually is diagnosed in Stages I and II, while postpartum patients frequently have extensive tumor.[4]

When carcinoma of the cervix is treated by irradiation, there is no way of protecting the fetus in utero from radiation damage and the nature and extent of this damage cannot be predicted. The pregnancy, therefore, must not be permitted to continue following any form of direct pelvic irradiation.

Treatment must be adjusted according to the duration of the pregnancy at the time the carcinoma is diagnosed. For patients with invasive carcinoma diagnosed during the first trimester of pregnancy, treatment should start with external irradiation. This should produce an abortion in 4 to 5 weeks. If this does not occur, surgical abortion is indicated because of the almost certain severe damage to the fetus. Following abortion, external irradiation can be completed and followed by standard intracavitary radium therapy.

If carcinoma is diagnosed during the second trimester of pregnancy, the uterus should be emptied by hysterotomy and treatment by external irradiation and intracavitary radium should follow.

If carcinoma is diagnosed during the third trimester and preservation of the fetus is greatly desired by the parents, sometimes it is possible to postpone initiation of treatment until the fetus is likely to be viable, so that it can be delivered by Caesarian section. (Although medical custom has encouraged delivery by Caesarian section, there are several recent reports that have stimulated doubts that vaginal delivery affects the prognosis of either the mother or the child.[4,24,40]) Then treatment can be initiated by external irradiation and followed by intracavitary therapy after the uterus has involuted. Whether such postponement is possible without unacceptable risks to the mother's life will depend on the extent of the carcinoma and consequent urgency of institution of treatment. However, it must be emphasized that continuation of pregnancy with hope to salvage a live baby is not permissible if radiation therapy is instituted.

Although many reports indicate a poorer prognosis for pregnant patients with carcinoma of the cervix, improved radiation application has resulted in a tumor-free survival incidence similar to that for all patients with cancer of the cervix.[4,8,24,40]

Lucci[24] and Creasman[8] have documented a remarkable improvement in survival incidence for patients with all stages of tumor concurrent with a change in radiation technique to emphasize initial total pelvic irradiation to high dosage. Such results, similar to those for nonpregnant patients with carcinoma of the cervix, compare favorably with reported results following primary surgery and would indicate that radiation therapy may be the usual method of choice.

REVIEW QUESTIONS

1. If carcinoma of the cervix is easy to diagnose, why are patients seen with extensive tumor? What impact does this delay have on prognosis? Why

2. What is the most frequent histological type of carcinoma of the cervix? What other type accounts for 5 to 10 percent of the cases?

3. What is the predominant route of spread of carcinoma of the cervix?

4. What intrapelvic lymph nodes must be included in any treatment plan for carcinoma of the cervix?

5. Define the clinical stages of carcinoma of the cervix. What is the basis for staging a patient? When is histological confirmation required? What are the shortcomings of clinical staging?

6. Which is of most value in treatment planning and estimation of prognosis, clinical staging, or histological tumor type?

7. Why has carcinoma-in-situ usually been treated by hysterectomy rather than irradiation?

8. What is the major problem in the treatment of a patient with invasive carcinoma of the cervix?

9. What are the two components of radiation treatment of patients with carcinoma of the cervix? What is the purpose of each? What is the sequence of application? If these procedures are not integrated by a single responsible physician, what difficulties may arise?

10. What is the significance of para-aortic adenopathy in patients with carcinoma of the cervix?

11. What levels of control are possible in each clinical stage with radiotherapy? How do the results for Stages III–IV compare with those for patients with carcinoma of the lung, esophagus, pancreas, stomach?

12. What is the evidence that radiation therapy can control pelvic adenopathy? How long has this evidence been available?

13. What are the potential advantages of surgery in the treatment of patients with cancer of the cervix?

14. In what special situations has surgery been useful?

15. What types of operation have been used? How do these procedures differ in technique, indication, morbidity?

16. Compare radiation therapy and surgery as to: applicability; results; morbidity; cost.

17. What are the "early" complications of properly conducted radiation therapy? Are these transitory? Do they prohibit normal daily activities of the patient?

18. What are the "late" complications of properly conducted radiation therapy? Are these transitory? Do they interfere with normal daily activities of the patient?

19. What is the clinical significance of lower ureteral obstruction following radiation therapy of a patient with carcinoma of the cervix?

20. If a patient develops a recto-vaginal fistula shortly after radiation therapy for cancer of the cervix, what is the most frequent cause?

21. Why does the definition of carcinoma of the stump of the cervix require a symptom-free interval between hysterectomy and symptoms related to the cancer? What is the usual interval?

22. How is radiation therapy compromised in carcinoma of the cervical stump? What are the results of treatment?

23. How frequent is adenocarcinoma of the cervix? What are the problems in determining optimum treatment?

24. How would you treat a pregnant (first trimester) patient with carcinoma of the cervix? How would the treatment vary with duration of the pregnancy? What if the patient was a primipara?

BIBLIOGRAPHY

1. ACKERMAN, L. V. and DEL REGATO, J. A. *Cancer: Diagnosis, Treatment and Progress*, Mosby, 4th ed. 1970.
2. American Cancer Society statistics. 1968 Cancer Facts and Figures.
3. BAUD, J. Carcinoma of the cervix (Stage I) treated intracavitarily with radium alone. *JAMA* 138:1138–1142, 1948.
4. BOSCH, A., and MARCIAL, V. A. Carcinoma of uterine cervix associated with pregnancy. *Amer J Roentgen* 96:92–99, 1966.

5. BUSCHKE, F., CANTRIL, S. T., and PARKER, H. M. *Supervoltage Roentgentherapy.* Charles C Thomas, Springfield, Ill., 1950.

6. CLEAVES, M. A. Radium therapy. *Chicago M. Recorder* 64:601–606, 1903.

7. COPELAND, M. (ed.) Clinical staging system for carcinoma of cervix. Amer. Joint Committee for Cancer Staging and End Results Reporting, Feb., 1964.

8. CREASMAN, W. T. Carcinoma of the cervix associated with pregnancy. (M. D. Anderson Hospital and Tumor Institute.) To be published.

9. CUCCIA, C. A., BLOEDORN, F. G., and ONAL, M. Treatment of primary adenocarcinoma of cervix. *Amer J Roentgen* 99:371–375, 1967.

10. CUTLER, M., BUSCHKE, F., and CANTRIL, S. T. In: *Cancer: Its Diagnosis and Treatment.* Saunders, Philadelphia, 1938, P. 399, table 42.

11. DEL REGATO, J. A., and COX, J. D. Transvaginal roentgen therapy in the conservative management of carcinoma in situ of the uterine cervix. *Radiol* 84:1090–1095, 1965.

12. FLETCHER, G. H. Radiation therapy for cancer of the uterine cervix. *Postgrad Med* 35:134–142, 1964.

13. FORSSELL, G. Übersicht über die Resultate der Krebsbehandlung an Radiumhein in Stockholm, 1910–1915. *Fortschr a d Geb d Röntgustr* 25:142–149, 1917.

14. FRICKE, R. E., and DECKER, D. G. Late results of radiation therapy for cancer of the cervical stump. *Amer J Roentgen* 79:32–35, 1958.

15. GRAHAM, J. B. Surgery or radiotherapy? Current Concepts in Cancer—No. 5. *JAMA* 193:13, 1965.

16. GRAY, M. J., and KOTTMEIER, H. L. Rectal and bladder injuries following radium therapy for carcinoma of the cervix at the Radiumhemmet. *Amer J Obstet Gynec* 74:1294–1303, 1957.

17. GUTTMANN, R. Effects of radiation on metastatic lymph nodes from various primary carcinomas. *Amer J Roentgen* 79:79–82, 1958.

18. HUTCHINSON, G. B. Leukemia in patients with cancer of the cervix uteri treated with radiation. A report covering the first five years of an International Study. *J Nat Cancer Inst* 40:951–982, 1968.

19. INGELMAN-SUNDBERG, A. Rectal injuries following the Stockholm method of treatment of cancer of the cervix uteri. *Acta Radiol* 28:760–764, 1947.

20. KOTTMEIER, H. L. Modern trends in the treatment of cancer of the cervix. *Acta Radiol suppl.* 116:405–414, 1954.

21. KOTTMEIER, H. L. Surgical and radiation treatment of carcinoma of the uterine cervix. *Acta Obstet Gynec Scand* 43 (suppl. 2):1–48, 1964.

22. KOTTMEIER, H. L. *Results in Treatment of Carcinoma of the Uterus and Vagina. Annual Report.* Vol. 14, 1966.

23. LACASSAGNE, A., BACLESSE, F., and REVERDY, J. Radiothérapie des cancers du col de l'utérus. Marson et Cie, Paris, 1941.

24. LUCCI, J. A., JR. Carcinoma of the cervix and pregnancy: An analysis of 111 cases. In: *M. D. Anderson Hospital Report: Carcinoma of the uterine cervix, endometrium and ovary.* Year Book, Chicago, 1962.

25. MEIGS, C. D. In: *Woman: Her Diseases and Remedies.* Blanchard and Lea, Philadelphia, 1854, p. 307.

26. MEIGS, J. V. Cancer of the cervix, an appraisal. *Amer J Obstet Gynec* 72:467–478, 1956.

27. MOSS, W. T. *Therapeutic Radiology,* Mosby, 3rd ed, 1969.

28. MUNNELL, E. W. Can recurrent cervical carcinoma be successfully managed? Current Concepts in Cancer—No. 8. *JAMA* 194:32, 1965.

29. PARSONS, L. Surgical treatment for cancer of the cervix, Stage I. Current Concepts in Cancer—No. 5 *JAMA* 193:14, 1965.

30. REGAUD, C. Traitement des cancers du col de l'utérus par les radiation: Idée soumaire des méthodes et des résultats; indications thérapeutiques. Rapport an VII Congres de la Soc. int. de chirurgie 1:35, 1926.

31. REGAUD, C. Comparaison des valeurs curatives de l'hysterectomie et des méthodes radiothérapiques dans le traitement des epithéliomas cervico-utérins du premier degré. *Bull Acad de méd,* Paris 107:611–625, 1932.

32. RUTLEDGE, F. N., and FLETCHER, G. H. Transperitoneal pelvic lymphadenectomy following supervoltage irradiation for squamous cell carcinoma of cervix. *Amer J Obstet Gynec* 76:321–334, 1958.

33. RUTLEDGE, F. N. The role of surgical resection in the management of cervical carcinoma. *Carcinoma of the uterine Cervix, Endometrium and Ovary.* Year Book, Chicago, 1962.

34. RUTLEDGE, F. N. Can irradiation destroy metastatic pelvic lymph nodes? Current Concepts in Cancer—No. 7. *JAMA* 193:24–25, 1965.

35. RUTLEDGE, F. N., FLETCHER, G. H., and MACDONALD, E. J. Pelvic lymphadenectomy as adjunct to radiotherapy in treatment for cancer of cervix. *Amer J Roentgen* 93:607–614, 1965.

36. SALA, J. N., and LEON, A. D. Treatment of carcinoma of the cervical stump. *Radiology* 81:300–306, 1963.

37. SANDLER, B. An investigation into the dosage delivered by certain techniques in the radiation therapy of carcinoma of the cervix. *Brit J Radiol* 11:623–636, 1938.

38. STANDER, R. W., and LEIN, J. N. Carcinoma of the cervix and pregnancy. *Amer J Obstet Gynec* 79:164–167, 1960.

39. Subcommittee on Radiotherapy of Cancer of the Committee on Hygiene of the League of Nations. Rules for the allocation of stages of cancer of the cervix. League of Nations Publ., Health, III:5, 1929.

40. WALDROP, G. M., and PALMER, J. P. Carcinoma of the cervix associated with pregnancy. *Amer J Obstet Gynec* 86:202–212, 1963.

41. WERTHEIM, E. The extended abdominal operation for carcinoma. *Amer J Obstet Gynec* 66:169–232, 1912.

CARCINOMA OF THE UTERINE CORPUS
(Adenocarcinoma of the Endometrium)

Management of patients with adenocarcinoma of the uterine corpus remains controversial. When possible, surgical removal of the uterus (with salpingo-oophorectomy) usually is the dominant therapeutic effort. Advocates of complementary radiation therapy disagree as to rationale, technique, and time of application.

Pathologic Findings

Most malignant tumors arising from the endometrium are adenocarcinomas, although some contain foci of metaplastic squamous epithelium and are called adenoacanthoma. Poorly differentiated tumors are more likely to invade the myometrium and to spread outside the uterus, particularly through the pelvic and vaginal lymphatics. Extension to the endocervix creates the potential of spread like cancer primary in the cervix.

Intrapelvic adenopathy has been documented in 17–28 percent[4,7] of surgical specimens. The incidence of metastases to any portion of the vaginal mucosa averages 10 percent[6] when hysterectomy is not complemented by radiation therapy. Such metastases can be nearly eliminated by preoperative irradiation (0.8 percent of 121 patients).[10] The tubes and ovaries may be involved in 4–10 percent[9] of patients, and distant metastases may involve nearly any organ.[5]

Clinical Evaluation

Patients with carcinoma of the uterine corpus are likely to be older than those with carcinoma of the cervix (80 percent over 50 years, 51.7 percent over 60 years).[10] They may be threatened by other major illnesses, particularly obesity, hypertension, diabetes mellitus, cirrhosis, and arteriosclerotic cardiovascular disease, with consequent limitation of surgery. Thus, Kottmeier[8] found only 53.1 percent of his patients eligible for panhysterectomy and Arneson[3] classified only 51 percent as clinical Stage I-A (tumor clinically confined to the uterus and operation advisable), compared to 40 percent clinical Stage I-B (tumor clinically confined to the uterus, but poor operative risk). Kottmeier[8] reported the intercurrent death rate in this group to be 9.4 percent at 5 years and 21.7 percent at 10 years following the diagnosis of adenocarcinoma of the corpus.

Clinical Staging

Treatment planning must be based on a clinical, rather than a surgical, appraisal of tumor extent. Although many staging schemes have been suggested, none has proved as useful as that used for cancer of the cervix. A workable clinical staging has been proposed by the American Joint Committee for Cancer Staging and End Results Reporting[2] (1964):

Stage O

Pre-invasive carcinoma, carcinoma-in-situ.

Stage I

Carcinoma strictly confined to the corpus uteri.

Stage II

Carcinoma involving the corpus uteri and cervix uteri.

Stage III

Carcinoma extending outside the uterus, but not outside the true pelvis.

Stage IVA

Carcinoma extending outside the true pelvis or obviously involving the mucosa of the bladder or rectum.

Stage IVB

Any of the above with evidence of metastasis outside the pelvis.

Treatment and Results

In tailoring treatment to the clinical extent of tumor in Stages O and I, hysterectomy is the main treatment component for medically operable patients because it is the most certain and easiest method of controlling tumor in the corpus, especially if there is deep invasion of the myometrium.

For patients with correctly diagnosed carcinoma-in-situ and for those with well-differentiated adenocarcinomas involving only a small site in the fundus of a normal sized uterus, panhysterectomy is complete treatment and complementary irradiation makes no contribution.

However, as the tumor becomes more extensive or less differentiated, or both, complementary radiation therapy (preferably preoperative) may contribute by controlling occult intrapelvic or vaginal spread. Experience with radical surgery, i.e., radical panhysterectomy plus pelvic lymph node dissection, has been limited.[1,12]

If the control of occult intrapelvic or vaginal spread of tumor is the objective of radiation therapy as a surgical adjuvant, the irradiation must include the entire pelvis and upper vagina. This is possible only with teletherapy. For reasons explained elsewhere, this treatment is more effective preoperatively than post-operatively. The required dose, if properly fractionated, is compatible with the necessary surgery. Although treatment has been effective with medium-voltage x-ray, supervoltage quality radiation is of great advantage in the "protection" of normal tissues. This biologically oriented use of radiation therapy as a complement to surgery surprisingly has been reported only by a few,[10,11] although the results reported[10] for the treatment of all patients classified as Stage I–A are better than those reported for highly selected surgical series. The effectiveness of this regimen can be measured both by tumor-free survival incidence (93.2 percent at five years for 121 patients) and by avoidance of vaginal metastases (1 of 121 = 0.8 percent).[10]

Packing of the uterine cavity with multiple radium sources has been used as preoperative treatment. However, this does not treat the pelvic and vaginal lymphatics, which may be tumor-bearing, but instead intensively treats only that tumor which is certain to be removed by hysterectomy. If preoperative "devitalization" of tumor cells in the corpus is a legitimate objective of radiation therapy, then more consistently homogeneous irradiation is possible, with teletherapy than with intra-uterine radium sources.

Effective preoperative use of radium would seem limited to treatment of the vagina, with an objective of controlling occult spread in that structure.

If patients with carcinoma in situ or invasive carcinoma limited to the corpus are judged medically inoperable, tumor control can be achieved with radiation therapy alone. Local control of intrauterine tumor will be less with irradiation than with surgery because of: decreased effectiveness of irradiation when there is deep tumor invasion of the myometrium; technical errors secondary to irradiation of an irregular cavity; and, in a few, an unsatisfactory radiation response for unknown biological reasons. In this group, intrauterine radiation (packing of the uterine cavity with multiple radium sources or other isotopes) replaces removal of the uterus. The rationale for complementary pelvic irradiation is unchanged. However, the combination increases the risk of radiation-related complications.

The crude survival rates for this group will be reduced by deaths from inter-current disease. Thus, in Arneson's study,[3] although only 1.5 percent of those patients with Stage I tumor treated by surgery died of intercurrent disease within five years, 21.6 percent of those with Stage I tumor considered medically inoperable died of intercurrent disease within five years. In this latter medically compromised group, Lampe[10] reported a 61.7 percent determinate 5-year survival rate with pelvic x-ray teletherapy plus intrauterine radium.

When tumor involves both the corpus and cervix (corpus et collum), treatment should be like that for primary carcinoma of the cervix (with spread to the corpus). Thus, standard panhysterectomy is not adequate, and radiation methods must include packing of the uterine cavity with multiple radiation sources in addition to vaginal apical radium and full pelvic teletherapy.

The results for this latter group, with more extensive tumor and high probability of intrapelvic spread, are modest compared with those for patients with tumor confined either to the corpus or cervix. Arneson's[3] 5-year survival rate was 31.5 percent.

When tumor has extended outside the uterus, but not outside the true pelvis, hysterectomy is not applicable, but control is possible by radiation methods. Using full pelvic teletherapy and intrauterine packing with multiple radium sources, Lampe[10] reported that 11 of 45 patients (24.4 percent) in this group were clinically tumor-free over five years.

When the carcinoma has extended outside the true pelvis, cure is not possible by current methods. However, local irradiation may accomplish specific palliative objectives, i.e., control of hemorrhage from the corpus or vagina or relief of pain from metastasis to bone.

REVIEW QUESTIONS

1. What is the major component of treatment of patients with adenocarcinoma of the uterine corpus? What are the restrictions of this treatment component? How frequent are these restrictions?

2. What medical problems frequently coexist with adenocarcinoma of the uterine corpus? How do these influence the cancer management?

3. Describe a clinical staging for patients with carcinoma of the corpus. Why has this staging been less useful than that for cancer of the cervix?

4. What are the objectives of complementary radiation therapy for the patient eligible for surgery?

5. What is the reported determinate survival of patients treated by complementary irradiation followed by hysterectomy? What is the incidence of death from intercurrent disease in this group?

6. If patients with adenocarcinoma limited to the corpus are inoperable for medical reasons, are they still curable? If so, by what method? If so, how often? How large is this group of patients (surgically operable, but medically inoperable) in reported series? What is the influence of death from intercurrent disease in this group?

7. When adenocarcinoma of the corpus spreads to the cervix, how may the biological behavior change? How does this affect treatment? prognosis?

8. When tumor has extended from the corpus into the pelvis or vagina, is the patient curable? If so, by what method? If so, how frequently? How does this survival incidence compare with that of patients with carcinoma of the lung?

BIBLIOGRAPHY

1. ALFORD, C. D., BETSON, J. R., JR., and DISANTI, N. Wertheim hysterectomy and pelvic lympha-denectomy for carcinoma of the uterine corpus. *Amer J Obstet Gynec*, 83:1306–1312, 1962.
2. American Joint Committee. Clinical staging system for carcinoma of the corpus uteri. American Joint Committee for Cancer Staging and End Results Reporting, 1964.
3. ARNESON, A. N. Long-term follow-up observations in corporeal cancer. *Amer J Roentgen*, 91:3–21, 1964.
4. BRUNSCHWIG, A., and MURPHY, A. I. Rationale for radical panhysterectomy and pelvic node excision in carcinoma of corpus uteri; clinical and pathological data on mode of spread of endometrial carcinoma. *Amer J Obstet Gynec*, 68:1482–1488, 1954.
5. HENRIKSEN, E. Lymphatic spread of carcinoma of cervix and of body of uterus; study of 420 necropsies. *Amer J Obstet Gynec*, 58:924–942, 1949.
6. HUNT, H. B. Comparative radiotherapeutic results in carcinoma of the endometrium as modified by prior surgery and post-irradiation hysterosalpingo-oophorectomy. *Radiology*, 66:653–665, 1956.
7. JAVERT, C. T., and HOFAMMANN, K. Observations on surgical pathology, selective lymphade-nectomy and classification of endometrial adenocarcinoma. *Cancer*, 5:485–498, 1952.
8. KOTTMEIER, H. L. Radiotherapy of carcinoma of the corpus uteri and carcinoma of the corpus and endocervix. pp. 96–131 in *Carcinoma of the Female Genitalia*, Williams & Wilkins, Baltimore, 1953.
9. KOTTMEIER, H. L. Carcinoma of corpus. Its classification and treatment. *Gynaecologia* (Basel), 138:287–310, 1954.
10. LAMPE, I. Endometrial carcinoma. *Amer J Roentgen*, 90:1011–1015, 1963.
11. SALA, J. M., and REGATO, J. A. Treatment of carcinoma of the endometrium. *Radiology*, 79:12–17, 1962.
12. SCHWARTZ, A. E., and BRUNSCHWIG, A. Radical panhysterectomy and pelvic node excision for carcinoma of corpus uteri. *Surg Gynec Obstet*, 105:675–680, 1957.

CARCINOMA OF THE OVARY

There is no consensus for the use of radiation therapy for patients with carcinoma of the ovary. This continuing uncertainty results from biological unpre-dictability of these tumors; difficulties in establishing a diagnosis of tumor when limited in extent; low radiation sensitivity of most ovarian carcinomas; problems of tolerance to radiation in adequate dosage delivered to the frequently required large tissue volume; and lack of planned studies which have provided meaningful answers.

Clinical Presentation

Ovarian cancer most frequently affects females in the 45- to 65-year range, although females of any age are vulnerable. Approximately 95 percent of ovarian growths in women younger than 30 years are benign, whereas two-thirds of ovarian growths in women over 60 years are malignant.[2] Thus, the detection of an enlarge-ment of the ovary leads to a difficult judgment, whether it is advisable to establish positive identification by laparotomy.

The clinical findings related to ovarian malignancy usually are based on tumor extension via direct invasion of other structures, peritoneal implantation, or lymphatic hematogenous metastases, and thus are indicative of advanced disease. The most common complaints, abdominal enlargement and abdominal pain, each affect over 50 percent of these patients.[7] Other nonhormonal findings include: vaginal bleeding or discharge, ill-defined gastrointestinal complaints, urinary disturbances, backache, and swelling of the lower limbs. About 5 percent of ovarian cancers cause endocrine-related changes[2] (i.e., feminizing effects of granulosa cell tumors, masculinizing effects of arrhenoblastoma).

Anatomical Staging

Extensive anatomical spread of ovarian cancer is the major deterrent to successful application of locally effective treatment (surgery, radiation therapy), and consequently is the primary prognostic indicator.

The staging classifications have not been pretreatment clinical assessments, but have been based on the findings at laparotomy when the diagnosis was established. A careful appraisal of tumor extent at the time of initial surgery is essential for optimal evaluation and therapeutic application.

The following staging, suggested by Moss,[6] is representative:

Stage I

Tumor limited to the ovaries.

Stage IA

Tumor limited to one ovary

Stage IB

Tumor limited to both ovaries

Stage II

Tumor of one or both ovaries with extension into the pelvis

Stage IIA

Extension/metastasis to the uterus and/or tubes only

Stage IIB

Extension to other pelvic structures

Stage III

Spread of tumor beyond the pelvis, but confined to the peritoneal cavity

Stage IV

Spread outside the peritoneal cavity

Special category

Unexplored patients with tumor thought to be from the ovary

Fluid with or without tumor cells does not influence the staging, but should be recorded.

Pathologic Findings

Although many detailed histological classifications of ovarian tumors may be of interest, clinical use requires simplicity and biological relevance. A lack of usefulness in the past can be documented by the large number of studies in which the histological type and grade of ovarian tumors were not mentioned.

Most tumors of the ovary are cystic and benign. About 20 percent are solid, and most of these are malignant.[2] The majority of malignant ovarian tumors are cystic or solid adenocarcinomas, and these must be emphasized in any classifications used by the clinician. Approximately 10 percent of malignant ovarian tumors are metastatic from other primary sites, and these often are bilateral.[2] About 5 percent of malignant ovarian tumors cause symptoms and signs of endocrine activity.[2]

Kottmeier[5] has emphasized the importance of stromal invasion, and others[4, 10] have emphasized the importance of histological grading. Using diagnostic criteria of stromal invasion and epithelial cellular changes of anaplasia, multilayering, and increased mitotic activity, 20 percent of ovarian tumors remain of borderline malignancy.[11] Inclusion or exclusion of this sizable group alters the results of any study.

A simplified, clinically usable classification of primary malignant tumors of the ovary follows:

   I. Cystadenocarcinoma
      A. Serous
      B. Mucinous
  II. Solid adenocarcinoma
 III. Endometrial-like adenocarcinoma (malignant endometrioma, adenocanthoma, other nonpapillary tumors)
 IV. Special tumors (dysgerminoma, granulosa cell tumor, arrhenoblastoma)

The following classification was proposed in 1961 by The Cancer Committee of the International Federation of Gynecologists and Obstetricians:

   I. Serous cystomas
      A. Serous cystadenoma (benign)
      B. Proliferating serous cystadenoma without stromal invasion (possibly malignant)
      C. Serous cystadenocarcinoma (malignant)
  II. Mucinous cystomas
      A. Mucinous cystadenoma (benign)
      B. Proliferating mucinous cystadenoma without stromal invasion (possibly malignant)
      C. Mucinous cystadenocarcinoma (malignant)
 III. Endometrioid tumors (resemble adenocarcinoma in the endometrium)
      A. Endometrioid cysts (benign)

    B. Proliferating endometrioid adenoma and cystadenoma (possibly malig-
nant)

    C. Endometrioid carcinoma (malignant)

IV. Undifferentiated and unclassified carcinoma

Treatment

The difficulties of management of patients with cancer of the ovary are related to frequent widespread tumor at the time of detection, with consequent lack of applicability of surgery or adequate irradiation.

Surgery

Surgery usually is necessary for establishment of the diagnosis and appraisal of tumor extent. Definitive surgical removal of tumor is the most effective treatment, but cannot be used with curative intent in patients with Stage III–IV and some Stage II tumors.

Radiation Therapy

Nearly all primary ovarian carcinomas arise from the germinal epithelium. This histogenesis might imply a high degree of radiosensitivity. However, except for dysgerminoma, ovarian carcinomas are, in general, of limited radiosensitivity. Thus, radiation therapy is severely handicapped by frequent widespread anatomic distribution of tumors of limited radiovulnerability.

Consequently, if the ovarian cancer is grossly limited to the pelvis, it seems preferable to irradiate this restricted tissue volume to a potentially cancerocidal dose rather than treat the entire peritoneal cavity, which is at risk, to a lower and likely ineffective dose, limited by patient tolerance.

The patient's intolerance to irradiation of the entire peritoneal cavity to adequate dosage is initially manifest by transitory nausea, diarrhea, and hemato-poietic depression. However, the most serious problems are nonreversible damage of the kidneys and liver by doses required to control tumor.

If the entire peritoneal cavity must be irradiated, a "moving-strip technique"[1] has been advocated in an attempt to improve the dose-time relationship. This is accomplished at the expense of inhomogeneity of irradation of anatomical structures and tumor due to daily variation in their position. A particular risk is "hot spots" of radiation causing damage to the intestine. After a trial, this technique has been abandoned at the University of California (San Francisco) because of the frequent associated morbidity.

Therefore, radiation therapy should have its optimal application for patients with Stage II cancer. Any usefulness for patients with Stage I disease is limited to those inaccurately staged because of undetected local extension of tumor. Use in patients with Stage III disease is compromised by necessary reduction of dosage to large tissue volumes. Local irradiation for palliative purposes occasionally is useful in patients with Stage III-IV disease.

Occasionally radiotherapy has been followed by complete clinical regression of apparently hopeless extensive tumor in the pelvis. In nearly all of these patients tumor again became clinically active after many years. Therefore, surgical removal of the ovaries, uterus, omentum and residual masses should follow irradiation regardless of the apparent excellent response. Most of our patients with excellent tumor response were premenopausal at the time of initial treatment, raising the question of the contribution of castration. Therefore, we suggest that both ovaries be removed, if possible, even from patients with extensive tumor.

Inasmuch as laparotomy is necessary for the diagnosis of tumor in situations in which radiation therapy is likely to be useful, irradiation usually has followed definitive surgery. Therefore, preoperative irradiation, frequently preferred in other clinical problems, has not been adequately evaluated.

In the past in some institutions, the uterus has not been removed so that it might be used as a container for radium. Currently available external radiation sources allow adequate dose distribution throughout the entire pelvis. Therefore, the uterus, which frequently is involved by ovarian cancer, should be removed at the time of initial definitive surgery.

If at the time of initial laparotomy, complete resection of tumor is not possible, we[12] advocate biopsy only, followed by radiation therapy. Following completion of adequate irradiation, especially if there has been detectable tumor response and no evidence of dissemination of tumor, a second laparotomy with intent to attempt radical resection is in order.

Dysgerminoma, the female counterpart of seminoma, is a special problem. This highly radioresponsive tumor frequently spreads to retroperitoneal, mediastinal, and supraclavicular lymph nodes. The indications for postoperative irradiation are the same as for seminoma in males, namely, the treatment of regional (pelvic and abdominal para-aortic) lymphatics. Such life-saving treatment should not be compromised by attempts to protect the remaining ovary, for such maneuvers risk the life of the patient and the genetic composition of any progeny. Dysgerminoma, like seminoma, still may be curable, with extensive metastatic spread to mediastinum, supraclavicular nodes, or even lung. Treatment of pulmonary metastases is justified because adequate radiation dosage may be within limits of lung tolerance.

The frequent problem of ascites in ovarian carcinoma has been treated by instillation of radioactive materials (colloids with ^{198}Au, ^{32}P). An early enthusiasm has waned because of difficulties of adequate administration, personnel radiation exposure, and cost, and the realization that other nonradioactive materials, i.e., chlorambucil and atabrine, are safer, cheaper, and at least as effective.

Chemotherapy

The frequent extensiveness of tumor with consequent inapplicability of surgery or radiation therapy has generated an interest in systemic treatment by chemicals. Alkylating agents have been used most frequently. Although there is no specificity for a particular alkylating agent, chlorambucil (Leukeran®), triethylenethiophosphoramide (Thiotepa®), cyclophosphamide (Cytoxan®), and L-phenylalanine mustard (Alkeran®) have been used with varying success. Some long-term remissions have resulted, thus favoring the use of the less toxic oral forms of these agents. In varying degrees, these medications are toxic to bone marrow and intestinal epithelium. Therefore, concurrent or consecutive use of chemotherapeutic agents and radiation therapy is difficult.

Table 14-10. Relationship of Survival, Tumor Extent, and Treatment

Tumor Extent	Surgery Only (5-year Survival Rate)	Surgery and Radiation Therapy (5-year Survival Rate)
Involvement of one or both ovaries	45/71 (63%)	43/74 (58%)
Removable local extension of tumor	14/29 (48%)	28/49 (57%)
Nonremovable local extension of tumor	3/26 (11.5%)	13/36 (36%)
Spread to abdomen or distant spread	1/132 (0.8%)	10/80 (13%)

Results

Tumor control by any treatment method can be related to both histological type and anatomical extent, although the latter is the best prognostic indicator.[8]

If tumor is limited to the ovaries (Stage I) or even has minimally extended locally, resection is curative, and adjuvant radiation therapy does not contribute. However, long-term tumor-free survivors with postoperative residual tumor in the pelvis or abdomen (Stages II, III) can be attributed to radiation therapy. Data substantiating the contribution of radiation therapy to patient survival are equivocal. The following data of Holme[3] and Rubin, Grise, and Terry[9] might substantiate a predictable contribution of local irradiation (Table 14-10).

The prognosis and the contributions of adjuvant irradiation vary with tumor type, as documented by data of Rubin, Grise, and Terry[9] (Table 14-11).

When tumor has spread beyond the pelvis, particularly if there is involvement of the liver, widespread seeding of the peritoneum, or spread beyond the peritoneal cavity, relief of special clinical problems, rather than cure, may be the reasonable objective.

Although the foregoing discussion is based on available, statistically supported data, it is important to remember that the response to treatment and, consequently, the prognosis for patients with ovarian cancer are erratic. Thus, it is imperative that the physician not abandon these patients even if the situation seems "hopeless."

Table 14-11. Relationship of Survival, Tumor Type, and Treatment

Tumor Type	Surgery Only (5-year Survival Rate)	Surgery and Radiation Therapy (5-year Survival Rate)
Well-differentiated cystadenocarcinoma	6/7 (86%)	11/15 (73%)
Poorly differentiated cystadenocarcinoma	1/14 (7%)	8/37 (22%)
Solid adenocarcinoma	1/13 (8%)	4/17 (24%)
Special tumors	4/12 (33%)	5/9 (56%)

REVIEW QUESTIONS

1. Why is a diagnosis difficult when cancer of the ovary is of limited extent? How does this influence the use of available treatment methods?

2. What are the basic divisions of any clinical staging of extent of ovarian carcinoma? How may the presence of tumor-bearing ascitic fluid influence this staging?

3. Although there are many interesting, special ovarian tumors, what malignant tumor is the most frequent and thus the major clinical problem?

4. How frequent are malignant tumors involving the ovary metastatic from another primary site? Are these tumors curable?

5. What is the potential importance of endocrine activity of ovarian cancers? How frequent are these tumors? What clinical findings might you expect from granulosa cell tumor? from arrhenoblastoma?

6. With current knowledge and available treatment, which is the better prognostic indicator—extent or type of tumor?

7. Is it surprising that ovarian carcinomas arising from germinal eptihelium are not highly radiation-responsive? How does the radiosensitivity of these tumors compare with that of carcinomas of the testis?

8. What are the major deterrents to effective radiation therapy for patients with ovarian carcinomas?

9. In what clinical situation (stage) may radiation therapy be a contributor to the cure of a patient with carcinoma of the ovary?

10. What problems of patient tolerance limit adequate irradiation of the entire peritoneal cavity? How does adjuvant chemotherapy affect this tolerance?

BIBLIOGRAPHY

1. DELCLOS, L., and MURPHY, M. Evaluation of tolerance during treatment, late tolerance and better evaluation of clinical effectiveness of the Co60 moving strip technique. *Amer J Roentgen*, 96:75–80, 1966.
2. DOCKERTY, M. B. Pathologic features of certain ovarian carcinomas. *Amer J Roentgen*, 88:841–845, 1962.
3. HOLME, G. M. Malignant ovarian tumours. *J Fac Radiol*, 8:394–401, 1956–1957.
4. KENT, S. W., and MCKAY, D. G. Primary cancer of ovary. *Amer J Obstet Gynec*, 80:430–438, 1960.
5. KOTTMEIER, H.-L. Classification and treatment of ovarian tumours. *Acta Obstet Gynec Scand*, 31:313–363, 1952.
6. MOSS, W. T. *Therapeutic Radiology*, 3rd ed. Mosby, St. Louis, 1969.
7. PEARSE, W. H., and BEHRMAN, S. J. Carcinoma of the ovary. *Obstet Gynec*, 3:32–45, 1954.
8. RAVENTOS, A., LEWIS, G. C., and CHIDIAC, J. Primary ovarian cancer: 25-year report of 275 patients. *Amer J Roentgen*, 89:524–532, 1963.
9. RUBIN, P., GRISE, J. W., and TERRY, R. Has post-operative irradiation proved itself? *Amer J Roentgen*, 88:849–866, 1962.

10. TURNER, J. C., JR., REMINE, W. H., and DOCKERTY, M. B. Clinicopathologic study of 172 patients with primary carcinoma of ovary. *Surg Gynec Obstet*, 109:198–206, 1959.

11. TWEEDDALE, D. N., and PEDERSON, B. L. Serous neoplasms of the ovary (with observations on related neoplasms). *Amer J Med Sci*, 249:701–717, 1965.

12. VAETH, J. M., and BUSCHKE, F. J. The role of preoperative irradiation in the treatment of carcinoma of the ovary. *Amer J Roentgen*, 105:614–617, 1969.

MALIGNANT TUMORS OF THE VAGINA AND VULVA

Vagina

Malignant tumors of the vagina are rare, being less frequent than those of the cervix (1:60), corpus (1:12), or vulva (1:3).[11] Primary vaginal tumors are less frequent than those secondary to neoplasms arising in the cervix, corpus, or ovary.[1] Therefore, it must be determined that the cervix, corpus, or ovary are not involved, or have not been recently involved by malignant tumors, before a diagnosis of primary vaginal cancer is established.

Most primary malignant tumors of the vagina are poorly differentiated epidermoid carcinomas,[1,11] although adenocarcinomas, sarcomas, and other tumors may occur.

The victims usually are 45 to 60 years of age and present with vaginal discharge and bleeding.[1]

Treatment

Management must be based on tumor type, a determination whether the neoplasm is primary or secondary, location and extent with consequent potential for lymphatic spread, and the condition of the patient. Primary malignant tumors of the upper vagina have the same potential to spread to iliac lymphatics as do cancers primary in the cervix. Thus, radiation therapy should consist of pelvic irradiation plus intracavitary (vaginal, cervical canal) irradiation. The surgical alternative should include vaginectomy and radical hysterectomy with pelvic lymph node dissection.

Tumors of the lower vagina may spread to pelvic nodes, particularly those adjacent to the hypogastric vessels, but also may extend to the vulva and, consequently, the inguinal nodes. Appropriate surgery, therefore, must be even more extensive than for tumors of the upper vagina.

Results

Most reported results have followed radiation therapy of some form, whereas the reported results of surgery have been less frequent.[2] Chau[5] emphasized the use of vaginal radium in controlling 12 of 15 "early" and 6 of 16 "late" vaginal tumors. Rutledge[11] reported a 35 percent tumor-free survival at five years following treatment dominated by radiation methods, with surgery limited to a few tumors of the upper vagina, some tumors that were "superficial," or those that were not controlled by irradiation. Murphy[9] had 35 five-year survivors from 135 patients treated. Buschke and Cantril[3] controlled primary vaginal carcinomas in 6 of 10 patients between 1939–1946, noting that "adequate external roentgen therapy directed toward and including the entire vagina and paravaginal area is an essential part of therapy. . . ."

Vulva

Carcinoma of the vulva may arise from the labia majora, labia minora, vestibule, or clitoris. Eighty-five percent of the patients are postmenopausal at the time of diagnosis.[10] Clinical complaints include: pruritus, lump, pain, ulcer, bleeding, and dysuria.

Most primary carcinomas arise on the labia, are well-differentiated epidermoid in type, and may spread submucosally and to inguinal and pelvic nodes. Tumors arising from the clitoris and vestibule may be less well-differentiated epidermoid carcinomas.[1]

Many vulvar cancers arise from compromised epithelium which may be dry and atrophic with patches of leukoplakia. Therefore, although the tumors might be responsive to irradiation, the surrounding normal tissues are a poor tumor bed. Nevertheless, for selected patients with extensive vulvar neoplasms, well-protracted external irradiation of adequate quality (not superficial radiation!) can be effective and is well tolerated.[4]

Vulvectomy with inguinal node dissection is advocated[6,12] as effective treatment, although the operative morbidity and mortality for a radical procedure may be distressingly high.[7]

The prognosis is relatively favorable. Green[6] reported the five-year survival of 25 of 29 patients with nodes free of tumor and of 17 of 36 patients with tumor-bearing lymph nodes using surgery. Merrill and Ross[8] advocated radical surgery and reported an absolute five-year survival of 42 percent of 83 patients.

REVIEW QUESTIONS

1. What is the primary consideration in establishing that a carcinoma in the vagina is primary there?

2. If a patient had been treated for carcinoma of the cervix one year prior to diagnosis of a squamous cell carcinoma involving the vaginal mucosa, would you consider the vaginal tumor primary or secondary? How would you substantiate this? What if the carcinoma of the cervix had been treated six years before?

3. What is the most likely pattern of spread from carcinoma primary in the vaginal mucosa? Does this vary with site of involvement? extent? Does this potential spread influence treatment?

4. What is the major deterrent to radiation therapy for squamous cell carcinoma of the vulva? Is this deterrent applicable in carcinoma of the vagina?

BIBLIOGRAPHY

1. ACKERMAN, L. V., and DEL REGATO, J. A. *Cancer: Diagnosis, Treatment, Prognosis,* 4th ed. Mosby, St. Louis, 1970.
2. BRACK, C. B., MERRITT, R. I., and DICKSON, R. J. Primary carcinoma of the vagina. *Obstet Gynec,* 12:104–109, 1958.
3. BUSCHKE, F., and CANTRIL, S. T. Radiation therapy of carcinoma of the vagina. *Radiology,* 56:193–201, 1951.
4. BUSCHKE, F., and CANTRIL, S. T. Roentgen therapy of carcinoma of female urethra and vulva. *Radiology,* 51:155–165, 1948.
5. CHAU, P. M. Radiotherapeutic management of malignant tumors of vagina. *Amer J Roentgen,* 89:502–523, 1963.
6. GREEN, T. H., JR., ULFELDER, H., and MEIGS, J. V. Epidermoid carcinoma of the vulva: An analysis of 238 cases. *Amer J Obstet Gynec,* 75:834–847; 848–864, 1958.
7. MCKELVEY, J. L. The treatment of carcinoma of the vulva. *Amer J Obstet Gynec,* 54:626–633, 1947.
8. MERRILL, J. A., and ROSS, N. L. Cancer of the vulva. *Cancer,* 14:13–20, 1961.
9. MURPHY, W. T. Primary vaginal cancer: Irradiation, management and end results. *Radiology,* 68:157–168, 1957.
10. PALMER, J. P., SADUCOR, M. G., and REINHARD, M. C. Carcinoma of the vulva. *Surg Gynec Obstet,* 88:435–440, 1949.
11. RUTLEDGE, F. Cancer of vagina. *Amer J Obstet Gynec,* 97:635–655, 1967.
12. WAY, S. Carcinoma of the vulva. *Amer J Obstet Gynec,* 79:692–697, 1960.

15

TUMORS
OF THE MALE REPRODUCTIVE
SYSTEM

MALIGNANT TUMORS OF THE TESTIS

The prognosis for patients with malignant tumors of the testis has improved dramatically in the past 40 years. This has resulted from greater knowledge of the biological behavior of these neoplasms and the resultant better directed and more effective therapy.

These tumors comprise less than 1 percent of all cancer. They commonly occur during the patient's reproductive years (25 to 40 years). The average age of patients with seminoma (40 years) is about 10 years higher than for patients with the other testicular neoplasms.[1]

Because of the varying biological behavior and the consequent difference in prognosis and therapeutic approach, the histologic determination of the tumor type is important.

The so-called "nongerminal" tumors represent only 3.5 percent of testicular tumors and are of little importance in this discussion. The major concern is with the "germinal" tumors which comprise the remaining 96.5 percent.[1]

"Germinal" tumors include four basic histologic patterns: seminoma; teratoma; embryonal carcinoma; and choriocarcinoma. Several of these histological components may be present in the same tumor with at least 15 possible combinations. However, only 5 varieties are of clinical importance:

1. Seminoma: 35–50 percent
2. Embryonal carcinoma: 20–25 percent
3. Teratoma: less than 10 percent
4. Teratocarcinoma, which is a combination of embryonal carcinoma or choriocarcinoma with teratoma: 20–30 percent
5. Choriocarcinoma (with or without seminoma and/or embryonal carcinoma): about 2 percent

Seminoma frequently is found in association with embryonal carcinoma, teratoma, or teratocarcinoma, but does not seem to alter the biological behavior of these other tumor components. The prognosis of embryonal carcinoma and choriocarcinoma, however, is improved by association with teratoma.

The prognosis becomes worse with increasing tumor size within each group;

with tumor extension through the tunica albuginea, into the epididymis or along the spermatic cord; in the presence of invasion of veins by tumor; with metastases; with Leidig cell hyperplasia in the remainder of the testis; and with elevated gonadotropins.[4,5,7] Survival rates in patients with seminoma are better in tumors with prominent lymphatic stroma.

Treatment

Treatment of the primary tumor is orchiectomy and dissection of the inguinal canal with ligation of the spermatic cord and vessels at the abdominal-inguinal ring. Preoperative irradiation of the testis, occasionally advocated, risks destruction of essential histologic evidence, and thus is contraindicated.

Although a few patients may survive following orchiectomy only, the prognosis for most patients depends on control of metastases, usually in the form of retroperitoneal adenopathy. The recent marked improvement in patient survival is related to more effective control of these regional metastases.

The lymphatics from the testicular parenchyma accompany the internal spermatic artery and vein to drain into the para-aortic nodes between the level of renal vessels and the aortic bifurcation. The nodes draining the right testis are located along the right lateral surface of the inferior vena cava and the front of the aorta and vena cava, whereas those draining the left testis are adjacent to the left lateral and anterior surfaces of the aorta. Communications between the lymphatic chains account for occasional involvement of both. The testis and epididymis also drain into ipsilateral external iliac nodes. Inguinal nodes may be involved following extension of tumor to involve the scrotum.

Involvement of retroperitoneal nodes may be followed by spread to mediastinal and supraclavicular nodes (more often the left). Occasionally the mediastinum may be bypassed when supraclavicular nodes become involved by spread of tumor through the thoracic duct.

Clinical methods for identifying tumor in para-aortic nodes are insensitive. Ureteral deviation requires sizable adenopathy. Inferior venacavagrams are likely to detect only sizable adenopathy from the right testis. Lymphograms may document much smaller tumor deposits, but to date testicular lymphograms have rarely been done, and the standard lymphogram may not be accurate at the critical level of the renal vessels (Figure 15–1).

Tumor may be found histologically in the abdominal para-aortic nodes of 15–50 percent of patients in whom the identification is not possible by current clinical methods. This incidence of adenopathy is higher with embryonal carcinoma than with seminoma.

Hematogenous metastases are most frequent with choriocarcinoma, less with embryonal carcinoma, and least with seminoma.

The histologic differentiation of tumor type is of particular importance in formulating treatment of the potentially or demonstrably involved lymphatics.

It is now universally agreed that, in the treatment of seminoma, postoperative irradiation of the regional lymphatics is an integral part of the therapeutic procedure whether or not lymph node involvement can be demonstrated clinically. In the absence of demonstrable retroperitoneal adenopathy, treatment should include at least the nodes adjacent to the ipsilateral external iliac vessels, abdominal aorta,

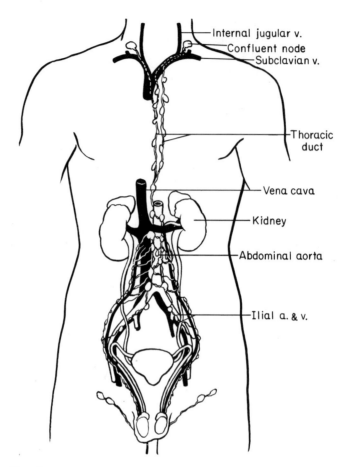

Fig. 15-1. Lymphatic drainage of the testes. Initial metastases may be at the level of the renal pedicle. Communication
exists between left and right para-aortic lymphatics. The
thoracic duct may empty into the right subclavian (or azygos)
vein. The scrotum drains to the inguinal nodes.

and vena cava to a level just above the renal pedicles. Seminoma is sufficiently
radioresponsive that the dose necessary for tumor eradication is well-tolerated
despite the large volume irradiated. If retroperitoneal involvement is demonstrated,
treatment to these nodes is followed by irradiation of the next relay, the mediastinum and supraclavicular nodes. Seminoma may be controlled even when widely
metastatic. Long-term survival or "cure" has been observed following treatment
of large retroperitoneal masses or large mediastinal and supraclavicular adenopathy
of an extent that, for most other tumors, would indicate incurability. Therefore,
vigorous treatment is imperative even in the presence of widespread neoplasm.
Because of the effectiveness of irradiation, retroperitoneal node dissection is unnecessary and, consequently, contraindicated in the treatment of seminoma.

In the treatment of patients with embryonal carcinomas and teratocarcinomas,
there is no such unanimous agreement in the choice between radiation therapy or

retroperitoneal dissection. These tumors are not so reliably treated by radiation therapy, as is seminoma because there is a considerable variation in radiation response, and for some tumors the dose necessary for sterilization may exceed intestinal tolerance. Retroperitoneal dissection is of limited effectiveness because a block dissection in this region is anatomically impossible, and therefore removal of all involved nodes cannot be expected.[7] The profit of such extensive operations has never been measured because, with rare exception, when the nodes have been found to contain tumor, postoperative irradiation has been added. The effectiveness and tolerance of radiation therapy are reduced by antecedent retroperitoneal dissection because of the interference of the blood supply with consequent reduction of tumor response and normal tissue repair. Preoperative radiation, in the high dose necessary for these tumors, may add to the complications of a difficult surgical procedure.

Interruption of radiation therapy of the regional lymphatics after modest dosage followed by retroperitoneal node dissection and postoperative resumption of the irradiation has been proposed. This technique violates current concepts of dose-time relationships, risks both the destruction and alteration of useful diagnostic information and seems unlikely to reduce the postoperative complications, thus failing in its primary objective. There is accumulating evidence that survival rates following orchitectomy plus retroperitoneal node irradiation are at least comparable to any other treatment method.

The use of any local treatment method, whether it be surgery or irradiation, must be tempered by recognition of the relatively high incidence of hematogenous metastases in patients with embryonal carcinomas. Therefore, newly defined effective chemotherapeutic agents will become an important component of treatment.

Although choriocarcinoma is moderately radiosensitive, the aggressive biological behavior manifested by early and widespread hematogenous metastases makes any regional treatment regimen unrewarding. Unfortunately, in contrast to its use in choriocarcinoma in the female, chemotherapy is ineffective.

A most important part of any treatment program is thorough post-treatment examination at regular intervals (every two months for the first two years, gradually becoming less frequent) because further treatment, such as that to the mediastinum and supraclavicular fossae may be life-saving, particularly for patients with seminomas.

Complications of Radiation Therapy

Irradiation of the required large tissue volume may be accompanied by undesirable side effects. These are likely to be more frequent and more severe for patients with embryonal carcinoma and teratocarcinoma than for patients with seminoma because of use of higher radiation doses.

Nausea should be minimized by reduction of the daily dose increment rather than obscured by medication. Our patients continue to live "normally" active lives during this period.

Many will have a moderate intestinal reaction manifest by looseness and frequency of stools, controllable by reduction of the daily dose increment and minimal use of medication.

A few will have substantial peripheral blood changes, reflecting the effect of radiation of a large marrow volume. These changes have never required discontinuation of treatment of our patients.

Late-appearing, serious sequelae, particularly of the intestinal tract, no longer should occur, although they formerly were associated with the development of various treatment techniques.

The remaining testis receives small doses of radiation, primarily from scatter from the body trunk, even with use of special metal gonad protectors, supervoltage equipment, and careful treatment technique. With our techniques,[5] this gonadal dose amounts to about 1.0–1.5 percent of the incident dose. This small dose has had no measurable effect on urge or apparent capacity to reproduce.[5] However, the potential genetic influence is not known.

Results

The great improvement in prognosis, related to effective treatment of regional lymphatics and possible earlier diagnosis, can be documented by comparing collected cases in the literature in 1922[6] (4 percent, four-year survival rate) with current reports[3-5] (overall five-year "tumor-free" survival incidences of 50–75 percent). Survival can be related to tumor type and extent (Table 15–1). Cure has followed treatment of massive regional and even widespread (for instance, pulmonary) metastases in patients with seminoma, embryonal carcinoma, or teratocarcinoma. Therefore, the philosophy of treatment should be different from that for most other malignant neoplasms in adults. Patients dying of cancer of the testis rarely are clinically tumor-free after treatment and nearly always succumb within 30 months. Clinical freedom from tumor for 24 to 30 months after treatment, therefore, has a high correlation with "cure," even though a few patients may die with tumor several years after treatment.

Table 15-1. Five-Year "Tumor-Free" Survival Rates
For "Germinal" Tumors of the Testis

	(Collected Reports) All Cases	Cases Without Clinically Detected Metastases on Initial Examination (Our Series[4])
Seminoma	64–84%	90%
Embryonal carcinoma	15–50%	75%
Teratocarcinoma	40–80%	86%
Total	50–64%	87%

REVIEW QUESTIONS

1. What are the basic histological patterns of "germinal" tumors of the testis? What are the clinically important combinations?

2. What is the biological significance of seminoma associated with other tumor types? What is the biological significance of teratoma associated with other tumor types?

3. What are the two components of treatment of patients with malignant tumors primary in the testis? Which component of treatment has been correlated with recent improvement in prognosis?

4. What is the primary drainage pathway for tumors arising in the testicular parenchyma? How does this affect the accuracy of the standard (nontesticular) lymphogram? of the IVP (intravenous pyelogram)? How does this inaccuracy of diagnostic examination affect treatment planning?

5. What is the implication of inguinal adenopathy in patients with primary tumors of the testicular parenchyma?

6. In which testicular tumors are the risks of hematogenous metastasis greatest? How does this influence treatment planning?

7. What is the current optimal treatment for patients with seminoma? What are the results of such treatment? What is the influence of regional adenopathy on each?

8. What is the optimal treatment of patients with embryonal carcinoma or teratocarcinoma of the testis? What uncertainties make treatment of these patients controversial?

9. In patients with embryonal carcinoma or teratocarcinoma of the testis, what are the limitations of irradiation in treatment of the regional tumor-bearing lymph nodes? What are the limitations of retroperitoneal dissection? How does the use of both modalities in a single patient affect the chance of tumor control and treatment-produced morbidity?

10. What is the order of tumor-free survival for patients treated for seminoma? embryonal carcinoma? teratocarcinoma? At what post-treatment interval can control of tumor be measured effectively?

BIBLIOGRAPHY

1. DIXON, F. J., and MOORE, R. A. Tumors of male sex organs. In: *Atlas of Tumor Pathology*, Fascicles 31b and 32. United States Armed Forces Institute of Pathology, Washington, D.C., 1952.
2. FRIEDMAN, H. B., and MOORE, R. A. Tumor of testis: Report on 922 cases. *Milit Surg*, 99:573, 1946.
3. HOST, H., and STOKKE, T. Treatment of malignant testicular tumors at Norwegian Radium Hospital. *Cancer*, 12:323–329, 1959.
4. NOTTER, G., and RANUDD, N. E. Treatment of malignant testicular tumors: A report on 355 patients. *Acta Radiol* [Ther] (Stockholm), 2:273–301, 1964.
5. PARKER, R. G., and HOLYOKE, J. B. Tumors of the testis. *Amer J Roentgen*, 83:43, 1960.
6. TANNER, C. V. Tumors of the testicle with analysis of 100 original cases. *Surg Gynec Obstet*, 35:565–572, 1922.
7. TAVEL, F. R., OSIUS, T. G., PARKER, J. W., GOODFRIEND, R. B., MC GONIGLE, D., JASSIE, M. P., SIMONS, E. L., TOBENKIN, M. I., and SCHULTE, J. W. Retroperitoneal lymph node dissection. *J Urol*, 89:241–245, 1963.

CARCINOMA OF THE PROSTATE

Carcinoma of the prostate is a major cause of death (about 17,000 deaths in 1967 in the United States[3]) and morbidity in men. The incidence increases with advancing age until it is the most frequent cancer in men over 75 years.[3] This neoplasm has been found at autopsy in about 20 percent of men over 40 years.[7]

Although occasionally biologically indolent (38 of 544 untreated patients survived five years[12]), the more frequent clinical course is that of rapid tumor progression. In a series reported by Bumpus,[2] prior to the therapeutic use of estrogens and castration, the average survival from the onset of symptoms and signs was 31 months, more than one-half of the patients developing metastases within one year of the clinical onset, and two-thirds of these dying within 9 months. Those without evidence of metastases on initial examination had an average survival of 12 months after diagnosis.

Nearly all cancers of the prostate are well-differentiated adenocarcinomas originating in subcapsular sites of glandular atrophy.[10] Seventy-five percent of these neoplasms arise in the posterior lobe, 10 percent are found in the lateral lobes, and 15 percent in the anterior lobe.[10] Ten to 20 percent may be multicentric when discovered.[7]

The prostatic capsule is nearly always invaded (in 204 of 232 patients,[10] 177 of 191 patients[16]), but the adjacent rectum (in 12 of 800[23]) and bladder rarely are involved.[7] The abundant venous and nerve plexuses are frequently invaded, and the high incidence of metastases to bony pelvis, lower vertebrae, and proximal femora is attributed to the communication of the prostatic and vertebral venous plexuses. With current methods of diagnosis and treatment, about 50 percent of these patients will develop metastases within one year of the onset of symptoms, and at death in excess of 80 percent will suffer metastases[7] (lymph nodes, 75 percent[17]; bone, 75 percent[21]; or viscera, 40 percent[21]).

Chemical and Hormonal Relationships

Acid phosphatase is a product of normal adult prostatic epithelium or its malignant variant.[7] A majority of patients suffering from metastatic cancer of the prostate have serum acid phosphatase levels in excess of 10 King-Armstrong units, although 20 to 25 percent may remain within normal limits.[5] A persistent elevation above 10 King-Armstrong units is an absolute indication of metastatic carcinoma of the prostate.[13] This secretion of acid phosphatase by normal and malignant prostatic epithelium depends on androgen stimulation, being sharply depressed by castration or estrogen administration.

The serum alkaline phosphatase also is elevated in most patients with metastases from carcinoma of the prostate, usually in response to osteoblastic metastases. Although this elevation is not specific for prostatic cancer, the serum alkaline phosphatase may decline to normal levels following orchiectomy or estrogen therapy if the metastases respond, only to rise with reactivation of the metastases.

Treatment

Since the introduction of definitive surgical treatment (perineal prostatectomy by H. H. Young in 1904[22]), the most significant therapeutic advances have been nonsurgical even though introduced by surgeons (use of estrogen and castration[15]). Unfortunately, in most reports[4, 7, 8] only about 5 percent of all patients are candidates for radical prostatectomy (operability rates as high as 22 percent have been reported[4]) while 40 to 60 percent have detectable metastases at the time of diagnosis.[8] Thus, in excess of 40 percent of these patients have localized tumor, but usually have been treated only with palliative methods. Beneficial effects of local irradiation long have been recognized by a few (external irradiation[20] or interstitial irradiation[9]), but more widespread enthusiasm for vigorous radiation therapy with "curative" intent, made possible by supervoltage and megavoltage equipment, has been recent.[1, 6, 11] Such treatment, if effective, might have greater impact than radical prostatectomy because of its more widespread applicability.

Results of Treatment

Bagshaw, Kaplan, and Sagerman[1] reported the results of radiation therapy of 73 patients selected because the primary tumor was considered too large for radical prostatectomy (or the patient refused operation), but was still localized to the "prostate, its capsule, or the immediately adjacent periprostatic tissue," and had not detectably metastasized. Thirteen of 30 patients followed for more than five years after treatment were alive without clinical evidence of tumor, but 16 had died, usually with metastatic tumor. It was estimated that most tumor-bearing prostate glands became smaller during treatment, usually returning to normal size after several months, although some remained enlarged, but stable.

Complications of Treatment

Because of the advocated high radiation dose (6,000–7,500 rads in six to ten weeks) and the proximity of the rectum and bladder, treatment-produced complications are expected. More than 50 percent of Bagshaw's[1] patients had rectal or bladder complications, but usually they were transitory. Such vigorous local irradiation did not seem to alter sexual potency.

Palliative Radiation Therapy

A major clinical problem results from the frequent and widespread bony metastases. These lesions, ultimately affecting the majority of patients with carcinoma of the prostate, are characteristically "blastic" and involve the axial skeleton. Pain relief can result in 50–65 percent of these victims[18] from local irradiation with adequate dosage (3,500–5,000 rads in three to four weeks).

Therapeutic Use of Hormones

Adenocarcinoma of the prostate, like adenocarcinoma of the breast, is hormone dependent. Huggins[15] and others[14] pioneered therapeutic hormone manipulation three decades ago. This has consisted of castration, administration of estrogens (usually oral diethylstilbestrol), or both. Inasmuch as only about 5 percent of all patients with prostatic cancer are eligible for "curative" prostatectomy, nearly all patients have been subjected to hormonal tumor-suppressive or palliative treatment. Indeed, even those few patients surgically treated for cure have received estrogens or have been subjected to orchiectomy. Despite a large and prolonged experience with documentation of favorable subjective and objective responses, no single approach (i.e., use of estrogens and castration consecutively or simultaneously) has been generally accepted.[19] Such routine use for all patients has been questioned on the basis that any lowered incidence of tumor-related deaths has been outweighed by an increased incidence of deaths from intercurrent diseases, especially those of the cardiovascular system.[19] This necessity to weigh the risks of treatment against the expected benefits encourages the withholding of therapeutic hormone manipulation until tumor-related problems require relief.

Summary

The treatment of men with adenocarcinomas of the prostate usually has been tumor-suppressive or palliative because even minimal tumor extension from the primary site has contraindicated radical prostatectomy, long considered the only "curative" method. Routine therapeutic hormone manipulation for this large patient group has been questioned[19] because of the associated increased incidence of intercurrent diseases. Therefore, radiation therapy, which may be curative for that large group of patients with minimal local tumor extension but no metastases and palliative for many tumor-related problems, should be used much more frequently than it has been in the past.

REVIEW QUESTIONS

1. What is the correlation between patient age and carcinoma of the prostate? How may this affect management of the patient?

2. What is the most common site of origin for adenocarcinoma of the prostate? How should this affect diagnosis by physical examination?

3. What are the common routes of spread of adenocarcinoma of the prostate? How does this affect treatment and prognosis?

4. How reliable is an elevated serum acid phosphatase in the diagnosis of adenocarcinoma of the prostate? How often does a patient with adenocarcinoma of the prostate have a normal serum acid phosphatase?

5. In what fraction of patients with adenocarcinoma of the prostate is radical prostatectomy *not* applicable? How many of these patients have localized tumor? If radiation therapy could control one-third of this group (limited regional tumor extension without metastases), how would its impact compare with radical prostatectomy?

6. What is the palliative role of radiation therapy for patients with adenocarcinoma of the prostate?

BIBLIOGRAPHY

1. BAGSHAW, M. A., KAPLAN, H. S., and SAGERMAN, R. H. Linear accelerator supervoltage radio-therapy. VII Carcinoma of prostate. *Radiology*, 85:121–129, 1965.

2. BUMPUS, H. C., JR. Carcinoma of the prostate. A clinical study. *Surg Gynec Obstet*, 43: 150–155, 1926.

3. Cancer facts and figures (1968), American Cancer Society, New York, N.Y.

4. COLSTON, J. A. C. Radical perineal prostatectomy for early cancer. Follow-up study of 108 personal cases. *JAMA*, 169:700–703, 1959.

5. COOK, W. B., FISHMAN, W. H., and CLARKE, B. G. Serum acid phosphatase of prostatic origin in the diagnosis of prostatic cancer: Clinical evaluation of 2,408 tests by the Fishman-Lerner method. *J Urol*, 88:281–287, 1962.

6. DEL REGATO, J. A. Radiotherapy in the conservative treatment of operable and locally inoperable carcinoma of the prostate. *Radiology* 88:761–766, 1967.

7. DIXON, F. J., and MOORE, R. A. Tumors of the Male Sex Organs. *Atlas of Tumor Pathology*, Section VIII, Fascicles 31b and 32. Armed Forces Institute of Pathology, Washington, D.C., 1952.

8. FLOCKS, R. H., CULP, D. A., and ELKINS, H. B. Present status of radioactive gold therapy in management of prostatic cancer. *J Urol*, 81:178–184, 1959.

9. FLOCKS, R. H., KERR, H. D., ELKINS, H. B., and CULP, D. A. Treatment of carcinoma of the prostate by interstitial radiation with radioactive gold (Au198): A preliminary report. *J Urol*, 68:510–522, 1952.

10. GAYNOR, E. P. Zur frage des prostatakrebses. *Virchow Arch [Path Anna]*, 301:602–652, 1938.

11. GEORGE, F. W., CARLTON, C. E., JR., DYKHUZIN, R. F., and DILLON, J. R. Cobalt60 telecurie-therapy in the definitive treatment of carcinoma of the prostate: A preliminary report. *J Urol*, 93:102–105, 1965.

12. GRISWOLD, M. H. Cancer of the prostate in Connecticut. *Conn Med*, 10:106–109, 1946.

13. GUTMAN, A. B., GUTMAN, E. B., and ROBINSON, J. N. Determination of serum "acid" phosphatase activity in differentiating skeletal metastases secondary to prostatic carcinoma from Paget's disease of bone. *Amer J Cancer*, 38:103–108, 1940.

14. HERBST, W. P. Effects of estradiol dipropionate and diethylstilbestrol on malignant prostatic tissue. *Trans Amer Ass Genitourin Surg* 34:195–202, 1941.

15. HUGGINS, C., and HODGES, C. V. Studies on prostatic cancer, effect of castration, of estrogen and of androgen injections on serum phosphatase in metastatic carcinoma of the prostate. *Cancer Res*, 1:293–297, 1941.

16. KAHLER, J. E. Carcinoma of the prostate gland: A pathologic study. *J Urol*, 41:557–574, 1939.

17. MUIR, E. G. Carcinoma of the prostate. *Lancet*, 1:667–672, 1934.

18. PARKER, R. G. and HARRIS, A. Unpublished data.

19. Veteran's Administration Cooperative Urological Group. Carcinoma of the prostate: Treatment comparisons. *J Urol* 98:516–522, 1967.

20. WIDMAN, B. P. Cancer of the prostate. The results of radium and roentgen-ray treatment. *Radiology*, 22:153–159, 1934.

21. WILLIS, R. A. *Pathology of Tumours*. Butterworth, London, 1948.

22. YOUNG, H. H. The early diagnosis and radical cure of carcinoma of the prostate. *Johns Hopkins Med J*, 16:315–321, 1905.

23. YOUNG, H. H. The cure of cancer of the prostate by radical perineal prostatectomy (prostatoseminal vesiculectomy): History, literature and statistics of Young's operation. *J Urol*, 53:188–252, 1945.

16

TUMORS
OF THE URINARY SYSTEM

CANCER OF THE KIDNEY

Radiation therapy has a minor role in the treatment of adenocarcinoma (hypernephroma, Grawitz's tumor) of the kidney. Resection is necessary for control of the primary tumor and often is used for removal of metastatic lesions and for palliative control of hemorrhage or pain. Nevertheless, local irradiation may be the optimal treatment method for certain metastatic lesions and may prove useful as an adjuvant to surgery in treatment of the primary tumor.

Malignant tumors arising from the epithelial lining of the renal pelvis and calyces are rare and are best managed surgically. Those malignant tumors arising from the immature renal parenchyma (Wilms' or nephroblastoma) are a major radiotherapeutic problem and are discussed separately.

Renal adenocarcinomas (hypernephroma, Grawitz's tumor) originate from the tubular epithelium. The misleading term hypernephroma should be discarded. These tumors are more frequent in males between 40 and 60 years.[2] The prognosis worsens with increasing anaplasia of the tumor, invasion of the renal capsule, and extension into renal veins. Metastases usually are lymphatic to regional lymph nodes and hematogenous, particularly to lungs, liver, bones, and brain.

In potentially "curable" patients, radiation therapy has been an ill-defined adjuvant to surgery. Limitation of use has been real, based on the tumor biology, with frequent, widespread metastases; and has been imaginary, based on an unfounded concept that renal adenocarcinomas are "radioresistant." "The dogma of radioresistance of cancer of the kidney is unacceptable."[8] In our experience response of the individual tumor is unpredictable but some have responded very significantly.

Postoperative radiotherapy has been directed to regional lymphatic extension or direct extension of tumor into the renal bed. Renal vein invasion with its implication of hematogenous spread would seem an unrealistic indication for postoperative treatment.

There has been a recent, renewed interest in preoperative irradiation with potential advantages of lessening of tumor dissemination during nephrectomy; reduction of tumor size, with resultant easier operation; and conversion of tumors from inoperable to operable.[8]

316

Radiotherapy may be used as primary treatment of inoperable renal carcinoma with palliative objectives of pain relief and diminution of hematuria. In a few patients, response has been sufficient that tumors, initially considered inoperable because of perirenal extension, have become removable.[7]

Local irradiation of destructive, bony metastases can be very effective in relieving pain and stopping bony destruction, thus preserving functional skeletal integrity. These well-documented achievements often have been obscured by the myth of "radioresistance" of renal carcinoma.

Documentation of the contributions of radiotherapy to those patients with renal adenocarcinoma is difficult. Several reports indicating an advantage of combined surgery and radiotherapy recently have been collected[10] (Table 16–1).

For patients with renal carcinoma removal of the primary tumor, if technically possible, may still be indicated in the presence of hematogenous spread. Metastases may remain solitary or few for a long period during which time the primary tumor may cause distressing symptoms and become nonremovable. Surgical removal or radical irradiation of solitary metastases may also be indicated, and occasionally may provide symptom-free survival for many years. Thus, every patient must be managed on an individual basis.

REVIEW QUESTIONS

1. What limits the effectiveness of radiation therapy for patients with adenocarcinoma of the kidney? How do these limitations vary for patients potentially curable and for patients in whom palliation is the objective?

2. In what primary renal malignant tumor has radiation therapy a major role?

3. What are the potential objectives of radiation therapy for the patient with potentially curable renal adenocarcinoma? Are there any data to substantiate effectiveness in achieving these aims?

BIBLIOGRAPHY

1. BRATHERTON, D. G. Tumors of the kidneys and suprarenals: III. The place of radiotherapy in the treatment of hypernephroma, *Brit J Radiol*, 37:141–146, 1964.
2. CARTER, R. L. The pathology of renal cancer. Current concepts in cancer—No. 18. *JAMA*, 204:221–222, 1968.
3. CHARTERIS, A. A. Radiotherapy in the treatment of kidney tumors, *Brit J Urol*, 23:361–363, 1951.
4. FLOCKS, R. H., and KADESKY, M. C. Malignant neoplasms of the kidney: In analysis of 353 patients followed for three years or more. *Trans Amer Ass Genitourin Surg*, 49:105–110, 1957.
5. MURPHY, G. P. and MOSTFI, F. K. The significance of cytoplasmic granularity in the prognosis of renal cancer. *J Urol*, 94:48–54, 1965.
6. OCHSNER, M. G. Renal cell carcinoma: Five-year followup study of 70 cases. *J Urol*, 93: 361–363, 1965.

Table 16-1. Evidence of Better Survival in Hypernephroma with Combined Nephrectomy and Irradiation[10]

Source	Survival, Years	Nephrectomy, %	Nephrectomy and Irradiation, %	Preoperative	Postoperative	
Riches, Griffiths, and Thackray[9]	5	30	49		+	Based on 1,746 cases gathered from 67 centers
	10	17	27		+	
Charteris[3]	5	26	36		+	Series of 46 patients
Flocks and Kadesky[4]	5	46	55		+	In a series of 305 cases 10-yr. survival figures present strong evidence for preoperative irradiation (especially in those patients with capsular and venous invasion)
	5	46	57	+		
	10	23	33.3		+	
	10	23	50	+		
Bratherton[1]	5	29	43		+	Provides radiation technique and results in 64 cases
	10	26	33		+	
Ochsner[6]	5	9	39		+	Analysis of 70 cases
Murphy and Mostfi[5]	Mean	3.1 years	5.4 years		+	Clear cell carcinoma (57 cases); granular cell carcinoma (97 cases)
		2.1 years	2.3 years		+	

7. RICHES, E. W. *Tumors of the Kidney and Ureter. Monographs on Neoplastic Disease*, Vol. V. Williams & Wilkins, Baltimore, 1964.

8. RICHES, E. W. The place of irradiation. Current concepts in cancer—No. 18. *JAMA*, 204: 230–231, 1968.

9. RICHES, E. W., GRIFFITHS, I. H., and THACKRAY, A. C. New growths of the kidney and ureter, *Brit J Urol*, 23:297–356, 1951.

10. RUBIN, P. Cancer of the urogenital tract: Kidney. Current concepts in cancer—No. 18. *JAMA*, 204:232–233, 1968.

CARCINOMA OF THE BLADDER

Carcinomas of the bladder have a great variety of anatomical patterns and a broad spectrum of biological behavior. Therefore, none of the many available surgical or radiological therapeutic modalities can be expected to be "the best" method of treatment for all situations. Selection of the most suitable treatment for the individual patient must be based on a thorough understanding of both the pathological processes and the therapeutic techniques.

Clinicopathological Considerations

Selection of the most suitable surgical or radiotherapeutic procedure is determined by the type and extent of tumor, the antomical and functional condition of the bladder, and the general condition of the patient. The necessary information about the tumor and the condition of the bladder is gained through examination of the urine, intravenous pyelography and cystography, cystoscopy, cystoscopic biopsy, and bimanual palpation of the pelvis with the patient anesthetized. The radiation therapist must join the urologist in this necessary, thorough evaluation.

Type and Extent of Tumor

The indications for radiation therapy and the choice of the most suitable radiological technique are based on the correlation of the microscopic details (histological differentiation and infiltration) with the gross pattern (papillary or solid) and the extent of invasion of tumor into the bladder wall or beyond as determined by cystoscopic examination and bimanual examination of the pelvis of the anesthetized patient.

There is a close correlation between the gross and histological patterns of cancers of the bladder and their biological behavior, as manifested by their clinical malignancy, their radiation responsiveness, and ultimately the prognosis.[27, 28]

Since the renal pelves, ureters, bladder, and part of the urethra are lined by a continuous layer of "transitional" epithelium, it is not surprising that 80 to 90 percent of the urothelial cancers of the bladder can be designated as "transitional cell" carcinomas. This diagnosis frequently submitted by the pathologist, is of little

prognostic or therapeutic meaning without correlation with: the degree of microscopic differentiation; the gross pattern of tumor; and the extent of invasion of the
bladder wall by tumor. In estimating the probable biological behavior of the tumor
as part of the evaluation for radiation therapy, it is useful to recognize the following varieties of epithelial neoplasms of the bladder: transitional cell carcinoma;
squamous cell carcinoma; and adenocarcinoma (Table 16–2).

Transitional cell carcinomas of the bladder have two characteristics which
have an important bearing on their management: (1) their frequent multiplicity,
and (2) their tendency to be papillary.

At least one-half of the epithelial tumors of the bladder are multiple, either
at the time of original investigation or following the treatment of an apparently
solitary lesion. In Melicow's series[24] of 2,500 initially "solitary" bladder tumors,
almost 70 percent of the patients returned with tumor, often in sites other than
that of the first recognized tumor. Controversy persists whether this multiplicity is
due to (1) multicentricity of origin resulting from stimulation by carcinogens;[2, 25]
(2) implantation metastases from seeding of tumor onto intact mucosa; or (3)
spread through the submucosal lymphatics from an originally unifocal carcinoma.
Any of these mechanisms might be operative. It is impossible to decide whether
tumors appearing locally after removal of a solitary growth (often called satellite
tumors) are new multiple tumors or clinical recurrences. Understanding of the
mechanisms responsible for this multiplicity may lead to a more rational therapeutic
approach.

Another important characteristic, influencing management, is the tendency of
many tumors to be papillary and extend into the lumen of the bladder. Corresponding to the experience with papillary, exophytic carcinomas originating from
other mucous membranes, these tumors are favorable objects for radiation therapy
if they are treated prior to deep invasion of the muscle of the bladder wall.

Table 16-2.   Types of Bladder Carcinoma in 2,500 Specimens[24]

Urothelial Tumors	
Papillary transitional cell carcinoma (histological grades I, II, III)	81.1%
Nonpapillary transitional cell carcinoma (usually grade IV)	7%
Metaplastic (usually squamous cell) carcinoma	11.4%
Adenocarcinoma	0.5%

Papillary Tumors (transitional cell)		
Papilloma	12.4%	} 37.6%
Grade I	25.2%	
Grade II	24.7%	} 44.9%
Grade III	20.2%	
Grade IV	17.5%	

Melicow, 1955

Table 16-3. Correlation of Histological Differentiation
and Gross Pattern (Solid or Papillary)
with Infiltration Rate and Prognosis (Wallace[32])
in Carcinoma of the Bladder

Gross and Histological type	Incidence of Infiltration (%)	5-Year Survival Rate (%)	Type (See Table 16–4)	Radio-vulnerability
Papilloma	0	72	I	+
Papillary differentiated carcinoma	19	52	(Grade I)	+
Papillary anaplastic carcinoma	62	21	II (Gr. II and III)	+ +
Solid differentiated carcinoma	82	18	III (Grade IV)	+
Solid anaplastic carcinoma	90	16		+ +

Column 4 is added for comparison with the corresponding histological grades as used in Table 16–4.
Column 5 is added to indicate the approximate degree of radiovulnerability.

In bladder carcinomas, there is a correlation between the epithelial differentiation and the papillary (intraluminal and exophytic) pattern of growth. With decreasing histological differentiation the incidence of solid tumors and invasion into the bladder wall increases. Correspondingly, the likelihood of control by any method of treatment, including radiotherapy, decreases. The correlation between histological differentiation, tendency toward solid or papillary growth, incidence of infiltration, and prognosis may be seen from Wallace's evaluation in Table 16–3. In the last column, the relative radiovulnerability of these tumors is estimated.

The importance of extent of tumor in planning and evaluating treatment has resulted in attempts to formulate meaningful staging systems (Jewett and Strong,[16] the International Union Against Cancer [UICC],[21] and the American Joint Committee[8]). These have been based on examinations of the patient and biopsies (clinical) and on examinations of the surgical specimen (surgical). In general, attempted distinctions include: infiltration of the submucosal connective tissue; invasion of the superficial muscle; invasion of the deep muscle; permeation of lymphatic or blood vessels; tumor fixation to or invasion of adjacent structures; regional and distant metastases. The accuracy of clinical staging based on physical examination and resection biopsy has been estimated from 40 to 80 percent.[1] The errors are due to underestimation of the tumor extent (understaging). The degree of understaging increases with increasing tumor extent, particularly with increasing depth of infiltration.[1] This inherent difficulty in clinical assessment should encourage more frequent thorough treatment. For the radiotherapist, this means irradiation of the whole bladder and immediately adjacent normal tissues, possible only with external high energy sources. This frequent underestimation of tumor extent unfavorably influences the reported results of radiation therapy, which must follow clinical assessment. Thus, comparison to surgical series based on study of the removed bladder and regional nodes is not valid.

Condition of the Bladder and General Condition
of the Patient

In addition to an analysis of the tumor, it is necessary to appraise the anatomical and functional condition of the bladder in order to answer two questions: (1) Is there any malignant or premalignant mucosal change beyond the demonstrable tumor? and (2) will the bladder tolerate radical radiation therapy?

Microscopic foci of neoplasm, metaplasia, and carcinoma-in-situ may be found in the mucosa near the gross tumor and also elsewhere in the bladder.[22-24] The demonstration of such changes requires that treatment include the entire bladder. Therefore, thorough inspection of the grossly uninvolved mucosa and biopsy of suspicious areas are necessary, and biopsies of grossly normal bladder mucosa occasionally may be indicated.

It is important to determine the presence of urinary tract infection and urethral obstruction (by tumor, prostatic hypertrophy, or urethral stricture), for these may lower the bladder's tolerance to radiation.

Radical radiation therapy of bladder carcinoma, regardless of technique, is a major procedure which may be associated with considerable unavoidable morbidity. Therefore, an evaluation of the patient's general condition and an estimate of his tolerance of treatment are necessary. In debilitated patients, a severe radiation reaction may cause frequency and dysuria, thus further weakening the patient.

Therapy

Surgery

Surgical procedures for the treatment of carcinoma of the bladder are:

1. *Endoscopic transurethral resection* or cystodiathermy for single or multiple papillomas and papillary carcinomas which have not deeply invaded the bladder wall.

2. *Partial cystectomy* (segmental resection) for solitary malignant tumors which are localized to the superior portion of the bladder where they do not encroach on the uretheral orifices and have a well-defined margin, and thus can be excised with an adequate margin of normal-appearing mucosa.

3. *Total cystectomy* with diversion of the urinary stream by ureterostomy, implantation of the ureters into the sigmoid colon (ureterosigmoidostomy) or into an "artificial" bladder, formed from isolated bowel that acts as a sterile reservoir (Bricker procedure). Surgery may be extended to an operation with an intent to "clear the pelvis" of all its contents except the rectum (radical cystoprostatectomy or exenteration).

As previously stated about one-half of the epithelial tumors of the bladder are multiple—either in space (growing simultaneously over different parts of the mucosa) or in time (originating successively as new lesions in untreated portions of the mucosa). The majority of vesicular tumors (about 80 percent) arise at the base of the bladder (trigone or lower lateral walls) where they may involve one or both ureters and/or the bladder neck. Therefore, in most instances, curative surgery requires total cystectomy. Many experienced urological surgeons avoid this radical procedure whenever possible because, apart from the functional impairment, the associated complications of ascending urinary tract infection and electrolyte imbalance may outweight the "curative" effect of total cystectomy, so that more conservatively treated patients may live longer and more comfortably. Sir Eric Riches (Middlesex Hospital) concluded: "We try and choose a simple method rather than an elaborate one if it is likely to be effective, to leave the patient with a satisfactory functioning bladder if possible and preferably with the same number of body orifices as he had when he started life.[29]

The extensive experience at the Royal Marsden Hospital (London)[31] has led to the policy: ". . . to try the most suitable form of radiotherapy, radiotherapy with surgery, or conservative surgery alone as the first step of a planned treatment, reserving radical cystectomy for the second stage should the treatment fail or the response be incomplete." There are two exceptions: (1) if at the time of surgery, preparatory to implantation of the radiation source, the tumor is found to be larger than expected, so that it has infiltrated the perivesical fat; or (2) in the presence of large bulky tumors filling the bladder, in order to avoid opening the bladder with the almost unavoidable risk of implantation of tumor cells in the scar, radical surgery is the primary treatment.

Radiation Therapy

1. *Basis:* The radiocurability of a carcinoma of the bladder is determined by the radiovulnerability of tumor in relation to the radiation tolerance of the normal bladder mucosa, the bladder wall and other pelvic structures. In general, deep infiltration of the bladder wall musculature demarcates curability of transitional cell carcinomas of moderate (Grade II and Grade III) and high degree (Grade I) of differentiation by external or intracavitary irradiation. Interstitial therapy may be effective and tolerable for infiltrating tumors of limited extent. This is consistent with experience in the treatment of other epithelial neoplasms (e.g., larynx). The advantage of the greater radiovulnerability of the less differentiated bladder tumors (column 5, Table 16–3) is outweighed by their greater frequency of deep extension into the bladder wall (column 2, Table 16–3), hence their poor prognosis (column 3, Table 16–3). Some undifferentiated tumors (Grade IV) are sufficiently radiovulnerable that they can be controlled even with massive invasion of muscle and spread to regional lymph nodes.

2. *Indications:* Based on these guiding principles, specific indications for radiation therapy of the different types of carcinoma of the bladder can be summarized (Table 16–4):

Papillomas and/or papillary carcinomas, Grade I are considered as one entity. This group represents about 30 to 40 percent of carcinomas of the bladder.[24] Some investigators do not recognize a sharp demarcation between benign and malignant bladder tumors, or they may consider every epithelial neoplasm in the bladder as potentially malignant. Tumors of this type are characterized by their low degree of radiovulnerability and their limitation to the mucosa. By definition, benign papillomas are limited to the mucosa. Eighty percent of tumors designated as papillary carcinoma Grade I do not invade bladder muscle. Both cystoscopically and microscopically these tumors exhibit an orderly structure. These lesions are not frequently controlled by external irradiation because the necessary very high

Table 16-4.   Radiation Therapy of Carcinoma of the Bladder. Choice of Techniques.

Type	Histology	Superficial	Infiltrating	Extravesicular
			Group	
I	Papilloma (Papillary carcinoma, Gr. I)	Intracavitary	—	—
II	Papillary carcinoma (Grades II and III)	—	External	External
III	Solid undifferentiated carcinoma (Grade IV)	—	External	External
IV	Epidermoid carcinoma	—	Interstitial	

dose is poorly tolerated by the bladder wall and other pelvic structures. However, these tumors may be suited for intracavitary irradiation, which provides a very high dose to the entire mucosal surface with a rapid fall-off of dose with increasing depth in tissue (to 50 percent of surface dose, or less, in 5 mm, depending on the radioactive source and the technique used). If lesions of this type are solitary or few in number, or if recurrences are separated by long remissions, transurethral resection of lesions as they are recognized at repeat cystoscopy may keep patients asymptomatic for many years or decades. If the lesions recur rapidly or are widespread over the bladder mucosa, intracavitary irradiation can be offered as an alternative to total cystectomy. In some of these patients new lesions assume a more malignant character. In the large Birmingham group, 9 percent of single papillomas and 26 percent of multiple papillomas underwent malignant change.[26] This documents the necessity for careful microscopic study of recurrent lesions so that treatment can be instituted prior to deep invasion of the bladder wall.

Lesions of this type, suitable for intracavitary irradiation, represent about 10 percent of all cancers of the bladder. Because of selection by referral of patients with more advanced lesions to medical centers this incidence is probably lower in larger centers than in private urological practice.

Papillary carcinomas, Grades II and III, comprise 40 to 50 percent of bladder carcinomas (Table 16–2).[24] This type of tumor can be recognized cystoscopically as "less orderly," may be attached with a thin pedicle, and may have some irregular, "floating" necrotic tissue. These lesions may be solitary or multiple, either as one larger lesion surrounded by smaller satellites, or as several apparently unrelated lesions in different portions of the bladder, or as multiple tumors developing as clinical recurrences following treatment of an apparently unifocal primary tumor. Microscopically this type of tumor has a much less orderly epithelium, with numerous abnormal cells and cells undergoing mitosis. These tumors start as papillary mucosal lesions which exhibit a spectrum of epithelial differentiation. In the moderately differentiated tumors, the central stalk of the papilla and the papillary structure itself are well preserved, whereas with lessening differentiation the papillary structure becomes less recognizable. Additional lesions may be less differentiated. Correlated to an increasing degree of anaplasia, the papillary structures become less distinct, and the lesions become more solid and invasive, and correspondingly more malignant.

Papillary carcinomas (Grade II–III) often are sufficiently radioresponsive to be controlled by external irradiation prior to extensive tumor invasion of the bladder wall. With the more differentiated lesions, substantial invasion of the bladder wall probably demarcates curability by external irradiation. Some of the less differentiated lesions have biological characteristics similar to anaplastic solid tumors (to be described as Type III below) and may be controlled by external irradiation in the presence of moderate invasion of the bladder muscle.

Solitary lesions of this type, in an otherwise normal bladder, may be best treated by local procedures, preferably transurethral resection deep enough to leave a clear base with the musculature of the bladder wall exposed. Infiltrating tumors in the fundus or high on the lateral or posterior walls can be removed by partial cystectomy if a sufficient margin can be obtained without encroaching on the trigone or ureter. Tumors of moderate size (diameter of base not more than 3 to 4 cm), which are not suitable for partial cystectomy because of location, have been successfully treated by interstitial implantation of radioactive materials. However, such interstitial irradiation with its necessary high dose, even though affecting only a segment of the bladder, may compromise radical external irradiation if it becomes necessary later.

If, following local therapy, new lesions become demonstrable, particularly if their location in other portions of the bladder and long intervals between appearances suggest the possibility of newly formed tumors rather than recurrences, repeated transurethral resections may be successful for a considerable time. It is important, however, to recognize when such local therapy should be discontinued and the entire bladder should be treated by total cystectomy or radical external radiation therapy. In this situation, many experienced urologists recommend initial radiation therapy, reserving total cystectomy for radiation therapy failures. It is essential that radiation therapy be instituted before deep invasion of the bladder wall occurs and that it not be restricted, as it too frequently is, to far advanced disease, when it is of little value. It has become our policy during recent years, at the suggestion of the urologists, that patients with "solitary" papillary carcinomas initially be treated by thorough transurethral fulguration and then followed by frequent cystoscopic examination, so that at the first evidence of tumor locally or elsewhere in the bladder, radical external radiation therapy can be started. If there are multiple lesions at the time of initial examination, external irradiation immediately follows biopsy. Since this change in policy, the three-year tumor control has doubled.[6, 15]

Undifferentiated or anaplastic transitional cell carcinomas (Grade IV) usually are solid, solitary lesions which involve a large portion of the bladder and which, by the time of recognition, have almost always extensively invaded the bladder muscle and extended beyond the bladder wall. At times, the impression at cystoscopy may be that the tumor is extravesicle with secondary involvement of the bladder because a large pelvic mass is fixed to the bladder wall and the mucosa is only minimally ulcerated. Even with such extensive tumor, the clinical history may be short, implying rapid tumor growth. About 7 percent of bladder cancers are in this group (Table 16–2).[24]

Because of its biological character, this type of carcinoma usually is not suitable for total cystectomy, even if the operation is technically possible. The high radioresponsiveness may result in permanent control of far-advanced bladder cancer of this type in a small percentage of patients.

Epidermoid carcinoma (not to be confused with epidermoid carcinoma that may develop in areas of squamous cell metaplasia in undifferentiated transitional cell carcinoma) is rare, grows slowly, and metastasizes late. It is insufficiently radioresponsive to be treated successfully by external irradiation while usually being too invasive by the time of diagnosis for effective intracavitary treatment. If located in a site where segmental resection is not possible, an epidermoid carcinoma of limited size (not larger than 4 cm in diameter) occasionally can be treated successfully by interstitial irradiation.

The rare *adencarcinoma* may arise either from the mucus-secreting glands at the base of the bladder or in the dome from remnants of the urachus. The latter type may be amenable to segmental resection; the former offers problems similar to epidermoid carcinoma.

3. *Radiotherapeutic Modalities*
  I. Intracavitary irradiation
      a. Central radioactive solid sources (i.e., radium-226 or cobalt-60) are maintained in the center of the bladder by a Foley-type catheter introduced transurethrally (or rarely through a perineal incision).
      b. The radioactive solution (cobalt-60, sodium-24, bromine-82) may be contained in the bag of a Foley-type catheter.
      c. The radioactive solution (colloidal gold-198, cobalt-60, yttrium-90) occasionally may be instilled directly into the bladder.
  II. Interstitial irradiation by means of radon seeds, radioactive gold seeds, removable radium needles, or removable radioactive tantallum wire.
  III. External irradiation by supervoltage or megavoltage x-ray or cobalt-60.

Intracavitary irradiation delivers a high dose to the entire bladder mucosa, but because of a rapid "fall-off" delivers only a small dose to the bladder wall and surrounding structures. Therefore, it is useful for the treatment of superficial mucosal lesions which do not infiltrate into muscle, but which involve a large surface and are not controllable by other procedures except total cystectomy.[11-14,20,32]

Interstitial implantation of removable radium needles[19] or tantallum wire[20] has been used successfully for the treatment of solitary, moderately differentiated tumors in an otherwise normal bladder. These tumors should involve only small portions of the bladder wall (base of tumor not larger than 4 cm diameter), may have infiltrated into muscle but not into perivesicular fat (as determined at operation), should not be more than 1 cm thick. In some institutions radon seeds or radioactive gold seeds have been implanted.[26] All of these implantations should be done with good exposure through a suprapubic cystostomy. Transurethral insertion, formerly done frequently, has been abandoned in situations in which more than temporary effects are hoped for.

External irradiation, using super- or megavoltage x-rays or cobalt-60, has assumed an increasingly important place in the treatment of patients with bladder carcinoma when radical treatment of larger tissue volumes is necessary, when the location or multiplicity of the lesions contraindicates partial resection or implantation, or when the volume of tumor contraindicates the use of an intracavitary source. Orthovoltage x-ray has no place in the treatment of patients with cancer of the bladder because adequate doses cannot be delivered without resultant serious problems of normal tissue intolerance.

External irradiation is indicated in the treatment of papillary carcinomas of a moderate degree of differentiation (Grades II and III), because a substantial proportion can be controlled with avoidance of cystectomy, and in the treatment of anaplastic carcinomas (Grade IV) which occasionally can be controlled even with extravesical extension, which would make radical surgery inappropriate.[3-6,15,20,26]

4. *Morbidity and Side Effects of Radiation Therapy:* A certain degree of radiation reaction of the bladder must be expected even with properly conducted therapy. Since repeated cystoscopies during treatment are not advisable, the reaction must be estimated from the symptoms of increased frequency and dysuria.

When external irradiation is used, these symptoms usually occur late in the treatment course. In patients with minimally infiltrating carcinomas, not complicated by infection or obstruction, the reaction may not become evident until about the end of the fifth to seventh week with a bladder dose of about 5,000 rads. The intensity of the reaction and the time of its appearance depend not only on the dose but on the rapidity of treatment, the size of the individual fraction, the location and extent of the tumor, the degree of infection, the adequacy of urethral drainage and the condition of the bladder. In the presence of infection or partial urethral obstruction, the reaction may become so severe that the patient's general condition may deteriorate because the urinary frequency and pain interfere with sleep. Such urethral obstruction must be corrected by transurethral resection of the obstructing prostate or a portion of the tumor prior to radiotherapy. Infection should be treated pharmacologically.

Treatment of tumors involving the trigone may be poorly tolerated and particularly severe reactions can be expected when the tumor involves the bladder neck and the vesicourethral junction.

With adequate protraction of treatment and absence of these complicating factors, treatment may be tolerated without symptoms of bladder reaction. However, there is an unpredictable variation of individual sensitivity and tolerance so that an incapacitating degree of reaction occasionally follows well-directed therapy that would be tolerated by most patients. In such instances a severe reaction does not necessarily indicate the likelihood of severe late tissue changes, as complete restitution of normal bladder function has been observed if the tumor is controlled.[6,15]

In patients who have been treated successfully by technically correct external irradiation, re-examination many years later may demonstrate normal bladder capacity and function, and the bladder mucosa may not have any recognizable late signs of irradiation, or there may be mild telangiectasia and scarring at the site of the lesion. Severe fibrosis of bladder and rectum has occurred in patients who were treated with excessive doses or too rapidly. With technically correct and biologically correlated external irradiation, we have not observed significant fibrosis of the bladder during the past 25 years.[6,15] The patients, many living into their eighth decade, have had bladder function considered within normal limits.*

---

* Some of these patients had a bladder function better than expected at their age because of the incidental favorable effect on the benign enlargement of the prostate.

Table 16-5. Carcinoma of the Bladder. Results.

Type of Tumor	Institution	Therapy	No. Patients	Alive 5 Years	% 5-year Survival
Papilloma and papillomatosis	Birmingham[26] 1936–1950		629	461	73
Carcinoma	Birmingham[26] 1946–1950	External irradiation	121	18	15
Carcinoma	Swedish Hosp.[6] 1934–1950	External irradiation	85	14*	16*
Carcinoma	U. Calif.[6 15] 1957–1962	External irradiation	29	8(4*)	28(14*)
Carcinoma	Presbyterian Hospital, New York[19] 1931–1941	Interstitial irradiation (needles)	44	9	20*
Carcinoma	Kligerman†[17]	Interstitial irradiation (needles)	63	24	38
Carcinoma	Walter Reed Hospital[12]	Intracavitary	34	19	56
"Gross infiltrating" carcinoma	Manchester[26] 1946–1949	External irradiation	66	17	25
Superficial and moderately infiltrating carcinoma‡	Manchester[26] 1946–1949	Interstitial# irradiation (seeds)	104	51	49

*5-year symptom-free (clinically and cystoscopically).
†Selected types, suitable for segmental resection.
‡Moderately infiltrating, confined to bladder wall.
Of 55 patients with "grossly noninfiltrating" tumors treated by interstitial therapy, 60% were living after 5 years; of 39 with gross infiltration, 15% were alive after interstitial irradiation.[7]

With intracavitary therapy, the usually transient radiation mucositis occurs about one month after treatment. Limits of bladder tolerance to intracavitary therapy are now well-recognized and, if respected, the more severe reactions usually can be avoided. In the early days of experimentation with this technique, excessive doses delivered too rapidly produced severe reactions which were followed by massive fibrotic changes of the bladder wall (contracted bladder). Occasionally, cystectomy was necessary to relieve the intolerable symptoms associated with severe radiation produced changes. These results have been misinterpreted as unavoidable effects of any form of radiation therapy for carcinoma of the bladder. Unfortunately, doses within limits of bladder tolerance frequently are inadequate to control the highly differentiated papillomas and papillary carcinomas (Grade I), and thus the technique is of limited value.

5. *Palliative Radiation Therapy:* Definite indications for palliative radiation therapy are based on three main considerations: (1) the need for relief of specific symptoms and signs; (2) the magnitude of the treatment in proportion to the expected result; and (3) the patient's life expectancy. By these criteria radiation therapy for palliation of the patient with incurable carcinoma of the bladder is much less frequently indicated than some urologists and radiologists believe. In order to obtain a satisfactory and reasonably sustained effect, doses approaching those used for curative therapy are required. In a debilitated patient and in the presence of infection and obstruction, such doses frequently aggravate rather than palliate by increasing urinary frequency and dysuria. With lesions likely to be responsive in a patient in reasonably good general condition, treatment may be carried to moderate doses, with continuation dependent on observed tolerance. A main palliative objective is cessation of tumor-incited gross hematuria. Pain due to involvement of pelvic nerves is rarely relieved. Dysuria and frequency, if due to tumor involvement of the bladder neck or reduced bladder capacity, may be aggravated by radiation therapy.

6. *Results:* Results of radiation treatment, as presented in Table 16–5, need qualification:

Reported results of treatment of patients with carcinoma of the bladder frequently are listed as "survival rates" rather than as "cure rates." The term *cure rate* should be reserved for patients surviving more than five years *without clinical or cystoscopic evidence of tumor at any time during the interval since treatment.* Low-grade, minimally infiltrating carcinomas reappearing after radiation therapy may be controlled for many years by repeated transurethral resections. Therefore, the five-year survival of this group is of no significance in judging the efficacy of radiotherapy, for it has failed. In our experience[6,15] with patients treated between 1957–1962, the five-year survival was 28 percent, and the "cure rate" was 14 percent (Table 16–5).

The histological type of carcinoma so influences the prognosis (Table 16–3) that results of treatment which include all types of bladder cancer can be misleading (summarized in Table 16–5). For example, in the large Birmingham group, the five-year survival of patients with papilloma and papillomatosis was 73 percent, whereas the survival of patients with carcinoma was only 15 percent.

The results of treatment are related to extent of tumor. However, the inaccuracies of clinical assessment negate any close correlation with radiation therapy. Examples of gross correlations are listed in Table 16–6.

**Table 16-6.   Relationship of Results of Radiation Therapy
and Tumor Extent**
(5-year Survival)

	Tumor Extent	
Authors	Involvement no Deeper than Superficial Muscle of Bladder Wall	Involvement of Deep Muscle of Bladder Wall or Perivesicle Fat
Caldwell, Bagshaw & Kaplan[7] 73 patients	50%	20%
Jack & Buschke[15] 56 patients	44%	14%
Ellis[10] 152 patients	36%	7%
Kurohara, Rubin & Silon[18] 61 patients	33%	13%
Crigler & Miller[9] 126 patients	32%	28%

Treatment of cancer of the bladder is still being investigated clinically. Some of the techniques are new so that their indications, limitations, and potential are not fully recognized, and their execution is not always optimal. These data, therefore, are not always based on long experience with well-established procedures which can be considered as standard accomplishments, as is possible with cancers of the cervix and larynx. Better understanding of tumor biology and physical details of treatment should result in better selection of patients and better treatment application, with consequent improvement in results.[6,15] In our own recent experience, the three-year control rate has doubled with better selection of patients (36 percent as compared with 16 percent).[15]

REVIEW QUESTIONS

1. What factors must be considered in selecting treatment for patients with carcinoma of the bladder?

2. What is the most frequent histological type of carcinoma of the bladder? What additional histological assessments are necessary for evaluation for treatment?

3. What gross characteristics of transitional cell carcinoma arising from the bladder epithelium are important in planning patient management?

4. How often does transitional cell carcinoma involve multiple sites of the bladder epithelium? What is the basis of this multiplicity? How does this characteristic influence treatment?

5. What is the clinical correlation between papillary form, histological differentiation, and invasion of the bladder wall musculature? How does this correlation relate to prognosis? Why?

6. Why is appraisal of the bladder important in evaluating a patient for radiation therapy? How would pretreatment determination of contraction of the bladder influence use of radiotherapy? What if the bladder is infected? What is the implication of widespread mucosal abnormality? of urethral obstruction?

7. In the treatment of the patient with carcinoma of the bladder, what are the limitations of transurethral fulgration? of partial cystectomy? of total cystectomy?

8. What site is most frequently involved by carcinoma of the bladder? How does this affect treatment?

9. What finding is the best indicator of the possibility of local radiotherapeutic control of carcinoma of the bladder? How does this correlate with carcinoma of the larynx? esophagus? oral tongue?

10. What radiotherapeutic modalities are available for patients with carcinoma of the bladder? What are the advantages and limitations for each modality? What is the optimal application of each?

11. What is the radiation treatment-related morbidity of patients with bladder cancer? How can this be assessed? Can this morbidity be related to tumor extent? condition of the bladder? treatment technique? Is there any treatment related mortality?

12. Can a normally functioning bladder be retained after proper irradiation of selected patients with carcinoma of the bladder? If so, how often?

13. What are the objectives of palliative radiation therapy of patients with bladder carcinoma?

14. What order of tumor control is possible for patients with carcinoma of the bladder? (Relate to tumor extent and tumor type.)

15. What are the potential advantages of combined radiation therapy and surgery? the disadvantages?

BIBLIOGRAPHY

1. BAKER, R. The accuracy of clinical vs surgical staging. Current Concepts in Cancer-22, *JAMA* 206:1770–1773, 1968.
2. BOYLAND, E. Biochemistry of bladder cancer. *Brit Med Bull*, 14:153–158, 1958.
3. BUSCHKE, F., and CANTRIL, S. T. Roentgentherapy of carcinoma of urinary bladder. An analysis of 52 patients treated with 800 kv roentgentherapy. *J Urol*, 48:368–383, 1942.
4. BUSCHKE, F., and CANTRIL, S. T. Indications for roentgen therapy of bladder carcinomas. Recognition of suitable cases. *Surg Gynec Obstet*, 82:29, 1946.
5. BUSCHKE, F., CANTRIL, S. T., and PARKER, H. Carcinoma of the bladder. Chapter VII in: *Supervoltage Roentgentherapy*, Charles C Thomas, Springfield, Ill., 1950.
6. BUSCHKE, F., and JACK, G. A. Twenty-five years' experience with supervoltage therapy in treatment of transitional cell carcinoma of the bladder. *Amer J Roentgen*, 99:387–392, 1967.
7. CALDWELL, W. L., BAGSHAW, M., and KAPLAN, H. S. Efficacy of linear accelerator X-ray therapy in cancer of the bladder. *J Urol* 97:294–303, 1967.
8. Clinical staging system for carcinoma of the urinary bladder, American Joint Committee on Cancer Staging and End Results Reporting, Feb. 1967.

9. CRIGLER, C. M., and MILLER, L. Radiotherapy for carcinoma of the bladder. *J. Urol.* 96:58–61, 1966.

10. ELLIS, F. Bladder neoplasms—the challenge to the radiotherapist. *Clin Radiol* 14:1–16, 1963.

11. FRIEDMAN, M., and LEWIS, L. G. Irradiation of carcinoma of the bladder by a central intra-cavitary radium or cobalt60 source (The Walter Reed Technique). *Amer J Roentgen,* 79:6–31, 1958.

12. FRIEDMAN, M., and LEWIS, L. G. A new technique for the radium treatment of carcinoma of the bladder. *Radiology,* 53:342–363, 1949.

13. HARRIS, W. Discussion. In: Friedman and Lewis, Reference 12, p. 361.

14. HINMAN, F., JR., SCHULTE, J. W., and LOW-BEER, B. V. A. Further experience with intracavi-tary radiocobalt for bladder tumors. *J Urol,* 73:285–291, 1955.

15. JACK, G. A. Improved results of irradiation for carcinoma of the bladder. *J Urol,* 102:330–332, 1969.

16. JEWETT, H. J., and STRONG, G. H. Infiltrating carcinoma of the bladder. Relation of depth of penetration of the bladder wall to incidence of local extension and metastases. *J Urol* 55:366–372, 1946.

17. KLIGERMAN, M. M., ROBINSON, J. N., FISH, G. W., and DAVID, I. Segmental resection and radium implantation in treatment of carcinoma of urinary bladder. *J Urol,* 68:706–713, 1952.

18. KUROHARA, S. S., RUBIN, P., and SILON, N. Analysis in depth of bladder cancer treated by supervoltage therapy. *Amer J Roentgenol* 95:458–467, 1965.

19. LENZ, M. The treatment of cancer of the bladder by radium needles. *Amer J Roentgen,* 58:486–492, 1947.

20. MACKAY, N. R., SMITHERS, D. W., and WALLACE, D. M. Radiotherapy of bladder tumours. Chapter 18 in: *Tumours of the Bladder.* D. W. Smithers, Ed, Livingstone, Edinburgh, 1959.

21. Malignant tumours of the urinary bladder: Clinical stage classification and presentation of results, Subcommittee on Clinical Stage Classification and Applied Statistics, Geneva: Union Internationale Contre le Cancrum, 1967.

22. MELAMED, M. R., KOSS, L. G., RICCI, A., and WHITMORE, W. F. Cytohistological observations on developing carcinoma of the urinary bladder in man. *Cancer,* 13:67–74, 1960.

23. MELICOW, M. M. Tumors of the urinary drainage tract: Urothelial tumors. *J Urol* 54:186–193, 1945.

24. ———— Tumors of the urinary bladder, etc. *J Urol,* 74:498–521, 1955.

25. ————Beta-glucuronidase activity in the urine of patients with bladder cancer and other conditions. *J Urol,* 86:89, 1961.

26. POOLE-WILSON, D. S., ASHWORTH, A., and BOLAND, J. The bladder. Chapter 28 in: *Treatment of Cancer in Clinical Practice.* P. B. Kunkler and A. J. H. Rains, Eds, Livingstone, Edin-burgh, 1959.

27. PUGH, R. C. B. The grading and staging of bladder tumours. *Brit J Urol,* 28:222–225, 1957.

28. PUGH, R. C. B. The pathology of bladder tumors. Chapter 10 in *Tumours of the Bladder,* D. W. Smithers (Ed.), Livingstone, Edinburgh, 1959.

29. RICHES, E. Choice of treatment in carcinoma of the bladder. *J Urol,* 84:472–480, 1960.

30. SCHULTE, J. W., HINMAN, F., JR., and LOW-BEER. B. V. A. Radiocobalt in the treatment of bladder tumors. *J Urol,* 67:916–924, 1952.

31. WALLACE, D. M. Surgery of bladder tumors. Chapter 16 in *Tumours of the Bladder,* D. W. Smithers (Ed.), Livingstone, Edinburgh, 1959.

32. ————. Clinico-pathological behavior of bladder tumors. Chapter 11 in *Tumours of the Bladder,* D. W. Smithers (Ed.), Livingstone, Edinburgh, 1959.

17

TUMORS OF BONE

The radiation treatment of tumor situated in bone can be divided into two categories: those lesions primary in bone and those lesions metastatic to it. In the former, use of radiation therapy is highly selective and of limited scope. Although it is the treatment of choice for Ewing's tumor, primary lymphoma (reticulum cell sarcoma), and myeloma, it has but modest effect on other primary malignant bone tumors such as osteosarcoma and chondrosarcoma, at least with tolerable doses. On the basis of current knowledge, benign tumors (e.g., giant cell tumors, osteoblastomas) should be irradiated only under very specific circumstances and with strict indications, although this restriction should be based on reasons other than that usually emphasized, namely, malignant change in irradiated bone. In contrast, local irradiation with rare exception is the palliative treatment of choice for metastatic lesions.

PRIMARY BONE TUMORS

Any meaningful study of the treatment of primary bone neoplasms requires a classification of these tumors, for the tumor types are numerous and the host tissue, bone, is dynamic. Proposed classifications are legion, and there is no consensus, for complicated classifications are little used and simple classifications have quickly apparent limitations. The classification shown in Table 17-1 has been used by Dahlin[1]:

333

Table 17-1. Classification of Primary Bone Tumors*

Histologic Type	Benign	Malignant
Hematopoietic		Myeloma[R] Reticulum cell sarcoma[R] Leukemic nodules[R]
Chondrogenic	Osteochondroma Chondroma Chondroblastoma Chondromyxoid fibroma	Chondrosarcoma (primary, secondary)
Osteogenic	Osteoma Osteoid-osteoma Benign osteoblastoma	Osteosarcoma
Unknown origin	Giant cell tumor[R]	Ewing's sarcoma[R] Giant cell tumor[R] Adamantinoma
Fibrogenic	Metaphyseal fibrous defect Desmoplastic fibroma	Fibrosarcoma
Notochordal		Chordoma
Vascular	Hemangioma[R] Lymphangioma Glomus tumor	Hemangiosarcoma Hemangiopericytoma
Lipogenic	Lipoma	Liposarcoma
Neurogenic	Neurilemoma	

*To give perspective, those tumors which have effectively been treated with local radiation have been designated[R].
After Dahlin.[1]

BIBLIOGRAPHY

1. DAHLIN, D. C. *Histogenesis and Classification of Bone Tumors. Tumors of Bone and Soft Tissue*. Year Book, Chicago, 1963.

Myeloma

Myeloma is a malignant tumor of plasmocytic derivation, usually involving multiple bone marrow sites at the time of diagnosis. Most of that minority of patients in whom only a solitary lesion can be defined initially ultimately suffer widespread distribution of tumor.[5]

Extramedullary myeloma may be "solitary" and usually appears in the upper air passages.[4,11] A minority of these patients develop multiple myeloma.[4] In part, this may be because many of the patients are elderly with a limited life span. We have had patients who suffered widespread dissemination of myeloma 16 years following treatment of a "solitary" myeloma of the maxillary sinus and 13 years following treatment of a similar lesion in the nasal fossa.

The diagnosis of myeloma usually is suspected on the basis of anemia, bone pain, and characteristic bone lesions, and is established on the additional basis of marrow abnormality and abnormality of the serum and/or urine.[9] However, Osserman[7] suggests that the characteristic protein abnormalities are unique and distinctive, justifying a diagnosis "within the disease spectrum of multiple myeloma" regardless of the constellation of clinical findings. Within this disease spectrum, he recognizes a "lymphomatous variant" and a para-amyloid phase.

Myeloma is an infrequent disease (4 new cases per 100,000 population per year[11]) although its incidence may be increasing, possibly related in part to increasing diagnostic sophistication.[4] Myeloma has been reported as the most frequent bone neoplasm.[4]

In a recent study,[9] compared with 185 patients with multiple myeloma, there were 2 patients with plasmocytic leukemia and 3 patients with "solitary" myeloma. However, in centers with special interest in this tumor, the proportion of "solitary" and extramedullary myelomas may be higher.[10]

Clinical Manifestations

Myeloma more frequently affects males (66[9]–73 percent[4]). The peak decade of clinical onset is 50 to 59 years with an average of 59.5 years.[4,9] Few under 40 years are afflicted.[4]

The most distressing manifestations are bone pain (68 percent), weakness and fatigue (16 percent), and anemia (10 percent[9]). These may be augmented by weight loss, infection, cardiopulmonary problems, neurological complications, uremia, and other complaints.

The diagnosis usually is established by bone marrow abnormality (88 percent), protein abnormalities in the serum and/or urine (31 percent), and characteristic bone lesions (12 percent[9]).

Myeloma most often involves the marrow of the vertebrae, skull, ribs, clavicle, and ilium.[4] Extramedullary plasmocytomas usually involve the upper airway.[4,10]

Pathologic Findings

Myeloma is a malignant proliferation of a family of cells in which the plasma cell is dominant.[7,11] A spectrum of cell variation ranges from mature plasma cells to foci resembling reticulum cell sarcoma or Hodgkin's disease.[4]

In addition to the bone marrow and upper airway, myeloma may involve lymph nodes, spleen, liver, kidneys, and other viscera. The distribution of amyloid resembles that of primary systemic amyloidosis.[4,7]

Roentgenologic Appearance

Myeloma may appear in several forms. The most frequent appearance is that of multiple, round, clean-cut foci of destruction of bone without surrounding sclerosis.[4,8,11] In the long bones, these destructive lesions may coalesce, with a consequent weakened bone which fractures. In some patients, the bones may appear normal or be diffusely decalcified and roentgenologically indistinguishable from the changes of senile or postmenopausal osteoporosis.[8] Other lesions, especially in the long bones and pelvis, may be trabeculated and "honeycombed" with expansion of the cortex. When these lesions are "solitary" and in the epiphysis of long bones, they may not be distinguished from giant cell tumors except by biopsy.[3] Any of these tumors may extend into the adjacent soft tissue and produce visible masses.

Laboratory Findings

Nearly all patients with myeloma have abnormal protein in the plasma and/or urine. Each patient seems to produce his own distinct abnormal protein.[7] In the urine, many of these proteins will yield a positive Bence-Jones test, although this test is subject to frequent false negative and occasional false positive results.[7] The characteristic electrophoretic myeloma pattern consists of a discrete increase in gamma globulin.

Treatment

In a recent survey,[9] the frequent objectives of treatment were relief of bone pain (57 percent), anemia (29 percent), known bone lesions (8 percent). One of every five patients was treated only because the diagnosis was established. Treatment methods included urethane (71 percent); radiation therapy (35 percent), corticosteroids (30 percent), specific chemotherapeutic agents (12 percent), and surgery (6 percent).

Radiation therapy, for many years, was the only effective treatment.[11] Localized tumors frequently can be controlled, making irradiation the treatment of choice for "solitary" neoplasms and tumor-produced local problems, i.e., pain and destruction of weight-bearing bone. Statements still found in some texts that myeloma always is very radiosensitive are not correct. There are few malignant tumors with such a wide variation of response to irradiation. Some large tumors disappear within a short time following doses of less than 300–400 rads. Others are little changed by subjective or objective measurement following doses of 4,000–5,000 rads. In our experience, the tumors which on x-ray appear multiloculated and expansive are the least responsive. The evaluation of subjective improvement following treatment often is difficult because of the variation in pattern and intensity of pain and the frequent simultaneous use of several agents, including pain-relieving drugs. The evaluation of objective evidence of response to treatment may be confused by the occasional lesion which does not progress for long periods without treatment. In a study of the response to irradiation objectively measured by (1) decrease in palpable tumor, (2) x-ray evidence of healing of skeletal destruction, and (3) decreased tumor-related paraplegia, Norin[6] documented improvement in 19 of 22 patients with "cumulative tumour doses"* in

---

* "Cumulative tumor dose" is an attempt to biologically equate a total radiation dose delivered in multiple increments over several days to a single dose.

excess of "1200 r" prompting a recommendation of "cumulative tumour doses" in excess of "1500 r" (3,400 R in 15 days, 4,000 R in 30 days).

Based on effectiveness of local tumor control and anatomical preservation, an attempt with radiation therapy is the preferable initial treatment for solitary plasmocytoma, whether extramedullary or in bone or for isolated symptomatic foci. Generalization of neoplasm many years later in many of these patients does not alter these initial therapeutic objectives. In a recent study of 30 patients with "solitary plasmocytoma,"[10] 16 lesions were in the upper airway and 9 were in bone. Thirteen of 14 lesions were controlled with doses in excess of 2,500 rads in 19 days (all 8 lesions receiving over 3,000 rads).

Surgery rarely is appropriate initial treatment even of a "solitary" lesion. However, it has proved valuable for rapid decompression of the compromised spinal cord and, on rare occasion, for removal of a specific lesion not controlled by radiation therapy.

Chemotherapy is appropriate for a disease which can be considered systemic. Urethan, glucocorticoids, fluorides, cyclophosphamide, and melphalan have been used with varying success for specific problems. In a recent study,[9] no data could be accumulated to support or deny the advisability of treating asymptomatic patients.

Prognosis

There is a wide range of survival for patients with myeloma. This variation is biological and cannot be closely related to treatment. Certain factors such as specific protein alterations, hypercalcemia, severe anemia, and widespread dissemination of tumor at the time of diagnosis are bad prognostic findings.

For patients with myeloma, there is no "initial event perfectly suited for measurement of survival."[9] Using current treatment methods, 50 percent of all patients can be expected to survive 14 to 20 months from the onset of symptoms and 5½ to 11 months from the time of diagnosis, and 10 percent of all patients may survive 38 to 84 (mean = 56) months from the onset of symptoms and 43 to 80 (mean = 58) months from the time of diagnosis.[9] Dahlin[4] documented an overall 53 percent five-year survival (18 of 34) for patients with "solitary" lesions, although 7 of these 18 later died with tumor. Eighteen of 51 patients with myeloma initially restricted to the vertebrae survived over five years.[2] Our longest survivor lived 16 years from the time of first treatment.

In Todd's report[10] of 30 patients with "solitary plasmocytoma," 18 (60 percent) survived over five years, and 11 of 16 patients (69 percent) with lesions of the upper airway were in this favorable group.

The most frequent causes of death in patients with myeloma are infection and noninfectious cardiopulmonary conditions, i.e., pulmonary edema and heart failure.[9]

REVIEW QUESTIONS

1. What is the clinical usefulness of the concept of a "solitary" myelomatous lesion? Have you ever seen a patient with such a lesion?

2. What is the most frequent clinical presentation of the patient with multiple myeloma?

3. What is the basic pathology of myeloma? What other neoplasms may be considered by the pathologist in the differential diagnosis?

4. What are the frequent roentgenographic findings in the patient with multiple myeloma? What diseases may be considered in the differential diagnosis?

5. What is the basic diagnostic abnormality in the serum of patients with multiple myeloma?

6. How can radiation therapy benefit patients with myeloma? Have you seen selective irradiation effectively used for these patients?

7. Why is surgery rarely indicated as definitive treatment for these patients?

8. What is an approximate incidence of survival at five years after treatment for patients with multiple myeloma? for patients with "solitary plasmocytoma"?

BIBLIOGRAPHY

1. ACKERMAN, L. V., and DEL REGATO, J. A. *Cancer: Diagnosis-Treatment-Prognosis*, 4th ed. Mosby, St. Louis, 1970.
2. COHEN, D. M., SVIEN, H. J., and DAHLIN, D. C. Long-term survival of patients with myeloma of vertebral column. *JAMA*, 187:914–917, 1964.
3. CUTLER, M., BUSCHKE, F., and CANTRIL, S. T. The course of single myeloma of bone. *Surg Gynec Obstet*, 62:918–932, 1936.
4. DAHLIN, D. C. *Bone Tumors*, 2nd ed. Charles C Thomas, Springfield, Ill., 1967.
5. INNES, J., and NEWALL, J. Myelomatosis. *Lancet*, 1:239–245, 1961.
6. NORIN, T. Roentgen treatment of myeloma with special consideration to the dosage. *Acta Radiol* [Ther] (Stockholm), 47:46–54, 1957.
7. OSSERMAN, E. F. Multiple myeloma. Current clinical and chemical concepts. *Amer J Med*, 23:283–309, 1957.
8. PAUL, L. W., and JUHL, J. H. *The Essentials of Roentgen Interpretation*, Hoeber-Harper, New York, 1965.
9. Study Committee of the Midwest Cooperative Chemotherapy Group. Multiple myeloma. General aspects of diagnosis, course and survival. *JAMA*, 188:741–745, 1964.
10. TODD, I. D. H. Treatment of solitary plasmocytoma. *Clin Radiol*, 16:385–399, 1965.
11. WALDENSTROM, J. *Diagnosis and Treatment of Multiple Myeloma*, Grune & Stratton, New York, 1970.

Malignant Lymphoma of Bone
(Reticulum-Cell Sarcoma)

Malignant lymphoma of any type may involve bone as part of a widespread process or as a soltiary lesion. In the latter situation, the tumor apparently arises within the bone marrow, may remain localized for substantial periods, and is potentially curable by currently available treatment.

Malignant lymphoma in bone comprises about 3.4 percent of all malignant tumors primary in bone.[3] In another perspective, in a review of 164 cases of lymphosarcoma,[2] bone involvement was discovered in 17 patients only one of which appeared to be primary in bone.

In a recent study[7] of 117 patients with malignant lymphoma of bone (exclusive of tumors causing spinal cord compression or involving the maxillary sinus), 59 had tumors apparently primary in bone. Of these 59 tumors, 42 were mixed cell type, 8 were pure reticulum-cell type, 2 were lymphocytic, and 7 were Hodgkin's disease.

The entity of malignant lymphoma primary in bone was first suggested by Oberling in 1928,[10] accepted by Ewing in 1939, and documented with a report of 17 cases by Parker and Jackson in 1939.[11] Recognition of this clinical entity is important because its prognosis is better than that of other primary malignant bone tumors and, of course, better than that of widespread lymphoma with bone involvement.

Pathologic Findings

These neoplasms are of a variable histology, even though frequently termed reticulum-cell sarcomas. In a recent review,[7] only 14 of 117 were dominantly reticulum-cell tumors, whereas 85 were of "mixed" cell type, and a few were lymphosarcoma[7] and Hodgkin's disease.[11] These histological patterns are indistinguishable from similar tumors arising elsewhere in lymphoid tissue. Occasionally, differentiation from other neoplasms, i.e., Ewing's tumor and metastatic neuroblastoma, may be difficult.

Lymphoma, when primary in bone, may spread to other bone (15 percent), lymph nodes (22 percent), lungs (10 percent), and other organs (47 percent).[1]

Clinical Manifestations

Primary lymphomas of bone usually affect young adults (average, 34 years)[9] and may be slightly more frequent in males. The insidious clinical onset often antedates diagnosis by many months (average, 9 months).[1,8] The most frequent symptom is localized, dull, aching, intermittent pain, often worse at night and unrelieved by rest.[8] Local swelling with minimal tenderness may be noted,[8,9] and fracture through tumor-altered bone has been identified in as many as one of four patients at the time of diagnosis.[13]

Systemic findings of fever and weight loss are infrequent.[7,8] Parker and Jackson[11] stated, "In no other bone sarcoma is the contrast between the comparative well-being of the patient and the size of the lesion so marked."

Roentgenograms

Malignant lymphoma primary in bone usually arises in the extremities, often adjacent to the knee. Sites of involvement have been listed in order of decreasing frequency by Medill[8] as femur (26.4 percent), tibia (19.9 percent), humerus (11.5 percent), scapula (9.17 percent), clavicle (6.6 percent), ilium, vertebrae, fibula, mandible, rib, ulna, skull, and sternum. The x-ray findings are not distinctive,[7] showing an ill-defined patchy destruction of bone often coexistent with patchy new bone. Most often the lesion starts in the medullary portion of the metaphysis. Endosteal spread may result in a fusiform enlargement of the shaft of a long bone. Although the bony cortex usually is destroyed, periosteal new bone seldom is prominent. Extension to adjacent soft tissue may be identified, although calcification is rare.[8,12]

Diagnosis

Diagnosis must be established by biopsy of the roentgenologically identified bone lesion in a patient without other known tumor. In those patients with involvement of multiple sites, the bone involvement is considered secondary. This arbitrary exclusion, as well as adherence to other rigid criteria, (i.e., long course with slow progression, very radioresponsive) preselects a group which may not be representative of a possible broad spectrum of behavior.[4]

The differential diagnosis includes Ewing's tumor, osteolytic osteosarcoma, metastatic neuroblastoma, and osteomyelitis.[8]

Treatment

Lymphoma in bone usually is dramatically responsive to irradiation. There may be early resolution of the tumor with sclerosis of the destroyed bone within a few months.[8] In the study of Ivins and Dahlin,[7] it was noted that the control of solitary lesions in the extremities was as good with radiation therapy as with amputation often supplemented by postoperative irradiation. This comparable effectiveness of tumor control with preservation of a functional limb makes radiation therapy the initial treatment of choice for tumor in any anatomical site. The irradiated volume should include the entire shaft of the involved bone and the adjacent soft tissue and the regional nodes. Doses should be extended to just within the limits of tolerance (i.e., 4,500–5,000 rads in five weeks) to minimize local tumor persistence.

Results

Although rigid diagnostic criteria may exclude biologically aggressive tumors primary in bone,[4] selection of a favorable group is useful clinically because, with proper treatment, the prognosis is better than that of other primary malignant tumors of bone. Seven of the 17 patients originally described by Parker and Jackson[11] were alive and well for more than ten years. Survival data have been recorded by Wilson and Pugh[13] (5-year survival rate = 42 percent of 33 patients), Francis et al.[6] (5-year survival rate = 48 percent; 10-year survival rate = 33 percent), and Ivins and Dahlin[7] (5-year survival rate for patients with "solitary" lesions = 35 percent; for those with regional adenopathy, survival = 26.7 percent). The latter authors[7] found no difference in prognosis for patients with pure reticulum-cell tumors and mixed cells tumors, but found the prognosis in Hodgkin's disease and lymphosarcoma to be less favorable.

REVIEW QUESTIONS

1. Of what clinical importance is the concept that malignant lymphomas may arise in and be confined to a single focus in bone?

2. What histological types of lymphoma arise in bone?

3. What are the criteria of diagnosis?

4. Why is radiation therapy the treatment of choice?

5. How does the prognosis of lymphomas primary in bone compare with that of other primary malignant tumors arising in bone?

BIBLIOGRAPHY

1. ACKERMAN, L. V., and SPJUT, H. J. Tumors of bone and cartilage. In: *Atlas of Tumor Pathology*, Sect. II, Fasc. 4, Washington, D.C., Armed Forces Institute of Pathology, June 1962.
2. CRAVER, L. F., and COPELAND, M. M. Lymphosarcoma in bone. *Arch Surg* (Chicago), 28: 809–824, 1934.
3. DAHLIN, D. C. *Bone Tumors*. 2nd ed. Charles C Thomas, Springfield, Ill., 1967.
4. DOLAN, P. A. Reticulum-cell sarcoma of bone. *Amer J Roentgen*, 87:121–127, 1962.
5. EWING, J. A review of the classification of bone tumors. *Surg Gynec Obstet*, 68:971–976, 1939.
6. FRANCIS, K. D., HIGINBOTHAM, N. L., and COLEY, B. L. Primary reticulum-cell sarcoma of bone; report of 44 cases. *Surg Gynec Obstet*, 99:143–146, 1954.
7. IVINS, J. C., and DAHLIN, D. C. Malignant lymphoma (reticulum-cell sarcoma) of bone. *Mayo Clin Proc*, 38:375–385, 1963.
8. MEDILL, E. V. Primary reticulum-cell sarcoma of bone. *J Fac Radiol*, 8:102–117, 1956.
9. MOSS, W. T. *Therapeutic Radiology*. Rationale, Technique, Results. 3rd ed., Mosby, St. Louis, 1969.
10. OBERLING, C. Les reticulosarcomes et les reticuloendotheliosarcomes de le moelle osseuse (sarcoma d'Ewing). *Bull Cancer*, 17:259–296, 1928.
11. PARKER, F., JR., and JACKSON, H., JR. Primary reticulum-cell sarcoma of bone. *Surg Gynec Obstet*, 68:45–53, 1939.
12. SHERMAN, R. S., and SNYDER, R. E. Roentgen appearance of primary reticulum-cell sarcoma of bone. *Amer J Roentgen*, 58:291–306, 1947.
13. WILSON, T. W., and PUGH, D. G. Primary reticulum-cell sarcoma of bone with emphasis on roentgen aspects. *Radiology*, 65:343–351, 1955.

Ewing's Tumor

Ewing's tumor (diffuse endothelioma of bone, endothelial myeloma, endothelial sarcoma[1]) is a clinicopathological entity consisting of a nonosteogenic, small round-cell tumor, apparently arising in the medullary portion of bone of a young subject. Ewing's initial report[5] in 1921 emphasized the frequent diaphyseal location, the regular histological appearance, the high degree of radioresponsiveness, and the desirability of differentiation from other bone tumors. Willis[19] cautioned against careless use of the diagnosis of Ewing's tumor, and noted that the clinical syndrome could be caused by several tumors, including metastatic neuroblastoma, small-cell osteosarcoma, metastases from carcinoma of the bronchus, and reticulum-cell sarcoma of bone. Nothing is known about the etiology or pathogenesis of this tumor which might aid in its definition.[17]

Clinical Manifestations

Ewing's tumor may comprise as many as 10 percent of all bone tumors,[4] afflicts males more frequently than females,[2, 17, 18] and usually is found in children and adolescents under 20 years of age.[18]

Two-thirds of these tumors are first detected in the pelvic girdle or long tubular bones of the lower limbs.[4, 10] In order of decreasing frequency, the apparent primary sites are femur, ilium, tibia, humerus, ribs, fibula, scapula, sacrum, vertebrae, and clavicle.[3] At least half of these patients will have metastases, usually to lung or bone, detected on initial examination.[10]

At the time of diagnosis, at the primary site there usually is a palpable, localized mass, which may have been noted for several months. Local pain, tenderness, and heat gradually increase despite fluctuations in their course of development.[17]

Other clinical findings may be related to tumor site and extent. These include the pain and disability of fracture, cough and dyspnea with pulmonary metastases and pleural effusion, pain and neurologic deficit with nerve involvement.

Fever, leukocytosis, malaise, anemia, and persistent elevation of the erythrocyte sedimentation rate may be present with either uncontrolled local or metastatic tumor.[17]

The duration of symptoms and signs has been found unrelated to survival,[2] and has not been correlated with the presence or absence of detected metastases at the time of diagnosis.[10] In a study of 45 patients during the period 1958–1963,[10] an increasing proportion of patients treated for cure was hopefully interpreted as an indication of diagnosis earlier in the course of disease.

Pathologic Findings

Grossly, Ewing's tumor is solid unless modified by hemorrhage or necrosis. The tumor growth rate varies from very rapid to slow, with apparent quiescent periods.[17] Histologically, the uniform, small round cells have scant cytoplasm and infrequent mitoses. Collars of tumor cells about vessels may simulate rosettes, but they are residua after necrosis.[17]

Ewing's tumor must be differentiated from reticulum-cell sarcoma, metastatic neuroblastoma, small round-cell osteosarcoma, small-cell carcinoma, and myeloma. In a recent study of the cellular ultrastructure,[8] a relationship to reticulum-cell sarcoma was again questioned.

Because of the frequency of response to radiation, if biopsy is contemplated treatment must be withheld.

Metastases, via either the lymphatics or the bloodstream, are frequent and may involve any organ, although the usual sites are bone and lung.

Roentgenologic Appearance

Although the x-ray appearance is variable, combinations of features can be suggestive of Ewing's tumor. These findings include a predominantly lytic destruction of bone without discrete margins; little evidence of defensive reaction in bone; spread along the shaft of a long bone from a central focus; expansion and perforation of the cortex with elevation of the periosteum and development of subperiosteal new bone, often appearing as linear laminations parallel to the shaft ("onionskin"); and a surrounding soft tissue mass.[14,17] At times a large, soft tissue mass may coexist with minimal radiographic changes in bone.

Treatment

Frequently, "a heterogenously treated population with less than optimal evaluation following an equivocal diagnosis" has been "offered in testimony to the efficacy of a particular form of therapy."[13]

In discussing his early experience with 37 patients, Ewing[6] recommended radiation treatment of the primary tumor. Despite intermittent surgical enthusiasm, this preference persists at the present time.[10,15,17,18] Phillips and Higinbotham[15] have stated that the appearance of distant metastases within 12 months of diagnosis in over half of their patients makes primary amputation an unattractive gamble. Boyer, Brickner, and Perry[2] state that not only is primary radical surgery futile and unnecessary, but it may be a disservice to the patient.

Radical surgery (amputation) and vigorous local irradiation are effective in locally controlling Ewing's tumor. Inasmuch as the prognosis usually is governed by the metastases, local irradiation is preferable because of anatomical and functional preservation.

Despite the reputation of a high order of responsiveness to irradiation, the incidence of local tumor control increases with increasing dose to the limits of normal tissue tolerance. Jenkin[10] noted local tumor reactivation in at least 7 of 20 primary lesions with doses in excess of 3,500 rads, although in all but 1 of the 7 there were concurrent metastases. Thus, if long-term local control is an objective, doses of about 5,500 rads in 6 weeks are suggested. The entire bone unit, such as the shaft of a long bone in an extremity, must be treated because of the likelihood of tumor spread within the bone.

For patients requiring palliative treatment, the frequent high order of radio-responsiveness can be exploited. Pulmonary metastases may resolve following tolerated doses to the entirety of both lungs. Our longest survivor is well seven years after treatment to the lungs (11 years since the initial treatment to bone) without chemotherapy. Specific clinical problems, e.g., cranial nerve paresis, headache, localized pain, and threatened fracture, may respond rapidly to minimal radiation doses which do not add to the systemic morbidity.

Inasmuch as most patients die with widespread dissemination of tumor within a short time after diagnosis, systemic treatment concurrent with vigorous irradiation of the primary tumor seems reasonable for those patients in whom only a single lesion can be identified at the time of diagnosis. Studies of such concurrent systemic treatment with cytotoxic drugs (e.g., cyclophosphamide and vincristine[9,11]) or with total body irradiation[13,16] are ongoing.

Results

Reported results of treatment may be expected to vary for a disease of ambiguous diagnostic criteria. Little has occurred to contradict Dahlin's[4] statement that Ewing's tumor is the most lethal of all bone tumors. However, documented survivors, perhaps more frequent with recent more vigorous treatment, contradict the myth of prognostic futility that if a patient with Ewing's is cured, the diagnosis is incorrect.

In studying 91 reported survivors, Falk and Alpert[7] noted that the prognosis was better if the clinical history was longer than three months; there were no metastases detected at the time of diagnosis; there was no associated extraosseous mass; and if the tumor apparently arose in either long bone or mandible. There is no obvious prognostic correlation with age or sex of the patient.[15]

Overall five-year tumor-free survival frequencies have been about 10 percent. In a recent study of the literature,[7] 78 of 987 patients (8 percent) survived five years. Boyer, Brickner, and Perry[2] reported an actuarial probability of a 12 percent five-year survival.

Seven of 50 patients (14 percent) reported by Wang and Schulz[18] were alive without evidence of tumor 6 to 13 years after treatment. Six of the 7 survivors were treated only with local irradiation. Six of 55 patients (10.9 percent) reported by McCormack et al.[12] were alive and well more than 10 years after treatment. Three of 24 patients surgically treated and 3 of 31 patients irradiated survived. Phillips and Higinbotham[15] reported 13 of 54 patients (24 percent) alive more than 5 years after treatment. Two of their patients were alive at 9 and 16 years following treatment of a metastasis. Others also have reported survivors after treatment of pulmonary metastases.[17,18] Of 39 patients irradiated with curative intent,[15] 13 (33 percent) survived longer than 5 years. Eleven of 24 patients (46 percent) survived at least 5 years when the entire involved bone was vigorously irradiated. These authors[15] emphasized the frequent similarity to reticulum-cell sarcoma of bone, and found an identical post-treatment survival rate for both tumors.

Although the tumor-related death rate within a year of treatment has been less in those programs with concurrent systemic treatment and irradiation of the primary tumor,[9,11,13,16] any early optimism needs to await the test of time.

Thirty-five percent of patients with Ewing's tumor die with uncontrolled tumor within 12 months of diagnosis.[15] This increases to 70–85 percent within 24 months.[7,15] Occasionally, patients may suffer reactivation of tumor many years after apparent control.[17,18]

These data accentuate the importance of palliative treatment, which is highly effective and minimally morbid. Radiation therapy to small doses frequently results in early, complete pain relief (27 of 36) and local tumor control (15–18 of 22).[18]

REVIEW QUESTIONS

1. What is your concept of Ewing's tumor? Is the histopathology characteristic?

2. What tumors may be confused with Ewing's tumor pathologically? clinically?

3. How frequent is Ewing's tumor?

4. What is the usual clinical presentation?

5. Is the x-ray appearance diagnostic? What are the usual features?

6. Why is local irradiation the treatment of choice for the primary tumor? How radio-sensitive is this tumor? What local growth characteristic of the tumor must be accounted for in treatment?

7. What is the overall survival for these patients? What is the usual course of this tumor?

BIBLIOGRAPHY

1. ACKERMAN, L. V., and SPJUT, H. J. Ewing's sarcoma in tumors of bone and cartilage. Armed Forces Institute of Pathology, Fasc. 4, 1962.
2. BOYER, C. W., JR., BRICKNER, T. J., JR., and PERRY, R. H. Ewing's sarcoma: Case against surgery. *Cancer*, 20:1602–1606, 1967.
3. DAHLIN, D. C. *Bone Tumors*, 2nd ed., Charles C Thomas, Springfield, Ill., 1967.
4. DAHLIN, D., COVENTRY, M., and SCANLON, P. Ewing's sarcoma. *J Bone Joint Surg*, [Amer], 43-A:185–192, 1961.
5. EWING, J. Diffuse endothelioma of bone. *Proc NY Path Soc*, 21:17–24, 1921.
6. EWING, J. Further report on endothelial myeloma of bone. *Proc NY Path Soc*, 24:93–101, 1924.
7. FALK, S., and ALPERT, M. Five-year survival of patients with Ewing's sarcoma. *Surg Gynec Obstet*, 124:319–324, 1967.
8. FRIEDMAN, B., and GOLD, H. Ultrastructure of Ewing's sarcoma of bone. *Cancer*, 22:307–322, 1968.
9. HUSTU, O., HOLTON, C. P., JAMES, D. JR., and PINKEL, D. Treatment of Ewing's sarcoma with concurrent radiotherapy and chemotherapy. *Pediatrics*, 73:249–251, August 1968.
10. JENKIN, R. D. T. Ewing's sarcoma: A study of treatment methods. *Clin Radiol*, 17:97−106, 1966.
11. JOHNSON, R. Personal communication, 1970.
12. MC CORMACK, L. J., DOCKERTY, M. B., and GHORMLEY, R. K. Ewing's sarcoma. *Cancer*, 5:85–99, 1952.
13. MILLBURN, L. F., O'GRADY, L., and HENDRICKSON, F. R. Radical radiation therapy and total body irradiation in the treatment of Ewing's sarcoma. *Cancer*, 22:919–925, 1968.
14. PAUL, L. W., and JUHL, J. H. *The Essentials of Roentgen Interpretation*. Hoeber-Harper, New York, 1962.
15. PHILLIPS, R., and HIGINBOTHAM, N. L. Curability of Ewing's endothelioma of bone in children. *J Pediat*, 70:391–397, 1967.
16. RIDER, W. D., and JENKIN, R. D. T. Preliminary observations on total-body radiation in the management of Ewing's tumor. Quoted by Millburn et al. and personal communication, 1970.
17. RIDINGS, G. R. Ewing's Tumor. *Radiol Clin N Amer*, 2:315–325, 1964.
18. WANG, C. C., and SCHULZ, M. D. Ewing's sarcoma: Study of fifty cases treated at Massachusetts General Hospital, 1930–1952. *New Eng J Med*, 248:571–576, 1953.
19. WILLIS, R. *The Pathology of the Tumours of Children*. Charles C Thomas, Springfield, Ill., 1962.

Osteosarcoma

Osteosarcoma is a primary malignant tumor of bone which "forms neoplastic osteoid or osseous tissue in the course of its evolution."[8] There is likely to be pronounced bone destruction even in the presence of new bone formation.[7] Older reports in the literature are of little value because the concepts of this disease have changed markedly since Ewing's[5] initial definiton, which included "all malignant tumors of bone cells."

Osteosarcomas comprised 21.9 percent of the bone sarcomas in the Mayo Clinic experience,[3] thus being second in frequency to myeloma.

Clinical Manifestations

Two-thirds of these patients are males. The peak incidence is between 10 and 19 years,[1,4] with a gradual decrease in incidence with increasing age.[3] Osteosarcomas arising in the jaws may affect a slightly older age group.[3]

Pain and swelling at the tumor site are the usual clinical findings.[1,4] Fracture through tumor-weakened bone is unusual.[3] Fever and weight loss apear only with extensive neoplasm.[7]

More than one-half of these tumors arise in the lower femur or upper tibia,[1,4,7] other frequent sites (in order of decreasing frequency) being the upper humerus, ilium, upper and mid femur, upper fibula, and skull.[4] Osteosarcoma in long bones of adolescents represents a rather specific clinical entity with a very poor prognosis.

Pathologic Findings

Osteosarcomas grossly may be predominantly osteoblastic (sclerosing), when ossification is prominent or osteolytic, when bone destruction is pronounced.[7]

Histologically they may be predominantly osteoblastic (54.7 percent), fibroblastic (23.3 percent), or chondroblastic (22.0 percent).[4] Most (85 percent) are poorly differentiated (Broder's grades 3 and 4).[4] Thus, there may be difficulty in differentiating pleomorphic tumors forming little osteoid from those nonosteoid-forming tumors classified as fibrosarcomas or chondrosarcomas.

Occasionally osteosarcomas may arise in bone altered by Paget's disease (3.3 percent), osteochondromas (0.3 percent), or prior irradiation (2.5 percent).[4]

Metastases usually are hematogenous, frequently going to the lungs. Occasionally metastases containing osteoid may properly identify primary tumors previously not considered osteogenic.[9] Metastases to other bones, often in unusual sites, may be mistakenly interpreted as multiple primary tumors. Lymphatic metastases are infrequent.[3,9]

Roentgenographic Appearance

There is great variation in the x-ray appearance of this tumor. The destructive process may appear predominantly lytic or sclerotic. The tumor borders are indistinct. Although the changes may start in and be limited to the medulla, most often the overlying cortex is involved, the periosteum is elevated, and there is a contiguous soft tissue mass. Although the primary site often is in the metaphysis, the epiphysis may be invaded.[3]

Treatment

The primary objectives of treatment are local control of tumor and patient survival.

Surgical amputation can provide effective local control of tumor if the margins are sufficiently proximal to the tumor in an extremity. Such removal is not possible for tumors arising in the skull, vertebrae, or ilium. Surgical ablation, immediately following identification of the neoplasm, has not saved the great majority of patients from an early death with lung metastases. Therefore, many surgeons are hesitant to produce the morbidity of extremity amputation in youngsters, most of whom simultaneously will be dying with widespread metastases, and attempting rehabilitation.

Radiation therapy has had a restricted role in the management of patients with osteosarcoma. However, many of these tumors are sufficiently radioresponsive that good palliation and occasional permanent local control will follow vigorous treatment of an adequate tissue volume.[9, 12]

If 75 percent of the pulmonary metastases become clinically apparent within five months of diagnosis,[9] a short delay of amputation might avoid much "totally futile mutilation."[9]

Thus, preoperative radiation therapy has been advocated[2, 9, 10, 12] because temporary local tumor control might allow selection of that "metastasis-free" minority of patients who ultimately could profit from amputation of an extremity. There is considerable recent evidence that such a policy does not further compromise the small group of survivors.[6, 9, 10, 12]

Doses between 6,000–7,000 rads are advisable and are tolerated with a moderate incidence of sequelae, including skin change, subcutaneous fibrosis with occasional restriction of movement at a joint,[9] and osteonecrosis.[12] Lee and MacKenzie,[9] in a study of their postirradiation specimens have noted that most tumors are either "totally destroyed" or "severely damaged."

On the assumption that some of the cells in osteosarcomas, large enough to be recognized clinically, are poorly oxygenated and, thus, unresponsive to conventional radiation doses, Suit[11] has attempted to reduce the preferential oxygenation of the remainder of the tumor and the adjacent normal tissues by application of a tourniquet on a tumor-bearing extremity. Total doses of 12,000–14,000 rads have then been tolerated, with some indication of consequent increased local tumor control.

Chemotherapy has not proved effective in destroying tumor locally and thus, to date, has not proved a useful agent even for palliation.

Prognosis

Considerable variation in reported survival data reflects variation in patient material, in part based on different diagnostic criteria. However, without exception, the frequency of long-term survival is low.

In those series in which surgery was the initial treatment, the five-year survival has varied only slightly, i.e., 12.7 percent (8 of 63),[1] 16–22 percent,[7] 20.3 percent.[4] The prognosis has not been correlated with age or sex of the patient or histological type or grade of the tumor, but it may be slightly better for lesions distal to the knees and elbows and worse for tumors arising in bone altered by previous irradiation or Paget's disease.[4]

Data reported by Lee and MacKenzie,[9] Phillips and Sheline,[10] Farrell and Raventos,[6] and Tudway[12] document that when amputation is selectively used several months after vigorous local irradiation, many patients are "spared unnecessary mutilation"[2] without compromise of their overall survival.

REVIEW QUESTIONS

1. What is the usual clinical course of osteosarcoma?

2. Is control of the primary tumor of value to those patients with distant metastases? Why?

3. What is the basis of preoperative irradiation of the primary tumor in a patient without clinically detected metastases?

4. What is the value of radiation therapy in palliative treatment of these patients?

BIBLIOGRAPHY

1. BRODY, G. L., and FRY, L. R. Osteogenic sarcoma: Experience at the University of Michigan. *Univ Mich Med Cent J*, 29:80–87, 1963.
2. CADE, S. Osteogenic sarcoma. A study based on 133 patients. *J Roy Coll Surg Edinb*, 1:79–111, 1955.
3. DAHLIN, D. C. *Bone Tumors.* Charles C Thomas, Springfield, Ill., 1967.
4. DAHLIN, D. C., and COVENTRY, M. B. Osteogenic sarcoma: A study of six hundred cases. *J Bone Joint Surg*, 49:101–110, 1967.
5. EWING, J. *Neoplastic Diseases.* 3rd ed., Saunders, Philadelphia, 1928.
6. FARRELL, C., and RAVENTOS, A. Experiences in treating osteosarcoma at the hospital of the University of Pennsylvania. *Radiology*, 83:1080–1083, 1964.
7. GESCHICKTER, C. F., and COPELAND, M. M. Osteogenic sarcoma. In: *Tumors of Bone and Soft Tissue.* Year Book, Chicago, 1965.
8. JAFFE, H. L. *Tumors and Tumorous Conditions of the Bones and Joints.* Lea & Febiger, Philadelphia, 1958.
9. LEE, E. S., and MACKENZIE, D. H. Osteosarcoma: A study of the value of preoperative megavoltage radiotherapy. *Brit J Surg*, 51:252–274, 1964.
10. PHILLIPS, T. L., and SHELINE, G. E. Radiation therapy of malignant bone tumors. *Radiology*, 92:1537–1545, 1969.
11. SUIT, H. D. Radiation therapy given under conditions of local tissue hypoxia for bone and soft tissue sarcoma. In: *Tumors of Bone and Soft Tissue.* Year Book, Chicago, 1965.
12. TUDWAY, R. C. Radiotherapy for osteogenic sarcoma. *J Bone Joint Surg*, 43:61–67, 1961.

**Giant-Cell Tumor of Bone
(Osteoclastoma)**

Giant-cell tumors of bone are autonomous neoplasms with a distinctive cellular composition and an unexplained etiology. Approximately 10 percent behave as malignant tumors.[1,5,20] Although current concepts of giant-cell tumors of bone date to the work of Jaffe, Lichtenstein, and Portis in 1940,[15] the subject remains controversial. Much confusion relates to lesions with a wide spectrum of biological behavior which have only slowly been recognized. These include osteitis fibrosa cystica, non-osteogenic fibroma, benign chondroblastoma, chondromyxoid fibroma, solitary unicameral bone cyst, solitary fibrous dysplasia, aneurysmal bone cyst, reparative granuloma (epulis), and even osteosarcoma.[4,20,24,25]

As of this time, there is little to alter the expression of Jaffe (1953)[14] that a giant-cell tumor of bone is a treacherous lesion that is difficult to assay, and of Lichtenstein (1956)[17] that the more he sees of giant-cell tumors of bone, the more wholesome is his respect for them.

Clinical Manifestations

In a Mayo Clinic study,[7] benign giant-cell tumors compromised 3.9 percent of all bone tumors and 15.1 percent of benign bone tumors, whereas the malignant counterpart comprised less than 0.5 percent of malignant bone tumors.

Ninety percent of giant-cell tumors occur in those older than 19 years,[1,7,19] with the peak incidence in the third decade.[7] Lichtenstein[18] has stated that "the odds are very much against anyone who ventures a diagnosis of giant-cell tumor in a child or adolescent. . . ." Females are affected more often than males.[1,7,19,27] Most giant-cell tumors involve the epiphyses of long bones with over 50 percent adjacent to the knee, in the distal femur or proximal tibia.[1,7,19,21] Other less frequently involved bones are the sacrum, distal radius, ilium, distal ulna, proximal femur, proximal fibula, distal tibia, and proximal humerus.[1,7,19,21]

Symptoms and signs often develop insidiously. Ultimately local pain is the major finding, although it is often accompanied by local swelling and reduced motion at a joint.[1,7,19] Fracture through altered bone is infrequent.[19]

Pathologic Findings

These well-vascularized tumors may have foci of hemorrhage and may contain cysts.[7,21] There often is a well-defined capsule,[1,7] but even benign tumors may aggressively replace adjacent bone.[7] The neoplasm my extend to the articular cartilage without affecting the joint.[1,7,19,27]

Giant-cell tumors are composed of basic, proliferating stromal cells plus giant cells, which may result from a fusion of these mononuclear cells with a resultant collection of 20–35 nuclei.[1,7,20] Microscopic diagnosis can be difficult, errors being due both to inexperience, because of the rarity of the lesion, and to a limited interest in and consequent knowledge of bone pathology.[20]

Johnson and Dahlin[16] found no correlation between histological grading and incidence of post-treatment recurrence or malignant change, whereas in the study of Mnaymneh, Dudley, and Mnaymneh,[19] post-treatment recurrence was more frequent in Grade II than in Grade I tumors. Murphy and Ackerman[20] related the frequency of post-treatment local recurrence to the number of mitoses and the degree of nuclear irregularity, but found no relationship to perforation of the cortex, number or size of the giant cells, or evidence of osteogenesis in the tumor.

Metastases, usually to the lung, have been found in patients with histologically "benign" tumors.

Russell[22] has suggested that there are two forms of malignant giant-cell tumor. In one, the microscopic appearance still resembles a giant-cell tumor. In the other, the stromal cells undergo metaplasia, and the tumor becomes indistinguishable from an osteosarcoma.

The correlation between unsuccessful radiation therapy and malignant transformation has been much discussed.[1,7,16,19,20] However, Hutter et al.[12] have emphasized that malignant transformation also has followed surgical treatment. The disproportionate use of radiation therapy for the unusual, the nonproved, and the histologically bothersome tumors makes any attempted correlation suspect. As stated by Murphy and Ackerman,[20] "We do not have any evidence that well-planned radiation therapy causes a benign giant-cell tumor to become malignant."

Giant-cell tumors occasionally complicate other bone lesions such as Paget's disease. Hutter et al.[13] noted a predilection for this combination to involve the bones of the face and skull, usual sites for giant-cell tumors.

Roentgenological Appearance

A benign giant-cell tumor is a well-defined, expansile, destructive lesion, usually involving the end of a long bone in which the epiphysis is closed.[1,7,21] Although initially eccentric in position, with enlargement the tumor may involve the entire end of the bone and extend to the articular surface, but spare the joint. Trabeculation may be detectable. Periosteal calcification is not present unless stimulated by fracture.[1,21]

An x-ray diagnosis of malignancy may be difficult, for rapid tumor enlargement, loss of cortex and extension into adjacent soft tissues may occur with benign tumors, while metastases have been noted with primary tumors that are considered "benign" histologically.

Thus, there is no pathognomonic x-ray appearance of giant-cell tumors of bone. Diagnostic errors have been committed in both directions, for microscopically confirmed tumors have lacked any telltale x-ray signs, and "typical-appearing" neoplasms have proved to be other lesions.[27]

In postirradiation roentgenographic evaluation, it is necessary to recognize an occasional "paradoxical" response.[3,4,11] This temporarily progressive osteolysis and aggravation of clinical findings, four to eight weeks following what we today would call rapid irradiation,[4] precedes ultimate healing, with recalcification of a bone which may remain expanded and even trabeculated.[21]

Diagnosis

Accurate identification of this tumor is a prerequisite for assessment of biological behavior and results of treatment. Giant-cell tumors of bone have been particularly plagued by variations in concept and inaccurate diagnosis. Correlation of the clinical data, the x-ray appearance, and the histology is essential.[4]

Those lesions requiring separation from true giant-cell tumors have been listed previously.

Treatment

As might be expected, there is considerable controversy regarding the appropriate treatment of a tumor about which there is lingering dispute. The rarity of giant-cell tumors and their capricious behavior lead physicians to become supporters of either conservative or radical treatment.

Many have supported selective or even liberal use of radiation therapy,[2,4,6,8,9,24,27] while others concurrently have disputed or even condemned such use.[7,19,20,23]

Surgical removal of giant-cell tumors of bone may be effective and expeditious, and can provide material for extensive study by pathologists. When such removal does not cause functional or serious cosmetic damage, it is preferable treatment. Continuing improvements in technique make nonmutilating surgical excision with a good margin of healthy bone possible in ever-increasing numbers of patients.

Curettage has proved rather ineffective because of frequent local recurrences (50–85 percent).[7,10,19]

Amputation, although effective, is not applicable for many tumors, and is objectionable as primary treatment even when possible.

The use of *radiation* in the treatment of giant-cell tumors of bone has become more sharply defined and more restricted as a consequence of the exclusion of variants and the improvement of surgical methods, which makes excision without serious disability possible for more patients.

The objective of radiation therapy is permanent control of the tumor accompanied by reconstruction of bone.[4] *Treatment with a "supervoltage" beam in a single course to a dose of 3,000–4,000 rads in 4 to 6 weeks is indicated instead of the use of repeated courses with small doses, as was previously fashionable!*

Necessary close post-treatment follow-up evaluation must include study of frequent, technically comparable x-rays. Initial objective evidence of therapeutic success may not be noted for several months and may follow the "paradoxical" or deteriorating response previously described. Cade[6] stated that "the full benefit of radiation is achieved in about 18 months." This delay in favorable change has been emphasized in nearly all reports advocating radiation therapy. Failure to recognize this delayed response may account for some opinions that radiation therapy is ineffective.

Although Murphy and Ackerman[20] stated in 1956 that "no series of genuine giant-cell tumors treated by irradiation has been reported that adequately shows the effectiveness of irradiation as the sole method of treatment," such effectiveness of treatment has been documented in many individual patients. Failures of local control can be minimized by thorough treatment of carefully diagnosed lesions. However, the success of radiation therapy depends on precise definition. For example Friedman and Pearlman[9] recently have reported a high level of control of tumors of the jaw of children (13 of 13), tumors of membranous bones (11 of 13), tumors of the vertebrae (8 of 12), and tumors associated with Paget's disease —those tumors most likely to be challenged as not being giant-cell tumors— although they had less success with controlling tumors of long bones in adults (7 of 15).

The risk of converting a giant-cell tumor of bone from benignancy to malignancy by use of radiation therapy, although often discussed, has not been measured. However, this risk is minimal with the single course technique described above, thus not constituting valid contraindication to treatment. As of December, 1969, Windeyer,[26] long an advocate of radiation therapy, stated: "I do not feel that there is a great risk of causing these tumors to become malignant by irradiation, as I think that those which have turned out to be malignant have been malignant from the beginning . . . the fear of causing malignant degeneration should not be a factor in the decision regarding therapy."

Prognosis

Inasmuch as local "recurrence" and malignant change may develop many years after treatment, long-term follow-up is important. Tumor size, specific bone involved, pretreatment duration of symptoms, and even cellular appearance have not been well correlated with frequency of recurrence.[7]

Curettage frequently is followed by local tumor growth (50–85 percent).[7, 10, 19] Excision with wide margins usually is successful (21 of 21 patients[19]), as is amputation.

The success of radiation therapy depends on the selection of patients and thoroughness of the application. Long-term control of giant-cell tumors of the long bones of adults may exceed 50 percent (7 of 15; 6 of 8[24]), but control of the more controversial tumors, e.g., those of the mandible and vertebrae, is better (jaws of children and young adults—13 of 13 patients[9]; vertebrae—8 of 12,[9] and 3 of 5 patients[2]). The outlook for patients with malignant giant-cell tumors has been gloomy. Only 2 of 10 patients, reported by Dahlin,[7] survived.

Therefore, we propose the following *indications for the treatment of benign giant-cell tumors of bone:*

1. Surgical removal with a wide margin is the treatment of choice when possible without serious functional or cosmetic change. In contrast, curettage is a poor procedure because of a high frequency of post-treatment recurrence.

2. For surgically inaccessible tumors (vertebrae) or for tumors which would require mutilating surgery, radiation therapy is the best choice.

3. For tumors in which there is question, e.g., identity or possible malignant change, the advantage of excision may license considerable resultant dysfunction.

If the tumor is malignant and there is no evidence of metastases, surgical removal is indicated, while local irradiation should be reserved for nonremovable tumors.

REVIEW QUESTIONS

1. What is your concept of giant-cell tumors of bone? What lesions must be considered in the differential diagnosis?

2. What factors enter into the diagnosis of giant-cell tumor of bone?

3. Can the diagnosis be established by x-ray examination? by histological examination?

4. What is the demarcation between benign and malignant giant-cell tumors of bone?

5. What is the "best" treatment for these tumors?

6. What is the role of radiation therapy for patients with these neoplasms? What are the advantages of radiation therapy? the dangers?

BIBLIOGRAPHY

1. ACKERMAN, L. V., and DEL REGATO, J. A. *Cancer: Diagnosis, Treatment and Prognosis.* 4th ed., Mosby, St. Louis, 1970.
2. BERMAN, H. L. The treatment of benign giant-cell tumors of the vertebrae by irradiation. *Radiology,* 83:202–207, 1964.
3. BRADSHAW, J. D. The value of x-ray therapy in the management of osteoclastoma. *Clin Radiol,* 15:70–74, 1964.
4. BUSCHKE, F., and CANTRIL, S. T. Roentgentherapy of benign giant-cell tumor of bone. *Cancer,* 2:293–315, 1959.
5. CADE, S. Giant-cell tumor of bone. *J Bone Joint Surg [Amer],* 31B:158–160, 1949.
6. CADE, S. In: *British Practice in Radiotherapy,* E. R. Carling, B. W. Windeyer, D. W. Smithers, Eds. Buterworth, London.
7. DAHLIN, D. C. *Bone Tumors.* 2nd ed. Charles C Thomas, Springfield, Ill., 1967.
8. ELLIS, F. Treatment of osteoclastoma by radiation. *J Bone Joint Surg [Amer],* 31B:268–280, 1949.
9. FRIEDMAN, M., and PEARLMAN, A. W. Benign giant-cell tumor of bone: Radiation dosage for each type *Radiology,* 91:1151–1158, 1968.
10. GOLDENBERG, R. R., CAMPBELL, C. J., and BONFIGLIO, M. Giant-cell tumor of bone. *J Bone Joint Surg [Amer]* 52A:619–664, 1970.
11. HERENDEEN, R. E. Results in röntgen-ray therapy of giant-cell tumors of bone. *Ann Surg,* 93:398–411, 1931.
12. HUTTER, R. V., WORCESTER, J. N., JR., FRANCIS, K. C., FOOTE, F. W., JR., and STEWART, F. W. Benign and malignant giant cell tumors of bone: A clinicopathological analysis of the natural history of the disease. *Cancer,* 15:653–690, 1962.
13. HUTTER, R. V., FOOTE, F. W., JR., FRAZELL, E. L., and FRANCIS, K. C. Giant-cell tumors complicating Paget's disease of bone. *Cancer,* 16:1044–1056, 1963.
14. JAFFE, H. L. Giant-cell tumour (osteoclastoma) of bone. Its pathologic delimitation and the inherent clinical implications (Moynihan Lecture). *Ann Roy Coll Surg Eng,* 13:343–355, 1953.
15. JAFFE, H. L., LICHTENSTEIN, L., and PORTIS, R. B. Giant-cell tumor of bone. Its pathologic appearance, grading supposed variants and treatments. *Arch Path* (Chicago), 30:993–1031, 1940.
16. JOHNSON, E. W., and DAHLIN, D. C. Treatment of giant-cell tumor of bone. *J Bone Joint Surg [Amer],* 41A:895–904, 1959.
17. LICHENSTEIN, L. Pathology: Diseases of bone. *New Eng J Med,* 255:427–433, 1956.
18. LICHENSTEIN, L. *Bone Tumors.* 3rd ed., Mosby, St. Louis, 1965.
19. MNAYMNEH, W. A., DUDLEY, H. R., and MNAYMNEH, L. G. Giant-cell tumor of bone. An analysis and follow-up study of the 41 cases observed at the Massachusetts General Hospital between 1925 and 1960. *J Bone Joint Surg,* 46A:63–75, 1964.
20. MURPHY, W. R., and ACKERMAN, L. V. Benign and malignant giant-cell tumors of bone. *Cancer,* 9:317–339, 1956.
21. PAUL, L. W., and JUHL, J. H. *The Essentials of Roentgen Interpretation.* 2nd ed., Harper & Row, New York, 1962.
22. RUSSELL, D. S. Malignant osteoclastoma; and the association of malignant osteoclastoma with Paget's osteitic deformans. *J Bone Joint Surg [Amer],* 31B:281–290, 1949.
23. STEWART, M. J., and RICHARDSON, T. R. Giant-cell tumor of bone. *J Bone Joint Surg [Amer]* 34A:372–386, 1952.

24. WALTER, J. Giant-cell lesions of bone, osteoclastoma and giant-cell tumour variants. Survey of a radiotherapeutic series. *Clin Radiol,* 11:114–124, 1960.
25. WILLIAMS, R. R., DAHLIN, D. C., and GHORMLEY, R. K. Giant-cell tumor of bone. *Cancer,* 7:764–773, 1954.
26. WINDEYER, B. W. Personal communication December 16, 1969.
27. WINDEYER, B. W., and WOODYATT, P. B. Osteoclastoma. *J Bone Joint Surg [Amer],* 31B:252–267, 1949.

Aneurysmal Bone Cyst

In 1942, Jaffe and Lichtenstein[2] emphasized the distinctiveness of a solitary cystic vascular lesion of bone by designating it "aneurysmal bone cyst." This lesion had been discussed in the literature as subperiosteal giant-cell tumor, atypical giant-cell tumor, aneurysmal giant-cell tumor, ossifying hematoma, and "hemorrhagic" bone cyst.[4] Aneurysmal bone cyst, better considered a vascular abnormality rather than a true tumor,[3] constitutes about 1.5 percent of primary bone tumors,[1] thus being less common than giant-cell tumors of bone. It is more frequent in adolescents, has no sex proponderance, and may be formed in practically any bone including the calvarium, although predominant in the diaphysis of long bones of the extremities or vertebrae.[1] Typical roentgenographic findings in lesions of long bones are eccentric position, diaphyseal location, ovoid configuration of an expanded, ballooned-out, rarified area containing fine septa. These findings allow diagnosis with confidence.[4]

Parosteal and symmetrical fusiform lesions of long bones also have been described.[4] In the vertebrae, the neural arch is the common site of involvement.

Microscopically, cavernous spaces containing blood are divided by fibrous septa, often containing osteoid. Giant cells may be present.[1]

Treatment and Results

Resection, curettage, or irradiation to modest dose have been highly effective. Therefore recognition is important, so that such treatment can prevent serious problems incident to progression of these vascular and, at times, rapidly expanding lesions.

Radiation to modest dosage, e.g., less than "2,000 R" (method of calculation not stated), reportedly has been successful in controlling aneurysmal bone cysts, with rare exception.[3] Such conservative treatment would seen preferable to either resection or curettage, particularly if any morbidity or disability would result from surgery. These uniformly good responses to irradiation, without a documented instance of "lytic thrust,"[4] without recurrence or malignancy (only a single exception reported by Lichtenstein),[3] probably account for a number of the favorable responses of "giant-cell tumors of bone," especially those involving vertebrae, reported in the earlier literature.

REVIEW QUESTIONS

1. What is the clinical importance of differentiating aneurysmal bone cyst from other lesions such as atypical giant cell tumor?

2. What is the advantage of radiation therapy for these lesions?

BIBLIOGRAPHY

1. BESSE, B. E., JR., DAHLIN, D. C., PUGH, D. G., and GHORMLY, R. K. Aneurysmal bone cysts: Additional considerations. *Clin Orthop*, 7:93–102, 1956.
2. JAFFE, H. L., and LICHTENSTEIN, L. Solitary unicameral bone cyst with emphasis on the roentgen picture, the pathologic appearance and the pathogenesis. *Arch Surg (Chicago)*, 44:1004–1025, 1942.
3. LICHTENSTEIN, L. Aneurysmal bone cyst. Observations on fifty cases. *J Bone Joint Surg [Amer]*, 39A:873–882, 1957.
4. SHERMAN, R. S., and SOONG, K. Y. Aneurysmal bone cyst; its roentgen diagnosis. *Radiology*, 68:54–64, 1957.

METASTASES TO BONE

Metastases, the most frequent malignant tumors involving bone, are a unique clinical problem because of their threat to the integrity of the skeleton. Involvement of the weight-bearing skeleton often is the most immediate concern in the care of these patients with disseminated cancer.

Most metastases, particularly those from malignant tumors arising in squamous epithelial structures (i.e., oral cavity, cervix) or from the thyroid or kidney, destroy bone without inciting much detectable reparative effort. Less frequently, metastases, particularly from carcinoma of the prostate, may provoke an osteoblastic response. Some metastases, particularly those from carcinoma of the breast, may be both lytic and blastic even in the same patient. The mechanism of lytic and blastic change is unknown, but is assumed to be related to the tumor's mechanically destructive effect on bone and to a consequent reparative attempt.

Most metastases to bone are from carcinomas rather than lymphomas. The primary sites of carcinomas metastasizing to bone in order of decreasing frequency are: in the male—prostate, lung, bladder, and stomach; in the female—breast, uterus, colon, and stomach.[1]

The most frequently associated clinical finding is pain. Often this pain antedates roentgenographic or more sensitive isotopic scanning[3] evidence of bone involvement. Therefore, in the patient known to have other metastases, characteristic, persistent, bone-related pain should prompt palliative treatment even in the absence of visual laboratory confirmation by x-ray or isotope scan.

In contrast, extensive bony metastases may be asymptomatic. Therefore, in these patients it is important to periodically assess the skeleton radiographically so that treatment can prevent fracture, particularly of the weight-bearing bones.

Radiographs are less likely to be falsely negative for metastases involving well-developed compact bone (skull, long-bone diaphyses) than for lesions in bones with a well-developed spongiosa (ribs, pelvis, vertebrae, long-bone metaphyses).

Most bony metastases are blood-borne. The bones most frequently involved have well-developed red marrow (skull, vertebrae, pelvis, proximal femur).[1] Metastases distal to the knee or elbow are comparably infrequent.

Although a clinically apparent solitary metastasis may stimulate a primary bone tumor, particularly if there is associated bone production, most metastases are multiple or occur in patients with known primary tumors, thus facilitating diagnosis.

Lymphomas frequently involve bone. Patients with Hodgkin's disease have an incidence of bone involvement exceeding 50 percent at autopsy and 15 percent on x-ray bone survey, while patients with lymphosarcoma have bone involvement about half as often.[6,8] A blastic response is more frequently incited by Hodgkin's disease than by lymphosarcoma. Patients with bone involved by Hodgkin's disease, despite advanced clinical staging, may survive for many years (average 6.5 years).[7]

Treatment

The single most effective therapeutic agent for patients with bony metastases is ionizing radiation. Localized irradiation can relieve pain, control tumor with consequent bony reconstruction, and prevent fracture of weight-bearing bone for most patients without the morbidity of systemic anticancer treatment or an operative procedure. Pain relief followed irradiation in more than 90 percent of our patients with bony metastases from carcinomas of the breast and lung and in 2 of every 3 patients with metastases from prostatic carcinoma.[4] Pain from bony involvement by lymphomas can be relieved with only infrequent failure. Although metastases from squamous epithelial carcinomas (i.e., oral cavity, cervix) may be less responsive, a trial of local irradiation often is worthwhile.[5]

A careful program of periodic reassessment by x-ray followed by selective local irradiation can prevent the disaster of fracture through the tumor-involved, structural skeleton. These patients rarely require "prophylactic" orthopedic procedures.

In contrast, fracture through the tumor-weakened, weight-bearing skeleton, i.e., the femur, may require operative internal fixation so that the patient need not be bedfast. Although these "pathologic" fractures may "heal" following only the surgical fixation, postoperative irradiation is indicated. In a recent laboratory study,[2] new bone quickly formed at the site of "pathologic fracture" after internal fixation plus irradiation, while the fracture site calcified after internal fixation alone.

Bony metastases such as those from primary renal and thyroid carcinomas have been controlled by resection. Such treatment, usually advised when the tumor is "slowly" progressive, has tacitly implied better control with resection than is possible with irradiation. There is no confirmatory evidence. Indeed usually such patients eventually are irradiated when additional bony metastases are not resectable.

REVIEW QUESTIONS

1. Why are metastases to bone clinically important?

2. What carcinomas frequently metastasize to bone?

3. Which bones are most frequently involved by metastases?

4. Are bony metastases usually lytic or blastic? Which carcinoma frequently has osteoblastic metastases?

5. Is x-ray examination a sensitive detector of bony metastases? How does this knowledge influence you in a patient with cancer who has persistent bone-related pain but a "normal" x-ray?

6. Why is local irradiation better than surgery or chemotherapy for most bony metastases?

7. Is the success of local irradiation in the treatment of patients with bony metastases related to tumor type? to specific bone site? to the presence of fracture?

8. How would you treat a patient with carcinoma of the breast with a lytic metastasis in the neck of the femur? What if there was a fracture through the abnormal bone?

BIBLIOGRAPHY

1. ACKERMAN, L. V., and SPJUT, H. J. *Tumors of Bone and Cartilage. Atlas of Tumor Pathology*, Section II, Fascicle 4, Armed Forces Institute of Pathology, 1961.
2. BONARIGO, B. C., and RUBIN, P. Nonunion of pathologic fracture after radiation therapy. *Radiology*, 88:889–898, 1967.
3. BRIGGS, R. C. Detection of osseous metastases: Evaluation of bone scanning with Strontium-85. *Cancer*, 20:392–395, 1967.
4. PARKER, R. G., and HARRIS, A. Unpublished data.
5. ROMINGER, C. J., and HAHN, G. A. Roentgen therapy in palliation of bony metastases from carcinoma of cervix uteri. *Amer J Obstet Gynec*, 85:169–175, 1963.
6. RUBENFELD, S. Osseous manifestations in the malignant lymphomas. *Bull Hosp Joint Dis*, 17:271–280, 1956.
7. STUHLBARG, J., and ELLIS, F. W. Hodgkin's disease of bone. Favorable prognostic significance? *Amer J Roentgen*, 93:568–572, 1965.
8. VIETA, J. O., FRIEDELL, H. L., and CRAVER, L. F. A survey of Hodgkin's disease and lymphosarcoma in bone. *Radiology*, 39:1–15, 1942.

18

TUMORS
AND TUMORLIKE LESIONS
OF SOFT TISSUES

Reliable experience in the radiotherapy of soft tissue tumors is scarce because of the continuing difficulty of identification of specific tumor types and the continuing lack of a cohesive effort to study their response to radical irradiation. However, contrary to widespread opinion, soft tissue sarcomas may be surprisingly radio-responsive, and this response is not closely related to morphology.[6]

The tumors to be considered are of mesenchymal origin and consequently can arise anywhere in the body. Their histogenetic relationship results in common histological features. Specific tumors usually can be recognized by the predominant line of cellular differentiation. However, in some instances precise identification is not possible because there may be no predominant cellular differentiation, or there may be differentiation along several lines.[8] This histologic variation may be present in various parts of the same tumor and in the same tumor over a period of time, and may be modified by local changes, i.e., necrosis, hemorrhage, edema, and metaplasia.

Clinical correlation is as necessary for the pathologist as is pathological correlation for the clinician. Awareness of the usual anatomical distribution, relative frequency, age predilections, and gross growth characteristics of these tumors may lead to the correct diagnosis. Such correlation can prevent confusion (and mistreatment) between entities such as nodular fasciitis and fibrosarcoma. It can lend comfort to a diagnosis of cutaneous smooth muscle tumor, which infrequently is malignant. It can aid in the management of children with liposarcomas, as these tumors are less malignant than in the adult; or, conversely, it may be the basis for early radical treatment of rhabdomyosarcoma, which is more aggressive in children.

BENIGN AND MALIGNANT TUMORS AND TUMORLIKE LESIONS OF FIBROUS TISSUE

Keloids are exuberant, hyperplastic scars, covered by thin atrophic epithelium, resulting from proliferation of cutaneous fibroblasts. Clinical problems may follow surgical procedures or trauma, i.e., burns, and are more frequent in dark-skinned races. The fibroblasts in a fresh wound are highly radiovulnerable, but the mature keloid with degenerative change, poor vascularity, and little cellular activity is not.

358

Therefore, optimal treatment is preventative. The fresh wound of a known keloid-former should be irradiated within a few days after excision. After 1,500 R in seven to ten days in three increments with superficial x-ray, Brown and Bromberg[1] noted no regrowth of keloid in 18 of 30 patients and only partial regrowth in 10 of 30.

Dupuytren's contracture, a flexion deformity associated with palmar fibromatosis, and *Peyronie's disease,* a deformity associated with fibrosis in the sheath of the corpora cavernosa of the penis, have been reported[2, 10] to be responsive to small radiation doses. Any such response would seem most likely in those growths which are richly cellular and proliferative. Our own experiences with these problems have been disappointing.

Fibrosarcoma is an uncommon tumor arising from fibroblasts (and histiocytes[23]), usually in males. Histological diagnosis can be difficult because of the similarity between cellular fibromatoses and fibrosarcoma.[8, 23] These growths usually are found in external soft tissues, i.e., head, neck, trunk, and extremities, rather than in retroperitoneum, mediastinum, and various internal organs.[23] In Stout's[20] study of 41 patients with poorly differentiated fibrosarcomas, there was local recurrence in 31 of 41 (75.6 percent), distant metastases in 10 of 41 (24.4 percent), and 21 of 41 patients (50.1 percent) died with uncontrolled tumor. In a later study,[22] he found fibrosarcoma less malignant in children than in adults.

Fibrosarcomas are not considered radiocurable. This may be as much related to the tumor biology and the size when recognized as to the radiovulnerability. Most of these tumors will regress following doses in excess of 3,500 rads in three weeks.[17] Windeyer, Dische, and Mansfield,[24] in a study of 44 patients with fibrosarcoma of the soft tissues, found a high incidence of grossly complete regression of tumor following doses of 6,000–8,000 rads in five to nine weeks, although several lesions eventually recurred locally. Half of the 34 patients radically irradiated, usually in conjunction with resection, were alive and well over five years.

The high incidence of local tumor regrowth after resection should prompt a study of "routine" postoperative irradiation to high doses. Selective palliative use of radiotherapy frequently can be gratifying. We have noted good pain relief following local irradiation to moderate dose and, in a patient with widespread tumor, have clinically controlled a biopsy-proved fibrosarcoma involving the larynx and threatening the airway.

TUMORS OF MUSCLE

Malignant tumors of smooth muscle *(leiomyosarcomas)* are most frequent in the uterus, but may arise wherever there is involuntary muscle. These tumors rarely are radiotherapeutic problems.

Malignant tumors of striated muscle *(rhabdomyosarcomas)* may occur in two different clinical circumstances. These tumors in children, and occasionally in young adults, have been called embryonal rhabdomyosarcomas, although they may be more histologically differentiated than pleomorphic tumors in adults.[23] Two-thirds of these tumors arise in the urogenital tract, orbit, pharynx, nasal cavity, and auditory canal.[23] In contrast, 75 percent of rhabdomyosarcomas in the adult arise deep in the extremities or torso.[23]

The rhabdomyosarcomas of adults metastasize rapidly via blood vessels and lymphatics, and thus are incurable by local treatment methods.

Embryonal rhabdomyosarcomas of the head and neck in children, particularly those involving the orbit, have been controlled for several years following local irradiation to doses in excess of 5,000 rads in five weeks.[3,7] In our limited experience, embryonal rhabdomyosarcomas of the urogenital tract in children have been very radioresponsive but have always regrown (in one instance as late as two years after treatment) in spite of pelvic irradiation to assumed normal tissue tolerance. We are not aware of permanent control of this type of tumor in a male child. Occasionally, however, there has been an apparent "cure" in females following surgery.

TUMORS OF ADIPOSE TISSUE

Liposarcomas most frequently appear in the retroperitoneal region and the lower limbs.[8,23] Poorly differentiated tumors metastasize in at least 40 percent of patients,[23] usually via the bloodstream, often to lungs, liver, and pleura.

Liposarcomas apparently have a wide range of radiovulnerability. Stout[19] and del Regato[6] have noted that the well-differentiated, infrequently metastasizing myxoid variety may be particularly radiovulnerable. Perry and Chu[17] reported gross responses in those tumors receiving in excess of 2,900 rads (fractionation?). Friedman and Egan[11] controlled some tumors with very high doses (9,000 rads in 31 to 49 days). However, the uncertainty of response and the sequelae of high dosage favor resection if feasible. Local radical irradiation is advisable for small liposarcomas which may not be resectable, and postoperatively when removal has been incomplete.

TUMORS OF VASCULAR TISSUE

Hemangiomas are tumors or malformations occurring in many clinical forms. Radiation therapy has been used primarily for cavernous or "strawberry" lesions, which usually are cutaneous but may be subcutaneous.[9] At first these involutional angiomas may be highly cellular. Lister[14] initially documented a characteristic growth pattern of untreated cavernous hemangiomas: (1) gross appearance at or shortly after birth; (2) enlargement during the first six months of life; and (3) ultimate spontaneous regression in 90 percent and complete disappearance in most youngsters.

Management of patients with this deformity requires that the physician educate the parents and grandparents so that aggressive treatment, with ultimate unnecessary sequelae, can be avoided. Small doses of radiation may "abort" the early growth and may be followed by early regression. This treatment may be useful for hemangiomas in critical locations that interfere with vision or mastication or remain ulcerated and infected in the diaper area. On occasion, irradiation can be lifesaving when growing hemangiomas threaten the upper airway.

Hemangiopericytomas[18] are uncommon, richly vascular tumors which may arise anywhere in the body,[23] but most frequently involve the superficial soft tissues of the head and neck and extremities, the oral cavity, pharynx, uterus, and retro-peritoneum.[8] About 10 percent occur in children.[13] Metastases may be vascular or lymphatic.[21]

The variation in biological behavior makes short-term studies of control of little value. Friedman and Egan[12] studied the response of 13 tumors to irradiation and suggested that the "lethal irradiation dose" probably is high, but that useful palliation may result from 3,000 rads in 18 days. We have seen a small hemangio-pericytoma involving the pharyngeal tongue controlled by 5,500 rads in 6 weeks, although a tumor of pelvic soft tissue only temporarily responded to a dose of 6,000 rads in 6½ weeks.

Kaposi's disease most commonly affects males 40 to 60 years of age, although even children may be involved.[8] The typical clinical presentation is the appearance of multiple, vascular nodules in the dermis of the distal extremities. These nodules grow, coalesce, form plaques, and ulcerate. Skin of the trunk and head and neck and sometimes the oral and pharyngeal mucosa may be involved. Although the skin is the usual dominant site of involvement, all organs, particularly the gastro-intestinal tract, may be affected. These nodules usually are highly radioresponsive. Cohen and associates[4 5] noted local control in 83 percent of patients treated with the single dose equivalent of 1,000 rads. Oswald and Stam[16] controlled deep lesions with 2,500 rads in 4 weeks.

Nasopharyngeal angiofibromas usually occur in pubescent males,[8] causing periodic epistaxis, upper airway obstruction, and soft palatal deformity. Sometimes these lesions regress as the patient matures. Local excision has prompted massive hemorrhage. Local irradiation by implantation has proved effective without serious morbidity. In seven patients with extensive lesions causing local bone destruction, Massoud and Awwad[15] noted disappearance of the mass in three and regression in two following doses of 4,000 rads in five weeks.

REVIEW QUESTIONS

1. How reliable is existing information about the use of radiation therapy for soft tissue tumors? Why?

2. Can you name a few benign soft tissue tumors which may be treated by radiation methods? What are the ground rules of use of radiation therapy in these patients?

3. Which malignant tumors of soft tissue may be controlled by local irradiation? under what conditions?

4. Why is surgery usually the preferred treatment of patients with malignant soft tissue tumors?

5. Why might local irradiation be a useful adjuvant to surgery in the treatment of these patients?

BIBLIOGRAPHY

1. BROWN, J. R., and BROMBERG, J. H. Preliminary studies on effect of time-dose patterns in treatment of keloids. *Radiology*, 80:298–300, 1963.
2. BURFORD, E. H., GLENN, J. E., and BURFORD, C. E. Therapy of Peyronie's disease. *Urol Cutan Rev*, 55:337–338, 1951.
3. CASSADY, J. R., SAGERMAN, R. H., TRETTER, P., and ELLSWORTH, R. M. Radiation therapy for rhabdomyosarcoma. *Radiology*, 91:116–120, 1968.
4. COHEN, L. Dose, time and volume parameters in irradiation therapy of Kaposi's sarcoma. *Brit J Radiol*, 35:485–488, 1962.
5. COHEN, L., PALMER, P. E. S., and NICKSON, J. J. Treatment of Kaposi's sarcoma by radiation. *Acta Union Internat contra Cancrum*, 18:502–508, 1962.
6. DEL REGATO, J. A. Radiotherapy of soft tissue sarcomas. *JAMA*, 185:216–218, 1963.
7. EDLAND, R. W. Embryonal rhabdomyosarcoma. *Amer J Roentgen*, 93:671–685, 1965.
8. EVANS, R. W. *Histological Appearances of Tumours*. Livingstone, Edinburgh, 1966.
9. FAYOS, J., and LAMPE, I. Treatment of angiomas in infants. *Ann Radiol* (Paris), 8:53–59, 1965.
10. FINNEY, R. Dupuytren's contracture. *Brit J Radiol*, 28:610–614, 1955.
11. FRIEDMAN, M., and EGAN, J. W. Irradiation of liposarcoma. *Acta Radiol* [*Ther*], 54:225–238, 1960.
12. FRIEDMAN, M., and EGAN, J. W. Irradiation of hemangiopericytoma of Stout. *Radiology*, 74:721–730, 1960.
13. KAUFFMAN, S. L., and STOUT, A. P. Hemangiopericytoma in children. *Cancer*, 13:695–710, 1960.
14. LISTER, W. A. The natural history of strawberry nevi. *Lancet*, 1:1429–1434, 1938.
15. MASSOUD, G. E., and AWWAD, H. K. Nasopharyngeal fibroma: Its malignant potentialities and radiation therapy. *Clin Radiol*, 11:156–161, 1960.
16. OSWALD, F. H., and STAM, H. C. Roentgen treatment of Kaposi's disease. *Dermatologica (Basel)*, 136:277–280, 1968.
17. PERRY, H., and CHU, F. C. Radiation therapy in the palliative management of soft tissue sarcomas. *Cancer*, 15:179–183, 1962.
18. STOUT, A. P., and MURRAY, M. R. Hemangiopericytoma. A vascular tumor featuring Zimmerman's pericytes. *Ann Surg*, 116:26–33, 1942.
19. STOUT, A. P. Liposarcoma—the malignant tumors of lipoblasts. *Ann Surg*, 119:86–107, 1944.
20. STOUT, A. P. Fibrosarcoma—the malignant tumor of fibroblasts. *Cancer*, 1:30–63, 1948.
21. STOUT, A. P. Hemangiopericytoma. A study of twenty-five new cases. *Cancer*, 2:1027–1054, 1949.
22. STOUT, A. P. Fibrosarcoma in infants and children. *Cancer*, 15:1028–1040, 1962.
23. STOUT, A. P., and LATTES, R. *Tumors of the Soft Tissues*. Atlas of Tumor Pathology, Fasc. 1, Armed Forces Institute of Pathology, Washington, D.C., 1966.
24. WINDEYER, B., DISCHE, S., and MANSFIELD, C. M. The place of radiotherapy in the management of fibrosarcoma of the soft tissues. *Clin Radiology*, 17:32–40, 1966.

19

PALLIATIVE RADIATION THERAPY OF THE PATIENT WITH INCURABLE CANCER

To cure sometimes
To relieve often
To comfort and support always
Trudeau

He is the best physician
who is the best inspirer of hope
W. S. Middleton

I die by the help of too many physicians
Alexander the Great
on his death bed—323 B.C.

Palliative treatment of the patient with incurable cancer must be directed to the relief of specific distressing symptoms caused by or associated with neoplasm. Although these symptoms usually are present at the time of evaluation of the patient, occasionally such clinical developments can be anticipated with sufficient assurance that "preventive" treatment is justified. Relief of suffering remains distinct and often exclusive from prolongation of life. Prolongation of life of the suffering patient with incurable cancer is not palliation—it is prolongation of the process of dying. Rather than prolonging life, palliative therapy is at its best when it succeeds in favorably changing the mechanism of dying.

This objective—relief of suffering—often becomes obscured. Confusion of objectives is frequent because palliative treatment requires greater medical judgment than does curative treatment. Heroic treatment administered at great cost, inconvenience, and even discomfort to patients with incurable cancer is a very costly tuition for the inexperienced and uncertain physician.

Even with great experience in the observation of the very tortuous and inexplicable course of uncontrolled cancer in the human, direct correlation of treatment with its effect frequently is very difficult. Nonetheless, the accomplishments of palliative treatment are very real, and are more frequent, long-lasting, and predictable for the patient with cancer than for victims of many cardiovascular, renal, or neurological disorders.

Radiation therapy, used discriminately, is a major force in producing comfort for the patient with incurable cancer. Sixty to 75 percent of all patients with cancer may receive radiation therapy at some time. However, no modality has been so misused. Some clinicians ask that radiation therapy be used in nearly all "hopeless situations." By this definition, every patient with incurable cancer who does not have convulsions and thus can lie still should be treated. Disappointment follows either the radiotherapist's justified refusal to treat or the unnecesarily frequent failure of accomplishment when treatment is applied in this indiscriminate fashion. Other clinicians so fear the potential complications of radiation therapy that its usefulness is rarely demonstrated. This unfortunate attitude may promote forms of treatment which have less potential reward and greater morbidity for the patient.

When cure is the objective, radiation therapy is a radical treatment form, and a modest complication rate is expected and licensed. If treatment fails, palliation often is a begrundgingly accepted bonus. This unscheduled palliation is not the issue in this discussion. When the initial objective of radiation therapy is palliation, new ground rules must be applied: Serious complications or slowly self-limiting side effects of treatment are no longer acceptable; overall treatment times must be short; cost to the patient must be minimized; convenience of treatment becomes a major consideration.

The therapeutic radiologist must have a clear concept of the potential accomplishments of other treatment modalities, such as neurosurgery, anesthesiology, chemotherapy, and pharmacology, so that he may use his own method in proper perspective.

Indications and contraindications for palliative radiation therapy can be based on performance records of the care of many patients over many years. These indications and contraindications will continue to change, however, for the understanding of the radiobiological response of tumors continues to increase; improvement in equipment permits the administration of larger doses with less treatment-produced discomfort in ever-increasing numbers of situations; and improved ancillary care makes palliative treatment reasonable in new situations.

Failure to insist on definite indications and contraindications for palliative, as well as radical, radiation therapy too often is shared by radiologists who have not developed competence in therapeutic radiology. As noted by Wangensteen,[5] "The limitation of a method constitutes no reflection upon its user, save insofar as he fails to recognize it."

OBJECTIVES OF PALLIATIVE RADIATION THERAPY

Relief of Pain

Pain is a most important symptom for the patient with incurable cancer. It may disrupt the life of an otherwise functional person. This pain may cover a broad spectrum of severity and characteristics. For treatment to be maximally effective, the underlying cause must be determined.

Metastatic tumor in bone is a frequent source of pain. Except when this pain is secondary to a specific structural change, such as verterbral collapse with nerve root compression, the response to radiation can be correlated reasonably well to tumor type. Carcinoma of the breast is the most frequent source of this clinical problem. If only a few sites of skeletal involvement require medical attention, local irradiation is the best available treatment, producing rapid, complete pain relief in at least 90 percent[3] of these patients. This favorable response is not related to anatomical site of involvement, histological or roentgenological appearance of the lesions, age or hormonal status of the patient, or to rate of progression of tumor. Only a minority of lytic metastatic lesions will recalcify or reossify following radiation,[3] but pain relief is independent of this objective sign of improvement. The clinical use of ionizing radiation reaches practical limitations when new sites of involvement appear with increased tempo, making it unreasonable to treat the great number of painful metastatic sites present. Although hormonal or chemical treatment is preferable in these situations, selective irradiation may be indicated for critical sites.

Bony metastases from many other tumors, such as neuroblastoma, lymphoma, and small-cell carcinoma of the bronchus, are radiation-sensitive. Rapid, complete pain relief and control of the local lesion can be expected with modest dosage delivered in a short time.

Bony metastases from more differentiated carcinomas, such as those of the prostate, thyroid, renal parenchyma, and bronchus, exhibit less predictable responses. However, in most instances treatment will be worthwhile.

The treatment of well-differentiated metastases from carcinoma of the endometrium, pancreas, and gastrointestinal tract often is disappointing. This is also true for bony metastases secondary to carcinoma of the cervix, in spite of the good response of the tumor within the pelvis. Use of radiation therapy in these circumstances rarely is preferable to more rapid and certain methods, such as cordotomy or nerve block.

Primary tumors of bone have a broad spectrum of radioresponsiveness. In general, osteosarcomas and chondrosarcomas are minimally responsive, although the response of certain components of these tumors can result in significant pain relief. In contrast, Ewing's tumor can be locally sterilized by irradiation, and pain relief following administration of modest doses should be rapid and complete. The responsiveness of myeloma varies markedly, and consequently is unpredictable in the individual patient. However, pain relief incident to myeloma occurs sufficiently often to justify vigorous therapeutic trial. It is not unusual for patients with wide-spread myeloma to resume useful, vigorous activity for many months, or even years, after irradiation of painful bony sites in the supporting skeleton.

When pain results from tumor directly involving peripheral nerves, relief following local irradiation is problematic, regardless of tumor type. For example, pain secondary to sacral plexus invasion in patients with carcinoma of the cervix or rectum, extensions into the pterygoid space in patients with cancer of the maxillary sinus, or involvement of cranial nerves from extension of carcinoma of the nasopharynx infrequently is relieved by irradiation. Therefore, when applicable, other methods of obtaining pain relief are preferable.

A tumor mass may produce severe pain because of its strategic location—beneath the liver capsule, in the pleura, in the axilla, or on the scalp. Indications for radiation therapy in these circumstances must be viewed in the perspective of the entire clinical problem. Such local treatment, however, is well-tolerated and avoids the systemic side effects of chemotherapy.

Unrelenting headache, associated with increased intracranial pressure in patients with cerebral gliomas, is not rapidly responsive to irradiation. Therefore, radiation therapy, if appropriate, best follows decompression, either by surgery or by adrenocortical steroids. Headache and neurologic symptoms and signs secondary to intracranial metastases (most commonly from bronchus or breast) often may be effectively palliated by irradiation. The response to irradiation usually parallels the response of the primary tumor or other metastases from the same primary. Indications for treatment of intracranial metastases should be based on an evaluation of the patient's entire clinical situation.

The severe, throbbing headache secondary to superior vena caval obstruction in patients with carcinoma of the bronchus usually can be relieved with radiation therapy. Mediastinal embarrassment rarely is caused by highly differentiated carcinomas which grow more slowly, but is more commonly related to rapidly growing, less differentiated types, such as oat-cell or small-cell carcinoma or undifferentiated carcinoma or lymphoma—tumor types which also respond readily to irradiation. Because of the greater likelihood of response to irradiation and the longer duration of effect, radiation therapy is superior to chemotherapy in this distressing clinical situation.

The excruciating pain of splenic infarction in the patient with leukemia may be quickly responsive to modest doses of local irradiation.

Prevention of Fracture

When bone is compromised by tumor, ordinary stress may produce fracture. If the bone is part of the weight-bearing skeleton, the resulting disability may be a major clinical problem throughout the remaining life of this unfortunate patient. Consequently, selective irradiation of sites where weight-bearing bone is structurally compromised, even in the absence of symptoms, can be considered palliative treatment through prevention of disability. Useful reconstruction of bone capable of bearing weight can follow irradiation of many of these lesions, whether they be primary, such as Ewing's tumor, or metastatic from various sites.

Once a pathologic fracture of a weight-bearing bone has occurred, if the general condition of the patient is good enough to assume a reasonably long life expectancy, irradiation usually should be preceded by fixation of the fractured bone so that the patient can be kept as active as possible.

Control of Blood Loss

Visible blood loss causes great anxiety for the patient, the relatives, nurses, and physicians. Although treatment to suppress blood loss may be medically beneficial, medical custom and emotion-clouded therapeutic decisions can, on occasion, lead to treatment that cannot be considered palliative. For example, this latter situation has occurred when the patient with incurable cancer of the cervix has been successfully treated for the supression of painless hemorrhage, only ultimately to suffer intractable pain from invasion of the sacral plexus by tumor.

The clinical problem of gross bleeding is frequent in patients with cancers of the uterine cervix, uterine corpus, oral cavity, pharynx, bronchus, or urinary bladder. Local irradiation of these lesions usually results in a decrease or cessation of gross blood loss. Because of the effectiveness and minimal morbidity, local radiation therapy is usually the treatment of choice in these situations. It must be realized, however, that the doses necessary for sustained supression of bleeding often approach those necessary for tumor control. In comparison, bleeding from cancer of the kidney is inconsistently and slowly responsive to radiation, often making resection the preferable treatment.

Blood loss from hemolysis, a frequent problem in patients with lymphoma, may cease after radiation-produced reduction of tumor masses or tumor-enlarged spleen.

Relief of Obstruction

Obstruction of organ lumina can cause severe distress. Ureteral obstruction, always a grave prognostic sign, is the most common cause of death of the patient with uncontrolled cancer of the cervix. Pelvic irradiation to high dosage may, on occasion, relieve ureteral obstruction and preserve renal function. However, in the previously treated patient with progressing and uncontrollable cancer of the cervix, uremia may be the least uncomfortable mode of exitus and should not be combated by definitive treatment. Tumors of the urinary bladder may cause ureteral obstruction at the ureterovesical junction. This finding alone would not seem an objective of palliative treatment.

Treatment of intestinal tract obstruction varies with specific anatomical sites and specific tumor types. In carcinoma of the esophagus, objectives of treatment with currently available methods must be based on the philosophy of the physician and the patient. With realization that by any treatment method only 5 to 10 percent of these patients are cured, relief of mechanical obstruction can be a worthwhile primary objective best accomplished with minimal treatment-produced morbidity. Establishment of normal or nearly normal esophageal passage can be accomplished by irradiation in at least 50 percent of patients, and once it is accomplished the esophagus tends to remain patent until the patient dies from progressing disease elsewhere. Because of a moderate degree of predictability of radiation response based on the gross and microscopic appearance of carcinoma of the esophagus, palliative radiation treatment should be selective. Bulky, exophytic squamous cell carcinomas, causing obstruction from protrusion into the esophageal lumen, usually will respond rapidly to irradiation, and will remain controlled locally while the tumor progresses elsewhere. In elderly patients, such treatment, on an outpatient basis, may be preferable to any other. When the carcinoma infiltrates the esophageal wall producing stenosis, relief of obstruction is not frequent even when the tumor is controlled by radiation therapy. In those lesions with deep ulceration, perforation secondary to uncontrolled tumor is probable, and may occur with dispatch following local irradiation. In the latter two situations, palliation may be more certain with surgical resection or bypass, or even intubaton. Lymphomas of the stomach may produce obstruction, in addition to discomfort, bleeding, and alteration of the digestive process. Radiation treatment may locally control the neoplasm with less morbidity than that associated with gastric resection. Inoperable esophageal adenocarcinoma involving the cardia, causing esophageal obstruction, responds rather predictably to irradiation so that the potency of the esophageal lumen can be re-established until the patient dies of other cause, i.e., hepatic metastases. Other intrinsic lesions obstructing the intestinal tract are rarely amenable to radiation treatment. Obstruction incident to compression from a radiation-responsive tumor adjacent to the intestine might be relieved by treatment, although this situation is infrequent.

Obstruction of the flow of cerebrospinal fluid is a major clinical problem caused by intracranial tumors. Surgical relief by shunting often is the definitive treatment of choice. When obstruction is produced by a radioresponsive lesion, irradiation may be indicated after surgical shunting.

Bronchial obstruction with peripheral pulmonary atelectasis and infection can cause major morbidity for the patient with nonremovable carcinoma of the bronchus. This peripheral pulmonary infection is rarely controlled by antibiotics unless adequate drainage through the bronchus can be established. Radiation therapy usually can provide patency of the lumen, making resolution of infection possible. Relief of broncial obstruction causing atelectasis may be followed by recovery of functional lung, an accomplishment of importance to the patient with borderline pulmonary function.

Malignant tumor infiltrating the mediastinum can cause distressing symptoms by compression of the trachea, major bronchi, or large vessels. Long-persistent misconceptions regarding mediastinal irradiation in this situation deserve clarification. Indiscriminate and technically incorrect radiation usage and lack of comprehension that rapidly growing neoplasm itself can close off the airway have propagated the myth that mediastinal irradiation will cause radiation edema and thus aggravate the condition, and that irradiation should therefore be preceded by chemotherapy. Properly conducted irradiation does not accentuate airway embarrassment. Mediastinal irradiation is preferable to chemotherapy because its desired tumoricidal effects may appear as rapidly, will be more long-lasting, and may be achieved without the unwelcome penalty of systemic reaction. Necessary dosage varies with type and volume of tumor. Leukemic or lymphosarcomatous masses and some thymomas may respond quickly to very small doses, while highly differentiated carcinomas (bronchus, breast) respond only to high dosage.

Mediastinal tumor of less extent but of strategic location may produce great morbidity from unrelenting cough. Relief following local irradiation may be obtained at the price of making tracheal and bronchial secretions viscid and sparse.

Tumor masses may compress and consequently obstruct blood and lymphatic vessels serving the extremities. This dire circumstance may be relieved by local irradiation. The rapid response of highly sensitive tumors, such as seminoma or lymphosarcoma in axillary, inguinal, or iliac nodes, has resulted in dramatic improvement of extremities in peril. In this situation, considerations of tissue tolerance and urgency for relief may dictate treatment of a small volume at the site of obstruction with a calculated indifference to adjacent tumor.

Healing of Ulcerated Lesions

Ulcerated, infected, bleeding surface lesions, even if no major threat, may be a concern to the patient and may result in a nursing problem. Such lesions on the chest wall of the patient with carcinoma of the breast, when they are not amenable to resection, may be controlled for the duration of the life of the victim by local irradiation. Tumor growing in the perineal scar following resection for carcinoma of the rectum may be controlled with judicious local irradiation. Ulcerated cancerous lesions involving the vaginal apex of the patient with incurable intrapelvic malignant tumor may likewise respond to local treatment, usually best accomplished with an intravaginal application.

Local Tumor Control for a Specific Purpose

Occasionally, a particular tumor mass may cause disproportionate distress to a patient with widespread cancer. This may result from tumor on the eyelid disturbing vision, or tumor in the orbit causing proptosis and diplopia or interfering with the motion of the eye. The latter situation, usually seen in patients with lymphoma, can be dramatically relieved by small doses of radiation. Tumor about the tracheostomy stoma may be the basis of apprehension before bleeding or obstruction is of concern. Sometimes a mass will cause difficulty by interfering with clothing, or it may cause a concern for appearance, or it may be on the scalp and repeatedly irritated by a comb. Local treatment, whether surgery or irradiation, need be decided in the overall perspective of the patient's illness, but often attention to seemingly small complaints results in a large measure of comfort.

Tumor Growth Restraint

Restraint of tumor growth, like palliation itself, is difficult to assess, for the natural history of tumors may include periods of quiescence. However, useful suppression of growth unequivocally may follow irradiation ("cancerostatic effect"). In his comprehensive observations on radiation therapy of gliomas, Bouchard[1] has emphasized that prolongation of useful life can be accomplished presumably by slowing the relentless progression of intracranial tumor. Growth suppression may be a major objective for the patient with carcinoma of the ovary or carcinoma of the breast, with chest wall recurrence or effusion from a serous surface; or in carcinoma of the thyroid with local extension or regional node metastases; or in malignancies of salivary gland origin.

Prevention of Fistula

Uncontrolled cancer in strategic sites may cause a fistula. The clinical problem is most frequent in patients with carcinoma of the cervix or vagina with involvement of the rectovaginal septum or base of the bladder, or in patients with neoplasms of the trachea, bronchus, or thoracic esophagus with local extension. If unsuccessful in these circumstances, radiation therapy, rather than uncontrolled tumor, may be incorrectly indicted as the cause of the fistula. If cancer of the cervix, bronchus, or esophagus is locally controlled by well-administered radiation therapy, fistulas are rare. In situations in which formation of a fistula is imminent and its avoidance is one of the purposes of treatment, it is important to treat slowly to avoid rapid dissolution of tumor and to allow for fibroblastic repair.

Relief of Neurologic Deficits

Strategically situated neoplasms may cause specific neurologic deficits of clinical importance. Retrobular tumor, most frequent in patients with leukemia or lymphosarcoma, may produce optic atrophy in addition to proptosis, diplopia, interference with eye motion, and corneal ulceration. Retinal metastases are at times seen in carcinoma of the breast. Promptly instituted local irradiation may relieve or avoid these problems so that vision is retained during the patient's lifetime. Cranial nerve palsy (most frequently the abducens nerve) from intracranial metastasis or direct tumor extension from the nasopharynx may be relieved by local irradiation. Encroachment on the spinal cord from metastasis or direct tumor extension initially should be relieved by surgical decompression in most instances. The effect of radiation therapy even on highly responsive tumors such as lymphomas, usually is too slow to avoid permanent cord damage once neurologic deficit has developed and is progressing. However, postdecompression irradiation is necessary as the definitive treatment to prevent progression of tumor and recurrence of the clinical problem. Some patients with lymphomas causing minimal spinal cord compression have been treated successfully by initial use of chemotherapy (i.e., nitrogen mustard), followed immediately by irradiation. This avoidance of laminectomy in very ill patients is possible only through close cooperation between neurosurgeon and radiotherapist, and is possible only during the very early period of threat to spinal cord viability.

Patients with cancer, usually primary in the bronchus, may be victims of remote effects on the nervous system. These clinical presentations include encephalopathies, myelopathies, neuropathies, and muscular disorders. They are not amenable to any known form of therapy except removal or destruction of the offending neoplasm.

Myasthenia gravis associated with thymic neoplasms is at times very effectively treated by irradiation.[2] In a number of our own patients, significant and continued improvement has been accomplished without surgery. It also appears that the operative risk is significantly smaller if surgery follows irradiation.

Relief of Systemic Symptoms and Signs

Patients with sizable tumor masses, particularly lymphoma or anaplastic carcinoma, may have fever, night sweats, maliase, anorexia, weight loss, and pruritus. Relief may follow local irradiation of the large masses, much as similar complaints associated with widespread tumor may respond to systemic therapy.

RADIATION THERAPY AS A PLACEBO

Requests for the use of radiation therapy as a placebo for the patient and/or the relatives or referring physician continue to plague the therapeutic radiologist, although the emergence of chemotherapy has undoubtedly lightened this burden. This deplorable practice has flourished because the radiologist has not exercised the equivalent of surgical judgment. Abdication of this responsibility has resulted in therapeutic gestures that are senseless, costly, and dangerous. To add needlessly the morbidity of futile treatment to the already overburdened patient is the trademark of an ineffective physician. Such a demonstration of therapeutic futility brings good radiation therapy into disrepute, with a consequent loss of opportunity to apply the method in a useful situation.

OPPORTUNITIES OF THE THERAPEUTIC RADIOLOGIST

Treatment of the patient with cancer demands more than technical excellence. Because of daily contact during treatment and continuing contact through follow-up examinations, the therapeutic radiologist has an unequalled opportunity to gain the confidence of the patient. If this opportunity is squandered, care of the patient during this very difficult time will be less than optimal. The patient, the family, and the referring physician will have reason to consider therapeutic radiology a technical specialty, far removed from clinical medicine.

CONCLUSION

Care of the patient with incurable cancer may be directed by physicians of various backgrounds and persuasions. If the involved physician has little experience in the care of such patients, he is likely to be influenced by the still prevalent attitude of therapeutic futility or by equally unjustified premature claims for widely publicized, but unproved methods recently on the scene. Surgery and radiation therapy remain the dominant therapeutic forces for the patient with cancer. It is unfortunate that a failure to demonstrate good radiation therapy has led to unjustified condemnation of the method rather than the user, with resultant loss to the patient's welfare. To obtain maximal benefits, radiation therapy must be allowed indications and contraindications like any other therapeutic modality. These choices must be the responsibility of the therapeutic radiologist, not of the referring physician. Application of realistically stringent indications and contraindications does not lessen but rather enhances useful accomplishment, and avoids unnecessary morbidity, waste of time, money, and effort, and sometimes, more importantly, delay in seeking more suitable treatment.

REVIEW QUESTIONS

1. What is the objective of palliative treatment of the patient with incurable cancer?

2. Has it been your experience that palliative treatment of patients with cancer has been of less interest to physicians than care of patients with incurable diseases of the heart, kidney, lung, and central nervous system?

3. What are the possible objectives of palliative radiotherapy of the patient with cancer? Can you give examples for each objective? Have you seen these yourself?

4. How radioresponsive is breast carcinoma metastatic in bone? How does this compare with breast carcinoma in its primary site or in lymph nodes?

5. Why should victims of breast carcinoma, especially those with bony metastases, have periodic roentgenologic assessments of the skeleton?

merit palliative radiotherapy?

6. What primary malignant tumors of bone may be sufficiently radiation-responsive to

7. For the patient with uncontrollable carcinoma of the cervix (post-treatment), is relief of tumor-produced ureteral obstruction a reasonable objective?

8. How often can tumor-produced esophageal obstruction be relieved by irradiation? What is the treatment-produced morbidity? How does this compare with surgery? How does accomplishment of this objective affect the patient's course?

9. Why is it unnecessary to precede radiation therapy by chemotherapy in the treatment of patients with malignant mediastinal tumors compressing vital structures?

10. What is the usual cause of vesicovaginal or rectovaginal fistula in patients with carcinoma of the cervix?

11. If a patient with radiosensitive tumor suffers quickly recognized and progressive neurological deficit of the lower limbs or bladder, what is the proper treatment?

12. Why is radiation therapy an illogical placebo for patients with incurable cancer?

13. Have you seen radiation therapy criticized as a treatment modality when it was misused, and thus the physician's responsibility? How does such an incorrect appraisal adversely affect care of the patient with cancer?

BIBLIOGRAPHY

1. BOUCHARD, J. Radiation therapy of malignant intracranial neoplasms. In: *Progress in Radiation Therapy*, Vol. I. F. Buschke, Ed, Grune & Stratton, New York, 1958, pp. 192–223.
2. PHILLIPS, T., and BUSCHKE, F. Role of radiation therapy in myasthenia gravis. *Calif Med*, 106:282–289, 1967.
3. PARKER, R. G., and HARRIS, A. Unpublished study on treatment of bony metastases, 1964.
4. PATERSON, R. Radiological achievement, 1937–1950. *Amer J Roentgen*, 66:521–526, 1951.
5. WANGENSTEEN, O., quoted by Ross, S. E. *JAMA*, 174:2224–2225, 1960.

20

SOME BASIC PRINCIPLES
OF RADIATION THERAPY
OF CANCER

1. For the cancer patient who is potentially "curable," the initial therapeutic procedure usually determines the outcome. In contrast to many other diseases, errors in initial management of the patient with cancer seldom can be corrected. At best, the patient may have one chance for "cure."

2. Cancer rarely is a medical emergency. With infrequent exception, there is time for thorough evaluation of the patient prior to starting treatment. A final decision regarding treatment must await the completion of careful diagnostic work-up. Sometimes it is advantageous to examine a patient several times in order to correctly appraise tumor extent as a proper basis for treatment planning. The damage resulting from a hasty, erroneous initial treatment is greater than that from a reasonable diagnostic delay. The anxieties of the patient, the relatives, and referring physician should not harrass the responsible radiotherapist into ill-considered decisions and premature institution of treatment. Two possible exceptions are patients with tumor-produced progressing mediastinal compression syndrome or spinal cord compression. In these circumstances, institution of proper treatment is an emergency, and exhaustive pre-treatment evaluation is unreasonable.

3. Definitive treatment of a patient with cancer should not be started where it cannot be continued and completed. Many potentially curable patients have become incurable because of injudicious initial management.

4. In the treatment of a patient with a specific cancer, all radiotherapeutic maneuvers are components of a single comprehensive treatment program, and must be the responsibility of a single qualified physician.

5. With current knowledge (or ignorance), no single therapeutic program (including those recommended in this book) is likely to be the only "correct" method. If there is a choice, the therapist should select the method best known to him.

6. The radiation therapist is more important than the equipment. However, good therapists and good equipment usually are found together.

7. Incurable cancer patients are penalized by physician disinterest. Palliative treatment of this appreciative group should be as rewarding as the treatment of those with incurable neurological, pulmonary, renal, and cardiovascular diseases.

8. Despite continued use, orthovoltage x-ray, with some exceptions, should be a part of our history. Both the tumor control and the tissue damage following

orthovoltage x-ray therapy, as previously conducted, should be disregarded in the evaluation of the efficacy of present-day radiation therapy.

9. Radiation therapy was born about 1900, and thus is a medical adolescent. Other specialties, even after a longer time for development, were practiced by tribal chiefs and barbers.

10. For some cancers, such as those of the bladder or esophagus, the radiation dose for effective palliation may approximate that for curative treatment. However, treatment-related morbidity may be minimized by irradiation of a smaller tissue volume when palliation is the objective.

11. One thousand rads per week to 6,000 rads total dose is not necessarily an optimal "cancerocidal" dose. Rather, it is an approximate limit of the tolerance of normal vasculo-connective tissues to radiation. Early and late tissue damage of clinical significance often can be minimized by restriction of dosage to 900 rads per week.

12. In evaluating a patient for radiation therapy, tumor type and histological differentiation may be relatively minor factors compared to tumor site, tumor extent, and condition of the patient.

13. A treatment method is not clinically useful if, in order to be effective against tumor, it causes serious early or late damage to normal tissues. It is unreasonable to subject nearly all patients to severe sequelae in an attempt to occasionally salvage a patient.

14. Radiation therapy, like surgery, is a local treatment method. Consequently, despite a desire for cure, local tumor control often is the best measure of therapeutic effectiveness.

15. Radiation therapy, like surgery, is a local treatment method. Therefore, treatment-produced complications tend to be local and can be related to treatment application. All adverse developments in a patient considered for, undergoing, or having completed radiation treatment are not radiation-related. For example, if during a course of pelvic irradiation, a patient develops the symptoms and signs of appendicitis, it may be appendicitis rather than "radiation reaction." Indiscriminate use of radiation therapy as a scapegoat by the ill-informed physican subjects the patient to unnecessary delay in establishment of the correct diagnosis and consequent institution of proper corrective measures.

16. In general, late-appearing radiation-produced damage of normal tissue is a reflection of damage detectable during or shortly after treatment. Therefore, minimization of reactions at the time of treatment will reduce unwelcome problems in survivors. ". . . Generally the patient who does not suffer during treatment rarely encounters complications after treatment." (Lederman).

17. Radiation damage to the vasculoconnective tissue not only is related to total dose, but also to the pattern of application.

18. Radical radiation therapy is a major procedure, and the resultant morbidity may be at least as great as with radical surgery. Therefore, such radiation treatment is not necessarily licensed by the surgeon's judgment that the patient would not tolerate surgery.

19. Failures of radiation therapy may be biological, or they may be secondary to human errors in application.

20. Adequate management of patients with many forms of cancer requires well-coordinated teamwork between all involved physicians, including the family

doctor, surgeon, radiotherapist, chemotherapist, and pathologist. This necessary teamwork means continued personal cooperation between members, not referral from one office to another. This cooperation includes pretreatment evaluation, re-evaluation during treatment and post-treatment follow-up. Such cooperative evaluation of the patient by members of the team is necessary even when one member, such as the surgeon or radiotherapist, accepts primary responsibility for treatment.

21. Although management of the patient with cancer should be based on a composite of qualified opinion, decisions of a tumor board at which all attendants have an equal vote often is bad medicine practiced democratically. The usefulness of a tumor board is proportional to the competence of its members. Regimented rotation of membership assignments is not conducive to optimal function. Lack of a tumor board is preferable to one with assigned members who are uninterested or incompetent in dealing with problems related to malignant tumors.

22. If the opinions of qualified consultants, such as the pathologist, are inconsistent with the clinical evidence, both their opinions and yours need be re-evaluated. The pathologist's report is not gospel. Interpretation of the report often requires an awareness, possible only with prolonged cooperation, of the pathologist's experience, philosophy, and prejudices. Often a definitive diagnosis is not possible by histological examination of the material available. In these circumstances, it is useless to send the material to judges residing at great distances. Sometimes integration of the pathologist's findings with the clinical findings leads to a seemingly proper diagnosis. If diagnostic conflict persists, carefully considered clinical evidence often must prevail.

23. The overall impact of slowly improving methods of definitive cancer treatment could be greatly enhanced by better initial clinical recognition of the protean manifestations of this group of neoplasms. This could be accomplished, despite current limitations of knowledge, by better educational programs for students and practitioners.

24. Therapeutic radiologists remain so scarce that they should minimize all physical risks by riding only on authorized commercial airplanes and avoiding violent arguments.

GLOSSARY

Abscopal Effect An effect produced at a site outside the irradiated volume in a living object.

Acanthosis Nigricans A pigmented regional papillomatosis of skin; in the adult usually related to the development of a carcinoma of internal organs.

Adenoacanthoma An adenocarcinoma containing foci of metaplastic squamous epithelium.

Adenocarcinoma A cancer of epithelial origin in which there is glandlike arrangement of cells.

Alkaloids Organic bases containing nitrogen; most important drugs from plants are in this category.

Alkylating Agents Heterogeneous chemical agents which contain alkyl radicals; frequently used in cancer chemotherapy; example is nitrogen mustard.

Alpha ray Stream of alpha particles, which are helium nuclei.

Anal Canal A channel of varying diameter extending 1–1.5 inches in the long axis from the anal orifice to the level of the puborectalis muscle.

Anal Margin (Anal Orifice) Terminal opening of the gastrointestinal tract starting at the level of the anal valves and extending 1.0–1.5 cm to include perianal skin.

Analogue Inhibitors These include agents which prevent the formation of nucleic acid bases (methotrexate, 5-FU) or interfere with utilization of preformed bases (6-mercaptopurine).

Astrocytoma A type of glioma arising from astrocytes.

Atrophy An acquired reduction in size of a cell, tissue, or organ.

Backscatter Ionizing radiation scattered backwards in the direction of the incident beam by an irradiated object.

Basal Cell Carcinoma A term for a group of tumors characterized by: (1) cells resembling immature cells of the epidermis and appendages; (2) a predominantly intradermal development; and (3) resemblance to various adnexal structures. Tumors are locally invasive but do not metastasize.

Bowen's Disease A cancer in situ of the skin clinically manifest as a dull red, scaly plaque; the histological appearance is not always distinctive; may become an invasive squamous cell carcinoma.

Cancer A term inclusive of a variety of malignant neoplasms; derived from the Latin word for "crab."

Cancer Incidence The number of patients newly diagnosed in a unit time from within a defined population; often expressed as the ratio of new cases per unit population (rate).

Cancer Prevalence The total number of patients (old or new) with cancer present during a unit time within a defined population.

Cancerocidal Destructive of cancer; used as an ill-defined description of radiation doses expected to destroy cancer.

Carcinogenesis Production of cancer.

Carcinoma A malignant neoplasm of epithelial origin.

376

Cell Reproductive or Replication Cycle   Progression of a cell through a series of orderly, repetitive events, including DNA synthesis and mitosis with consequent reproduction of the cell.

Cesium-137   A radioactive isotope with a half-life of 30 years which decays to 137Ba which emits gamma radiations with an energy of 660 kev; used as a teletherapy source and in interstitial and intracavitary applicators.

Cobalt-60   A radioactive isotope with a half-life of 5.3 years which emits beta and gamma (1.17 and 1.33 Mev) radiations; used as a teletherapy source and in interstitial and intracavitary applicators.

Corpuscular Radiation   Subatomic particles such as protons, electrons, neutrons, alphas traveling together at high velocities.

"Coutard's Law"   The point of origin of a carcinoma of a mucous membrane is the last to heal following radiation therapy.

Coutard's Method   The clinical application of ionizing, photon radiation in daily increments for several weeks in an attempt to favorably exploit differences in postirradiation recovery of tumor and normal cells. Popularized by Henri Coutard (1876–1950), a French radio-therapist.

Critical Volume of Tissue   That tissue volume containing the entire cancer and minimal adjacent normal tissues, which must be irradiated to a "cancerocidal" dose if the tumor is to be controlled locally.

Cure   Actually implies complete restitution to the pre-disease status; may be used for that situation when, after a disease-free post-treatment interval, the survivors have a progressive death rate from *all* causes similar to that of a normal population of the same age.

Cyclotron   A particle accelerator in which ions, such as protons or deuterons, while traveling in a circular path, are subjected to a series of "pushes" of relatively low voltage by a combination of a constant, powerful magnetic field and an alternating high frequency electric charge.

Deep X-ray   The range of orthovoltage x-ray which is most energetic and formerly was used to treat tumors deep to the body surface.

Depth Dose   See relative depth dose.

Direct Effect   A radiation effect resulting from the absorption of energy directly in critical sites or targets.

DNA (Deoxyribonucleic Acid)   A macromolecule composed of deoxynucleotides which carries the genetic information to direct the synthesis of RNA and, ultimately, specific proteins.

D_0 Dose   That dose of ionizing radiation which results in a surviving fraction of 0.37 on the exponential portion of the dose-survival curve.

Electromagnetic Radiation   Rhythmic electric and magnetic oscillations or wave motions traveling at the same speed. Examples: radio waves, infrared rays, visible light, ultraviolet light, roentgen rays, gamma rays.

Electron   An atomic particle with a negative electric charge of 4.803×10^{-10} e.s.u. and a mass of 9.107×10^{-28} gram.

Ependymoma   A glioma arising from the ependymal cells lining the ventricular system of the brain, the central canal of the spinal cord, and the ventriculus terminalis of the conus medullaris of the spinal cord.

Epidermoid Carcinoma   A cancer arising from stratified squamous epithelial surfaces; usually used interchangeably with squamous cell carcinoma, although occasionally the term is used to include both squamous cell and basal cell carcinomas.

Erythroplasia of Queyrat   A dyskeratotic, disorderly proliferative change of the epithelium of the glans penis (or inner prepuce) which is analagous to Bowen's disease and can be considered carcinoma in situ.

Esthesioneuroepithelioma, Olfactory (Olfactory Neuroblastoma, Esthesioneuroblastoma, Esthesioneurocytoma)   A rare, distinctive malignant tumor arising high in the nasal cavity, usually above the middle turbinate; probably arises from neuroepithelial elements of olfactory membrane; has histological features of neuroblastoma; usually is slow-growing and radiosensitive.

Ewing's Tumor   A controversial, highly anaplastic, small, round cell sarcoma considered to arise in bone.

Excitation A means of absorption of energy by an atom or molecule in which the electrons are not ejected from the orbits of the atom.

External Irradiation Irradiation from a source separated from the absorber.

Extraneous Volume of Tissue That tissue volume which surrounds the critical volume and can be selectively avoided while adequately irradiating the cancer.

Fractionation Delivery of a total radiation dose in multiple increments.

Gamma Ray Electromagnetic (photon) radiation which is emited from an unstable atomic nucleus and travels nearly at the speed of light in free space. Examples: radiations from radium-226, cobalt-60, cesium-137.

Glioblastoma Multiforme A biologically aggressive, histologically poorly differentiated glioma of astrocytic origin.

Glioma A tumor originating in cells of the neuroglia or their antecedents.

Glottis The voice-producing apparatus consisting of the true vocal cords and the intervening space.

Gold, Radioactive (^{198}Au) A radioactive isotope with a half-life of 2.7 days which emits beta (960 kev) and gamma (412 kev) radiation; used in small sources (grains) as a permanent interstitial implant and in colloidal form to suppress malignant serous effusions.

Half value layer (HVL) The thickness of a specific material which reduces the flux of radiation by one-half; a function of voltage, filtration, and target material; used as a rough gauge of radiation quality.

Hand-Schüller-Christian Syndrome A chronic, disseminated, nonlipid reticuloendotheliosis classically characterized by osteolytic lesions of the membranous bones, diabetes insipidus, and exophthalmos.

Hemangioma A benign tumor composed of dilated blood vessels; may be congenital or acquired, simple or hyperplastic, capillary or cavernous, superficial or deep; names such as naevus flammeus, port wine mark, strawberry mark based on gross appearance; distinction from telangiectasia and varicosities may be vague.

Histiocytosis X A term including solitary (eosinophilic granuloma of bone), disseminated (Hand-Schuller-Christian syndrome), and malignant (Letter-Siwe syndrome) nonlipid reticuloendothelioses.

Hodgkin's Disease A malignant tumor of lymphoid tissue with considerable histological variation and protean clinical manifestations; the hallmark of diagnosis is the histological identification of the Reed-Sternberg cell.

Indirect Effect A radiation effect resulting from energy absorbed in the solvent surrounding a site or target.

Interphase That interval in the life of a cell separating one mitotic period from the next one.

Interphase Death Structural or metabolic degeneration of a cell in interphase; thus is independent of progression through the cell replication cycle.

Interstitial Irradiation Radiation from sources placed in the tissue. Example: a radium-containing needle implantation of the oral tongue.

Intracavitary Irradiation Radiation from sources within special applicators placed within body cavities. Example: irradiation of the uterine corpus by applicators placed in the uterine cavity.

Ionizing Radiation Radiant energy which is absorbed by a process of imparting its energy to atoms through the removal of orbital electrons.

Iridium-192 A radioactive isotope with a half-life of 74.4 days which emits beta and gamma (300–600 kev) radiation; used in discrete stainless steel-sheathed sources in nylon ribbon for interstitial application.

Kaposi's Disease (Idiopathic Hemorrhagic Sarcoma of Kaposi) A sarcoma of multicentric origin; typically purple, vascular nodules within the dermis over distal extremities, especially the legs; primarily involves skin but may affect all organs, especially the intestine.

Keratoacanthoma (Molluscum Sebaceum; "Self-healing Primary Squamous Cell Carcinoma of Skin") A rapidly developing (4–6 weeks), self-healing skin lesion with hemispherical mass, rolled edges, thin atrophic margins, a central keratin core, and characteristic histological appearance; most occur on face, ears, and dorsal surfaces of the hands of those middle-aged or older; formerly considered a low-grade squamous cell carcinoma.

Keratosis   Any horny growth; may be qualified by descriptive or etiological terms such as seborrheic, senile, solar.

Larynx, Extrinsic   Term formerly used to include the upper surface of ventricular bands, the epiglottis and its appendages, and the external surface of the larynx, e.g., postcricoid portion and medial wall of the piriform sinus.

Larynx, Intrinsic   Term formerly used to include the vocal cords, ventricles, lower surfaces of the ventricular bands, and subglottic region.

"Law" of Bergonie and Tribondeau (1906)   "X-rays are more effective on cells which have a greater reproductive activity; the effectiveness is greater on those cells which have a larger dividing future ahead, on those cells the morphology and function of which are least fixed" (translated by G. H. Fletcher, 1959).

Letterer-Siwe Syndrome   A rare, disseminated, acute, proliferative reticuloendothelial reaction characterized by eczematous hemorrhagic rash, hepatosplenomegaly, osteolytic lesions, usually affecting infants and often resulting in death.

Leukemia   Cancer of the hematopoietic tissue characterized by widespread proliferation of leukocytes and their precursors.

Linear accelerator   A device in which particles, i.e., electrons, protons, can be accelerated to high velocities along a straight path by repeated "kicks" by means of a fixed, high-frequency alternating voltage.

Linear Energy Transfer (L.E.T.)   A measure of the average rate of energy loss along the track of an ionizing particle, expressed as energy units per unit track length.

Lymphoepithelioma (Described Simultaneously by Regaud and Schmincke in 1921)   A poorly-differentiated malignant tumor of epithelial origin with characteristic lymphocytic infiltration and clinical behavior, usually arising in the tonsil, pharyngeal tongue, nasopharynx, or paranasal sinuses.

Lymphoma   Primary malignant tumors of lymphoid tissue, including Hodgkin's disease, lymphosarcoma, giant follicular lymphoma, reticulum-cell sarcoma, and several anaplastic variants.

Lymphosarcoma   A primary malignant tumor of lymphoid tissue composed predominantly of lymphocytes of varying maturity.

Manchester Technic   A system of radium therapy for cancer of the cervix developed at the Holt Radium Institute, Manchester, England; it is an adaptation of the Paris Technique with special applicators and administration of precalculated doses to specific anatomical reference points.

Mean Linear Ion Density   The average number of ions formed per micron of path of a charged particle in an absorber. Used as a gross characterization of physical events in the process of absorption of radiation energy.

Medium-voltage X-ray   X-rays generated by voltages approximately between 180 and 400 kv.

Medulloblastoma   A glioma usually arising in the midline of the cerebellum of infants and children and characterized by a propensity for tumor cells to be carried by the cerebrospinal fluid and implant along the CNS axis.

Megavoltage Radiation   An ill-defined but frequently used arbitrary term for ionizing radiation with energy greater than that included under "Supervoltage."

Melanoma, Malignant   The malignant counterpart of the pigmented nevus; apparently arises from epidermal melanocytes or their antecedents; frequently a very biologically aggressive tumor with a high incidence of hematogenous metastases.

Metastasis   The transfer of tumor from one tissue or organ to another not directly connected with it. This capability is characteristic of cancer.

Moh's Method   A chemosurgical method of treatment of surface cancers based on histopathological control following repeated applications of escharotics; this "method . . . would be justified if other methods did not accomplish the same aims with greater certainty and with greater ease" (del Regato).

Multihit Survival Curve   A sigmoidal survival curve which results when each cell in a population contains one or more targets which must be hit more than once to be inactivated and thus kill the cell.

Multitarget Survival Curve   A sigmoidal survival curve which results when each cell in a population contains two or more targets which must be hit to be inactivated and, thus, kill the cell.

Mycosis Fungoides   An inept designation for a confusing condition; a progressive dermatosis which becomes tumorlike; considered of reticuloendothelial origin and thus classified with the lymphomas; considered a distinctive entity by some and as a manifestation of lymphoma by others.

Neuroblastoma (Neurocytoma, Sympathicoblastoma, Sympathicogonioma, Sympathicocytoma)   A malignant, embryonic, non-chromaffin tumor arising from sympathogonia. Primary sites include adrenal; intrathoracic, paravertebral, pelvic, and retroperitoneal sympathetic nerves.

Neutron   An uncharged particle with a mass nearly the same as that of a proton. A building block of all nuclei except hydrogen.

Neutron Beam   A stream of neutrons usually characterized by their energy as: (1) *fast*—above 500 kev (0.5 Mev); (2) *intermediate*—between 1 kev and 500 kev; and (3) *slow*—less than 1 kev.

Nuclear Reactor (Atomic Pile)   An apparatus for starting and maintaining a controlled nuclear fission chain reaction.

Oncology   The study of tumors; no specific relationship to medical discipline or physician special interest; therefore applies to surgery, radiology, medicine, biochemistry et al., and use of term should not be restricted to medical oncology or chemotherapy.

Orthovoltage X-ray   A term which applies to x-rays of insufficient energy to be "skin-sparing" or to avoid preferential absorption in bone. May be divided into superficial and deep x-ray. Sometimes has been used interchangeably with deep x-ray.

Oxygen Effect   The ability of molecular oxygen, present during irradiation, to potentiate radiation effect.

Oxygen Enhancement Ratio (OER)   The ratio of the radiation dose under anoxic conditions to the dose under fully oxygenated conditions required to produce an equivalent effect.

Palliation   Relief of symptoms or signs caused by disease; in clinical medicine, the antithesis of treatment with curative intent.

Paris Technic   A system of radium therapy for cancer of the cervix developed by Regaud and Lacassagne at the Institut du Radium in Paris prior to 1922; relatively small amounts of filtered radium are placed in the endocervical canal and vaginal apex for relatively long periods (100 hours) in one to two applications.

Paterson-Parker System of Radium Dosage (Manchester System)   A system with an objective of uniform dosage throughout the volume of interest resulting from a planned non-uniform radium distribution; introduced by R. Paterson, M.D., and H. M. Parker, Ph.D., in 1934.

Pectinate Line (Dentate Line, Dentate Margin)   The serrated line where the skin of the anus unites with and overlaps the mucous membrane.

Penumbra   That radiation just outside and adjacent to the full beam arising from the finite size of the source; in usage usually includes components from scatter in tissue or from incomplete beam collimation.

Phosphorus, Radioactive (^{32}P)   A beta emitter with a maximal energy of 1.7 Mev and a half-life of 14.2 days; may be administered orally or intravenously; is maximally incorporated into cells with short turnover times, that is, certain tumors, intestinal mucosa, bone marrow; used to treat leukemia and metastases to bone from cancers of the breast and prostate.

Photon (Quantum)   An assumed, minute, discrete packet of electromagnetic radiation.

Positron   A positively charged electron.

"Prophylactic" Neck Dissection   A misnomer applied to the surgical removal of the soft tissues of the neck in the hope of removing clinically nondetected metastases and possibly improving the prognosis beyond that achieved by operation after metastases are detected; this operation does not prevent metastases to the neck or ensure their control if present.

Proton   An elementary, tiny, positively charged particle, weighing 1,800 times as much as an electron; ordinarily found only in the nucleus.

Protraction   Spreading of a total dose of radiation over a period of time.

Quimby System of Radium Dosage   A system based on uniform distribution of radioactive material throughout an area or volume.

Rad   A unit of absorbed dose of ionizing radiation equivalent to the absorption of 100 ergs per gram of irradiated material.

Radiation Cataract A nonspecific lens opacity attributed to absorption of ionizing radiation; usually clinically apparent after a latent period of many years following treatment, and can be managed like a cataract of any etiology.

Radiation Dose Energy imparted per unit mass of absorber at a specific site under certain conditions (absorbed d.; threshold d.; tumor d.; depth d.; permissible d.).

Radiation Exposure Energy deposited by an ionizing photon beam per unit mass of air as measured by the electrical charges on ions of one sign released in air at that point. The unit is the roentgen.

Radiation Hazards Risks of clinically unacceptable tissue damage.

Radiation Reactions Tolerable constitutional responses and local tissue changes associated with the absorption of ionizing radiation; these may be early (at the time of treatment) or late (months or years later).

Radiation Therapy (Radiotherapy, Therapeutic Radiology) A clinical medical specialty in which ionizing radiation is used in the treatment of patients with neoplastic diseases.

Radiation Sickness A clinical syndrome including various degrees of nausea, vomiting, anorexia, headache, and lassitude freely attributed to the therapeutic application of ionizing radiation, but often "contacted" from the referring physician, friends, or relatives.

Radical Radiation Therapy Treatment to just within the usual limits of normal tissue tolerance (high dose and/or large tissue volume) with acceptance of an increased risk of radiation-produced sequelae to maximize the chance of cure.

Radioactivity, Artificial Emission of radiant energy arising from the breakdown of nuclei which have been made energetically unstable. Examples: ^{60}Co, ^{137}Cs.

Radioactivity, Natural Emission of radiant energy arising from the breakdown of nuclei which are unstable in their natural state. Example: radium.

Radiocurability The potential for cure by radiation therapy; not synonymous with radiosensitivity, for the majority of frequently radiocurable cancers are only moderately radiosensitive.

Radiology A medical specialty characterized by use of ionizing radiation for diagnosis and treatment of disease. Currently defined subdivisions include: diagnostic radiology, therapeutic radiology, nuclear medicine, radiation biology, medical radiation physics, and radiation safety.

Radiomimetic Agent A substance (e.g., nitrogen mustard) capable of producing some, if not all, of the biological effects produced by ionizing radiation.

Radioresistance A relative term, being the antithesis of radioresponsive; actually, no tissue is absolutely resistant to ionizing radiation.

Radiosensitivity Susceptibility to injury by ionizing radiation; often imprecisely used to generally characterize the response of a normal tissue or of a cancer to ionizing radiation; in radiobiology, must be precisely used with respect to a biological endpoint, e.g., the D_0 dose on the radiation dose-cell survival curve.

Radiovulnerability An ill-defined term sometimes interchangeably used with radiosensitivity; a measure of susceptibility to damage by ionizing radiation.

Radium-226 A natural element, discovered by Marie and Pierre Curie in 1898, which emits penetrating radiation (alpha and beta particles and gamma rays with energies up to 2.2 Mev) as it disintegrates with a half-life of about 1,600 years; a heavy metal with an atomic number of 88 and an atomic weight of 226, which behaves chemically like barium or calcium.

Recovery Return to a less damaged state and rarely to be unperturbed state; may refer to repair of radiation injury.

"Recurrent" Cancer A frequently used misnomer for cancer which becomes detected clinically because of growth after a latent period following treatment.

Reed-Sternberg Cell A usually identifiable form of reticulum cell which is the hallmark of histological diagnosis of Hodgkin's disease; originally described by Greenfield (1878), but attributed to Sternberg (1898) and Reed (1902).

Regeneration Renewal of tissue identical with or closely similar to that which was destroyed through the mechanism of multiplication of surviving cells.

Relative Biological Effectiveness (RBE) The ratio of absorbed doses of two radiations required to produce the same biological effect; it is customary to use orthovoltage x-rays as the standard.

Relative Depth Dose   Radiation dose at a specific location compared to a standard point of reference; usually the dose at a depth in an absorber expressed as a percentage of the dose at the site of maximal ionization.

Rem (Rad-Equivalent-Man)   A unit of radiation dose equivalent (DE) which accounts for variations in biological effectiveness of different types of radiation; obtained by multiplying the dose in rads by a quality factor (QF) and by distribution factors (DF); DE (rems) = D (rads) × (QF) × (DF)$_1$.

Rep (Roentgen-Equivalent-Physical)   A convenient short-hand statement of dose of ionizing radiation not covered by the definition of the roentgen; represents approximately 93 ergs per cm^3 of tissue.

Repair   (1) Those intracellular processes which relate specifically to lessening of sublethal damage; (2) restitution of damaged tissue, often incomplete with replacement by a scar.

Reproductive Death   The suppression of the proliferative ability of a cell which otherwise could divide indefinitely.

Reticulum-Cell Sarcoma   A primary malignant tumor of lymphoid tissue composed predominantly of reticulum cells, usually with a characteristic diffuse intercellular network of reticulin fibers.

Retinoblastoma   A frequently hereditary malignant tumor probably arising from the glial cells of the retina in children.

RNA (Ribonucleic Acid)   A heterogenous group of macromolecules, composed of nucleotides, which direct and function in the synthesis of proteins by transcribing and translating the specific information of DNA.

Roentgen (R)   An internationally accepted unit of radiation quantity; "the quantity of x- or gamma radiation such that the associated corpuscular emission per 0.001293 grams of air produces, in air, ions carrying 1 e.s.u. of quantity of electricity of either sign" (National Bureau of Standards); equivalent to 2.58 × 10^{-4} coulombs per kilogram.

Sarcoma   Malignant tumor of connective tissue origin.

Skin-sparing   Radiation-induced skin reactions can be minimized by use of those types of radiation which produce maximal ionization beneath the skin; examples: ^{60}Co, ^{137}Cs.

Split-dose Technique   Planned division of a course of radiation therapy into two discrete periods (e.g., 2 weeks of daily increments each) separated by an interval of at least several days with an objective of improving the therapeutic ratio.

Squamous Cell Carcinoma   (Epidermoid Carcinoma, Spinocellular Carcinoma)   Malignant tumors arising from and histologically imitating the epidermis; locally invasive and may metastasize, usually via the lymphatics.

Stem (Primitive) Cell   A cell which is capable of proliferation and may give rise to differentiated cells.

Stockholm Technic   A system of radium therapy for cancer of the cervix developed by Forssell and Heyman. Relatively large amounts (130–160 mg) of well-filtered (3.0 mm lead) radium within customized applicators are placed in the endocervical canal and vaginal apex for short periods (20 to 24 hours) on 2 to 3 occasions separated by 2 to 3 weeks.

Strontium-90   A radioactive isotope with a half-life of 28 years which emits beta (0.54 Mev) radiation; used in a contact applicator for ophthalmologic work.

Subglottis   That portion of the upper airway immediately below the true vocal cords.

"Superficial" X-ray   Minimally penetrating x-rays of low peak energy generated by voltages in the range up to 85–140 kv. Used to treat lesions on the body surface.

Supervoltage Radiation   High energy radiation with ill-defined limits usually extending beyond energies which no longer are preferentially absorbed in bone (e.g., 500 kv) to peak energies of several Mev.

Supraglottis   That section of the larynx above or proximal to the true vocal cords, thus including the ventricles, false cords, arytenoids, aryepiglottic folds, and laryngeal surface of the epiglottis.

Synergism   Positive summation of desired effect; the potential advantage of synergistic therapeutic agents is the dispersion of toxic effects.

Telangiectasia   Dilatation of small-caliber blood vessels; a late effect of ionizing radiation.

Tantalum-182 A radioactive isotope emitting both beta and gamma (70 kev–1.29 Mev) rays and having a half-life of 115 days; used in therapy in the form of a thin (0.2 mm diameter) flexible wire coated by platinum.

Teletherapy Treatment with the radiation source at a distance from the body.

Therapeutic Neck Dissection A neck dissection performed after the detection of regional metastases.

Therapeutic Ratio A favorable relationship of purposeful damage to tumor and unavoidable, but often repairable, damage to adjacent normal tissues.

Thoraeus Filter (Named after Robert Thoraeus, a Swedish Medical Physicist) A compound filter for orthovoltage x-rays; consists of tin, copper, and aluminum, in that order, from tube to patient; transmits an x-ray beam of similar half value layer with less attenuation than that transmitted by an equivalent filter of copper and aluminum.

Tumor A mass of tissue which grows independently of its surrounding structures; subdivided into benign (usually not a threat to the host) and malignant (potentially lethal to the host).

Tumor Bed Those adjacent normal tissues supporting a tumor.

Undifferentiated Carcinoma A malignant tumor with features adequate to determine its origin as epithelial rather than mesenchymal (size, shape, and color of cells), but without identifying features such as squamous cell, basal cell or glandular.

Vermilion Red; used in reference to the epithelium of the lips which is in continuity with the adjacent oral cavity mucosa.

Waldeyer's Ring A ring of lymphoid (adenoid) tissue formed by the lingual, pharyngeal, and faucial tonsils (W. von Waldeyer, a German anatomist, 1836–1921).

Wilms' Tumor A highly malignant neoplasm arising from embryonic remnants within the renal parenchyma and containing epithelial structures and mesenchymal tissues of varying degrees of maturation.

Xeroderma Pigmentosum A congenital disease with the skin changes aggravated by light; characterized by progressive pigmentary and atrophic cutaneous change, with eventual development of basal or squamous cell carcinomas.

X-ray (Roentgen Ray) Electromagnetic radiation of short wavelength (i.e., from 0.0001 to about 100 Angstroms) produced by the impingement of high energy electrons on various materials, particularly metal; used in medicine because they affect photographic film, cause certain materials to fluoresce, and produce physiological change through ionization of tissue.

X-ray "Burn" A misnomer for a severe radiation-induced change manifest by necrosis and ulceration of the epidermis and vascular damage, edema, and fibrosis of underlying dermis.

INDEX

Page numbers in *italics* refer to illustrations; page numbers followed by *t* refer to tables.